A HANDBOOK OF PSYCHIATRIC NURSING

A Handbook of Psychiatric Nursing

Compiled and edited by

Lloyd A. Wells, Ph.D., M.D.

Head of Section
Child and Adolescent Psychiatry
Mayo Clinic
and
Associate Professor
Mayo Medical School

WARREN H. GREEN, INC.
St. Louis, Missouri, U.S.A.

Published by

WARREN H. GREEN, INC.
8356 Olive Boulevard
St. Louis, Missouri 63132, U.S.A.

ISBN No. 0–87527–295--9

Printed in the United States of America

Contributors

BARBARA CHAMBERLIN, M.D., is in private practice of psychiatry in Memphis, Tennessee.

J. RAMON de la FUENTE, M.D., is a consultant in the Department of Psychological Medicine at the Instituto Nacional de la Nutricion and Associate Professor in the Department of Psychiatry and Medical Psychology of the Faculty of Medicine, Universidad Nacional Autonoma de Mexico, Mexico City, Mexico.

DIANE GOODLUND, M.S.W., is a social worker in LaCrosse, Wisconsin.

LARRY GOODLUND, M.D., heads the Section of Child and Adolescent Psychiatry at Gundersen Clinic, LaCrosse, Wisconsin.

RICHARD C.W. HALL, M.D., is Professor of Psychiatry and Internal Medicine at the University of Tennessee Center for the Health Sciences, and Chief of Staff of the V.A. Medical Center in Memphis, Tennessee.

MARY JANE ISLAND is a chemical dependency counselor in the Department of Psychiatry, Mayo Clinic, Rochester, Minnesota.

RAYMOND ISLAND is a chemical dependency counselor in the Department of Psychiatry, Mayo Clinic, Rochester, Minnesota.

MARCIA JUSTIC, R.N., B.S.N., M.S.N., is an Assistant Professor in the Department of Nursing at Winona State University, Winona, Minnesota.

JOYCE KEEN, Ph.D., is a psychologist at Iowa Methodist Medical Center, Des Moines, Iowa.

JUDITH R. KYCEK-NISHIMURA, R.N., B.S.N., is a community mental health nurse at Zumbro Valley Mental Health Center, Rochester Minnesota.

DONNIS LASSIG, R.N., is Clinical Director of Nursing, St. Mary's Hospital, Rochester, Minnesota.

ERIC K. MILLINER, M.D., is Consultant in Psychiatry, Mayo Clinic, Rochester, Minnesota.

PAMELA PETERS, R.N., B.S.N., M.S., is Clinical Specialist at St, Mary's Hospital, Rochester, Minnesota.

GERALD PETERSON, M.D., is Associate Dean of Mayo Medical School, Rochester, Minnesota.

LEONARD I. STEIN, M.D., is Professor of Psychiatry, University of Wisconsin Medical School. He directs community psychiatry training and is involved in interdisciplinary work.

KARLA SCHROEDER, R.N., B.S.N., M.S., is assistant head nurse in Psychiatry at St. Mary's Hospital, Rochester, Minnesota.

SONDRA K. STICKNEY, R.N., is psychiatric liaison nurse at Hermann Hospital, Houston, Texas

PAMELA W. WALLACE, M.D., is engaged in the private practice of Psychiatry in Lynchburg, Virginia.

DENISE M. WELLS, R.N., B.S.N., is a psychiatric nurse and writer in Rochester, Minnesota.

LLOYD A. WELLS, Ph.D., M.D., heads the Section of Child and Adolescent Psychiatry at Mayo Clinic, Rochester, Minnesota.

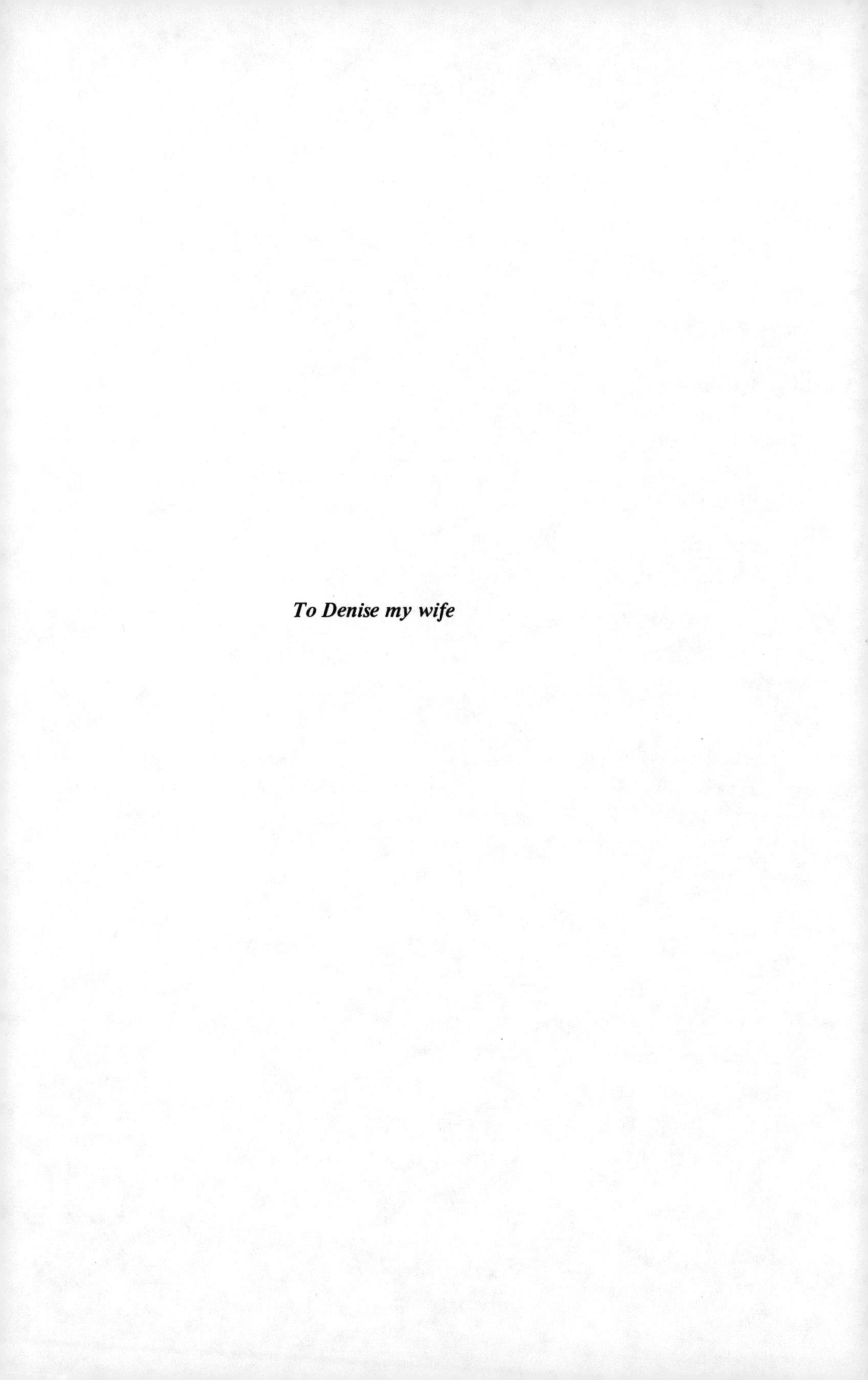

To Denise my wife

Foreword

This book represents the efforts of many people. To all the contributors I express my sincere thanks for their devotion to detail and deadlines. Lorraine Heenan diligently typed and retyped the manuscript. Mr. Green of Warren Green Publishing was gracious and helpful in his liaison efforts. The *Archives of General Psychiatry* and *Psychosomatics* graciously granted permission to reprint articles that had appeared in their pages. Finally, my wife Denise not only made major contributions to the text, taking time from her own history of rural psychiatry to write three chapters, but she also served as an invaluable editorial consultant. Her impact on the book was enormous, as was the enthusiastic support of Aynslee, Llyd and Ethan Wells.

Contents

A HANDBOOK OF PSYCHIATRIC NURSING

PART 1

SOME PERSPECTIVES IN PSYCHIATRIC NURSING

1 Introduction

Lloyd A. Wells

Nurses are no longer handmaidens to physicians. It has been very exciting during the past ten years to watch the evolution of psychiatric nursing as a distinct mental health profession. Because nursing is such a young profession, however, there continues to be a great deal of controversy about what constitutes a well-trained psychiatric nurse, what duties that person can perform, and what education is necessary for that position. One can argue at great length about all of these questions, but more to the immediate point is the fact that there continue to be nurses from a great diversity of levels and types of training and experience who call themselves psychiatric nurses.

In this text, I shall attempt to provide an overview of several mental health disciplines and topics which I feel any psychiatric nurse should be acquainted with. This is not a textbook in the formal sense. It will address itself minimally to such technical questions as where to place the electrodes when doing electroconvulsive therapy and how to put a patient in four-point restraints. Such matters are for other books and belong more to the technique of psychiatric nursing than to its intellectual substance.

Another feature of this book is the fact that its contributors come from a variety of mental health disciplines. Most books about nursing are written by nurses, and this is as it should be. In the psychiatric disciplines, however, there is a great need for more input from all mental health professionals about what each does. This book attempts to provide such a viewpoint.

Two of the great hazards of current methodology in psychiatric nursing are that because of the emphasis on planning for the patient there is sometimes an unnecessary rigidity and because of the perceived need for a nursing plan, a definitive plan is often developed without any comprehensive understanding of the patient and his problems. One must maintain flexibility and spontaneity and always be well aware that the patient being treated is an individual. Though he or she may represent a particular syndrome or a particular set of behavioral problems, he is nevertheless unique and needs to be treated as a unique individual. It is all very well and commendable to make a detailed plan of how to deal with the vagaries of this person's behavior, but that plan must not become cast in stone. It is necessary for the nurse and all other treating professionals to be able to switch techniques when necessary.

The nurse, no matter what his or her skills and training may be, is not better than his or her ability to recognize and deal with feelings and reactions to patients. There are many examples of the nurse using the defense mechanism of projective identification with a patient. Such an identification can lead to rejection or rescue of the patient by the nurse, and both of these alternatives are potentially disastrous to the welfare of the patient. Throughout this book there will be an emphasis on mechanisms by which the nurse can recognize his coutertransferential reactions to patients.

W.C. Menninger wrote eloquently in 1936 about the role of the psychiatric nurse (1,2). He felt that the psychiatric nurse needed to be committed to the work of psychiatric nursing, reasonably stable, capable of creating an accepting environment for the patient, and with both theoretical and functional understanding of psychiatry. Menninger felt that the greatest hazard to psychiatric patients from psychiatric nurses was that nurses would tend to standardize their care and not be flexible enough to individualize the care. This remains a hazard today.

Menninger also felt that all psychiatric personnel, including nurses, should have several general aims in treating an individual patient. These included the encouragement of direct expression of anger toward real and substitute objects — and the nurse often is a substitute object for anger; encouraging the relief of a sense of guilt for introjected hostility or projected hostility; encouraging displacements from disadvantageous objects; providing the patient with opportunities to obtain some narcissistic gratification; encouraging an opportunity to be cared for and accepted; and affording the patient a chance to care about and accept others. While some of these six aims may seem somewhat simplistic, they are essential to the care of a great many psychiatric patients.

Within this general framework, then, this book has been organized to give an overview of psychiatric nursing followed by attention to specific areas and disciplines, some intervention strategies, and a series of discussions of nursing roles. After a retrospective look at the history of psychiatric nursing with particular emphasis on its development in 19th century mid-America, the book considers descriptions of disease entities, including schizophrenia, affective disorders, organic brain syndromes, neuroses, personality disorders, adjustment reactions, chemical dependence and disorders of childhood. These descriptive accounts are followed by a section on nursing theory in general, including the very important topic of relationships with patients and the nursing examination of patients. This is followed by a discussion of specific types of techniques used in treating specific patients. The book ends with a discussion of more philosophic issues, including the future of psychiatric nursing and the relationship of psychiatric nursing to psychiatry and other mental health professions.

The future of psychiatric nursing is bright, though perils regarding its development abound. It is my hope that this book will contribute to the avoidance of those perils in the pursuit of that bright future.

REFERENCES

1. Menninger, W.C.: Psychiatric hospital therapy designed to meet unconscious needs, Am J Psychiat, *93*:347 (1936).

2. Menninger, W.C.: Individualization in the prescriptions for nursing care of the psychiatric patient, JAMA, *106:*756 (1936).

2 Overview

Lloyd A. Wells

It is always frustrating to write any kind of a paper which attempts to cover a vast subject of great scope in just a few pages. It is equally frustrating to cover a very speculative subject or a very subjective one. Psychiatric nursing is certainly all three of these and, thus, a brief chapter about an overview of psychiatric nursing is difficult and frustrating to write.

Perhaps a good way to keep cohesiveness in such an essay is to recall the old lines of Kipling:

"I keep six honest serving men,
They taught me all I knew;
Their names are What and Why and When
And How and Where and Who." (1)

In addition to asking these six questions it is impossible to provide an overview without some information about the past status of these questions as well as their present status. This book will end by addressing their future status.

What is a psychiatric nurse? What has a psychiatric nurse been? Psychiatric nursing is a relatively new field. From time immemorial people have had to take care of mentally ill fellow beings. There was no particular profession involved, however. Through the Middle Ages, people who were mentally ill were either cared for in large, public prisons by jailers or, occasionally, for the wealthy, by physicians, often in their homes. The profession of nursing, which was in its infancy in the Renaissance, was considered totally inappropriate for any well-bred person and mainly attracted to it the dregs of society. Even here the psychiatric field greatly lagged behind other branches of nursing. Many people in the Middle Ages and Renaissance who became mentally ill were merely turned out of their homes and not taken into any institutional kind of care. They frequently banded together at the periphery of society and often were considered to be possessed by the devil rather than mentally ill. These people, in caring for one another, would often seek the expertise of a suspected witch or wise-woman, who often attempted to treat them with various herbs. Thus, the psychiatric nurse can trace her professional ancestory to witches and prostitutes, and this underlines the point that the psychiatric nurse must be willing to use whatever resource is available, regardless of its origin or theoretical implications, in order to help the patient.

With the great era of large public mental hospitals in the United States in the late 19th century, the profession of psychiatric nurse was upgraded, and several institutions started hospital training programs. In fact, in some areas of the country, including the mid-west, training programs in hospitals for the mentally ill actually provided the bulk of nurses' training available, and many nurses trained in mental institutions went on to become great non-psychiatric nurses. The psychiatric nurse began to play an increasingly prominent role in the actual day-to-day care of patients. She — and psychiatric nursing was certainly dominated by "shes" up until recently — had very little status and was not looked on as a colleague but rather as a sometimes intelligent paraprofessional who could carry out orders. With the dearth of physicians in psychiatric care, especially in large institutions, it became necessary for the responsibilities of nurses to increase. With that increase the profession of psychiatric nursing gradually saw itself as more autonomous and began to develop its own philosophies and its own procedures of credentials. Today, psychiatric nurses are involved in the independent practice of psychotherapy and nursing, and they have certainly arrived as professionals who see themselves as such and are usually perceived as colleagues by physicians, social workers and other mental health professionals.

What do they do? They continue to provide an enormous amount of in-hospital care to mentally ill people. They do this using the most ancient techniques of nursing up to and including the most modern techniques of nursing. In addition to this age-old role, they also participate in independent practice, they teach, they do research, they develop programs, they serve as coordinators of groups and do group therapy, they do marital therapy, and the list is indeed endless. The duties, responsibilities and options available to psychiatric nurses are growing almost on a daily basis with the expansion of this relatively new profession.

The next question in the list is *why*. Why, indeed? The motivations for the choice of nursing as a career and particularly psychiatric nursing are as numerous as the number of people who are psychiatric nurses. In the past, the primary reason for people to enter the profession was probably economic. Certainly before the last 30 years, when training was poor and conditions were worse, a combination of necessity and the altruistic urge probably was the primary motivation.

Today, the field is one which is expanding rapidly and many people who enter it do so in part because of a wish to be successful in a rather new profession. Many people who go up the ranks in psychiatric nursing, however, are people who got there by serendipity. A young nurse from a two-year training program gets a job in a hospital and is assigned to a psychiatric ward. She finds, to her surprise, that she likes it. She begins to attend continuing nursing education courses. She becomes more interested in the subject and goes back for her baccalaureate. She finds that she continues to enjoy psychiatric nursing but wants more autonomy, so she returns to get a Master's degree or above. She achieves certification in the field and becomes a specialist. At no single point of her life did she say, "Tomorrow I am going to be a psychiatric nurse." She drifted into the field but gradually made it her own. This is probably a very common experience for people in the profession of psychiatric nursing.

If there is a generalization one can make about psychiatric nurses, it is that they often have a strong need to care for others. While this is an admirable trait, it is one which can sometimes interfere with the effective performance of one's work in this field. Thus, psychiatric nurses should be cognizant of the possibility that they will do too much for patients and that they will not respect the patient's own individuality and sense of responsibility. Several people who go into any of the mental health professions have a strong scotophilic characteristic — thay are interested in the trials and tribulations of others and derive some unconscious satisfaction from those trials and tribulations. This is certainly not as admirable as caring too much, but at the same time it often can interfere with the professional's work. The professional can insist that the patient go over every detail endlessly rather than getting on to the business of helping the patient to get better.

A final reason why people choose psychiatric nursing is that, as in all the mental health professions, it is a tremendous amount of fun.

The third question Kipling posed, *when*, is more difficult to address. The relevance of this question to psychiatric nursing, however, is to emphasize the fact that this is not by any means a static mental health profession, but one which has a relatively brief history replete with a great deal of change, (some of which has been perceived as revolutionary by other mental health professions), and with a future which is certain to be exciting. Any psychiatric nurse who attempts to consider the field just as it is today is bound to educate himself or herself poorly because the field is changing extremely rapidly. For this reason, this book is concerned with the past of the field, its present and especially its future.

How is an even more imponderable question. First, how does one become a psychiatric nurse? There are many routes open to the accomplishment of this venture, and indeed this is one of the attractions of nursing as a profession. It is much less institutionally rigid in terms of how one acquires roles than are most other health professions. People come to psychiatric nursing from extremely diverse backgrounds. One can call oneself a psychiatric nurse after working on a psychiatric unit with an A.D. degree. Similarly, one can be a psychiatric nurse with certification in the field and a Ph.D. degree. As nursing evolves, standards for education in this specialty will become much more uniform.

How does one function as a psychiatric nurse? There are many techniques to be learned, and some of them will be reviewed in this book. More important are the personal attributes one brings to the job, and these also will be addressed in the book.

The question of *where* again will be covered implicitly throughout the book. While most psychiatric nurses work in hospital settings — private or public psychiatric hospitals or psychiatric units on general hospitals — many psychiatric nurses work in other settings, including community mental health centers, psychiatrists' offices, liaison units of general hospitals, private practices and a great many more. In terms of geographical location, the question where may be answered by saying throughout the United States, although there are areas that are certainly greatly underserved in psychiatric nurses. Nevertheless, psychiatric nurses function highly effectively in many areas which are poorly served by all other mental health professionals.

The final question: *who*. The answer: you — and thousands of others who all bring to this field whatever education, expertise, and talent they may have.

Whatever techniques they may learn and wherever the profession of psychiatric nursing goes, their dedication and altruism, which need to be merged into a stream of professional caring, are the prerequisites for their task.

REFERENCES

1. Kipling, R.: "The Elephant's Child." *Just So Stories,* London, MacMillan and Company (1902).

3 Historical Notes

Denise M. Wells

Some of the higher primates attempt to care for ill members of their troop. Thus, the role of nursing goes back in all probability to a period before civilization as we know it. Certainly, through the ages certain people have learned primarily on their own to care for sick people. The actual establishment of a profession of nursing, however, occurred very late and in fact thousands of years after the emergence of medicine as a profession. Thus, nursing is a relatively new discipline and is suffering many of the growing pains which occur with new professions.

The work of a nurse has always been multifaceted and involves dealing with the person in depth and at length. Thus, it is no surprise that many of the people who select nursing as a profession have major needs to care for others and tend to be altruistic. Sometimes this altruism is *bona fide* while at other times it is self-serving. It is no surprise given the altruistic coping mechanism of so many nurses that religious orders have historically been very involved in providing nursing care and this was certainly true through the Middle Ages and Renaissance although the nuns were not considered to be nursing professionals. This continues today in many ways — for example, non-religious professional nurses in Britain are often called "sister."

In the 17th century, various orders of nuns began to view their social role as to provide care for the sick and I suppose that these nuns could be considered among the first professional nurses. Certainly, the nuns of the 17th century who began to work in workhouses and asylums for psychiatrically ill patients can be considered the first psychiatric nurses.

The first major attempt to upgrade the status of the psychiatric nurse occurred in the 18th century when Pinel, the man who had removed the shackles from French psychiatric patients developed a program in which nurses would work with healthier patients with the goal of rehabilitiating them. The program did not survive Pinel's own enthusiasm for it unfortunately.

The first psychiatric nursing program in the United States was begun by William Cowles working at McLean Hospital in 1882. This was the establishment of a training school for nurses, specifically to teach them to care for mentally ill patients. The program that Cowles began was helpful and provided staff who could work well with psychiatrically ill patients. At that time, most of the workers in hospitals for the insane were either physicians — of whom there were few — or completely untrained attendants. Thus, the trained nurse working in the psychiatric hospital setting was a major boon to the physicians there and to the well-being of the patients and the number of programs grew quite rapidly from one to 19 within the first decade of this movement. In spite of this fairly rapid growth, psychiatric nursing was not officially required by licensing boards until 1952.

The Rochester State Hospital which was founded in 1879 as the second Minnesota hospital for the insane was among the first psychiatric hospitals to institute a nursing program and a training program. This school was warmly welcomed by Dr. Jacob Bowers, the first superintendent of the hospital and by his successor, Dr. Arthur Kilbourne. Its actual institution and success, however, were largely due to the efforts of Dr. Robert M. Phelps, assistant superintendent at that hospital and later superintendent at the St. Peter State Hospital and also president of the American Psychiatric Association, and his wife, Dr. Sarah Linton Phelps, who was an assistant physician at the Rochester State Hospital. The two of them developed the nursing program and wrote a book for the nursing students (1). I thought it would be interesting to share some of the insights and comments from that book. It indicates that the role of psychiatric nurses has changed greatly in the past 90 years but that though the role is different it was a very great role in the last decade of the 19th century.

At the very start of the book, the two physicians addressed themselves to the importance of the character of the nurse stressing the need for "staid, well balanced, good work . . and stability of character . . . while we want you enthusiastic, we do not want you deceived. All is not smooth and easy in the path; indeed, if it were, the course would be of no value, for only by overcoming can you gain strength." They also addressed themselves to the effect that a trained nurse has on the entire medical staff and predict that gradually psychiatric nursing will become a specialty. They suggest that the salary for psychiatric nurses is rather low but that the perquisites including the chance for learning about human nature as well as such mandane items as board and free laundry lift the nurses' compensation "nearly up to the average of wages for ordinary school teaching . . ." They repeatedly stress the importance of a trained nurse to the care of mentally ill patients: "Again, through the nurse, the patient has been decidedly affected. From the careless, ignorant attendant, knowing very little of her patient's condition and caring less, we have passed to the careful, painstaking trained nurse, who observes the bodily and mental condition of each of her patients. She is quick to notice any change, either physical or mental, in those under her care, and reports such to the physician. She notes carefully any change of importance upon a chart provided for each of her patients. In her, the patient finds a sympathetic friend, who often speaks an encouraging word. We believe that the enthusiastic nurse can see something more than drudgery in her work today. We also believe that her place in the hospital force is a very important one, for to her earnest effort and good judgment is due much of the success in the care of our patients. One of the greatest movements in this work is the change from untutored attendant to the careful nurse."

The Phelps' textbook went on to outline anatomy, digestion, the circulatory system, respiration, the musculo-skeletal system and the special senses. It then turns to the central nervous system, the mind, and "insanity as a treatable disease." They divide the elements of the mind into intellect, sensibility and will roughly equivalent to ego, id and superego, interestingly. They make a strong effort to impress on the nursing students that insanity is an illness rather than a moral weakness and describe such elements of different types of mental illness as delusions, hallucinations, illusions, incoherence of speech and loss of memory. They strongly suggest that nurses pay careful attention to the patients' moral and mental keenness, power of attention, affective state, trains of thought which might be delusional or exalted. They strongly caution the psychiatric nurse to be against judging "too hastily . . . it is hardly appropriate, when a patient has been but a few days upon the ward, to say that he or she is alright. The older of you likely know many patients that seemed alright, and only after a considerable time found that these patients made a very extra amount of trouble. Don't be hasty, then, in making remarks. Simply say that you have 'seen nothing out of the way in the behavior of the patient' and then leave the judgment to others. The patient is not necessarily sane because you find no delusion, or because, during some ordinary conversation, he seems to answer questions alright."

They go on to divide insanity into three general types: mania, melancholia and dementia. They add that imbecility and idiocy should also be considered and that general paresis if very common. The Phelps' go on to discuss hours and wages for the nursing students. The nursing students were to receive $8 per month and worked 12 hours per day 6 days per week.

The authors then considered the necessary attributes and qualities needed in psychiatric nurses. They pay particular attention to the need of the nurse to subordinate her personality in her professional role and not to work for personal gratification: "The individual is sunk in the nurse, and there is steadily brought to the front effort for the sick, and a quiet disregard for her own personal convenience." They also discuss the need of the psychiatric nurse to have "even tempered endurance and quietness." In addition, the nurse needed to be reliable, industrious, kind to patients, truthful and obedient to institutional rules. A nurse should never be careless. The nurse should be respectful to the physician and willing to be of whatever assistance she can to him and should realize what her role in the hospital is. The head nurse is in the "position of having charge of the wards. They are to have the most complete and extensive knowledge of all the ward affairs, and be ready to give information and, to some extent, opinions concerning all matters connected with this work. The other nurses, each in her place, are expected to be as faithful and as intelligent as possible in their work."

The authors also address themselves to the complaint of some nurses that not enough is done to insure their own protection. This continues to be a complaint in the last fifth of the 20th century. "Our standard is that there is nothing to be done in the way of physical penalty. To in some way remove ugly patients out of the way to harm anyone, we, of course, admit is proper. We do not want to risk the lives and safety of nurses, and in general there is not severe risk to run. We do feel a regret when one gets injured, and a strong desire to hold the dangerous patient out of the power to harm anyone. And yet, as workers here, we all know that a great many patients would have to be tied up to render everybody *perfectly* safe, and we would be back to the standard of 100 years ago. We know, moreover, that they cannot be tied up without degenerating into dirtiness and neglect, and that the possible injuries and chafing of the patients in restraint are not second to possible injuries which they may receive when out and watched. Therefore, if we decide against penalties and punishment in the way of force, or against mechanical restraint as a penalty, we do it with a feeling that we are conforming to customs more humanitarian and best for the patients; and that, if we discard restraints, we are not discarding any means that are of special value in reforming the behavior of the patient and making him better." They go on to urge the nurses, however, to be aware of the proper use of force and that sometimes one can be forceful with a patient who is out of control without needing to resort to violence. They emphasize to the nurses that mentally ill people are not always responsible for their actions. Ways of forcefully controlling a patient who is out of control were listed and these included:

1. Holding the patient's hands behind him. This should not include twisting the patient's arm.

2. Holding a patient by the hair. This is only to be done if the nurse is in serious danger and needs to do it for self-defense.

3. Taking hold of the arm. The authors point out the hazards of grabbing the patient's arms since it does not control the patient and often causes some harm to old people and weak people.

4. Holding the back of the neck of patients. This is recommended only when the patient is attempting to bite the nurse.

5. Choking a patient. The authors cite this as "inexcusable."

6. Taking a patient down on the floor. The authors urge nurses to avoid this but says that it can be helpful when a patient and nurse are alone. The nurses are urged to avoid this method since often the patient will win such a struggle.

7. Shaking a patient. The authors state that this is never helpful.

8. Striking a patient. The authors state that this is assault.

Some of the rules for the nurses and nursing students are next discussed in the book. Nurses and attendants are not allowed to work for themselves while on duty; this includes making clothing and other sewing type of work. Furthermore, nurses are not to employ patients or sell things to them — nor are they to buy things from them. They are not to visit other wards except when they are on their time off. They must never go to their own rooms to read, write, sew or nap when they are supposed to be on duty. They may not take friends through the wards without permission. They are to be neat in person, should get up in the morning on time, should not force feed patients or rush the patients through their meals, should attempt to get the patients to take their medicine willingly and should not take advantage of amusements such as dances and concerts specifically arranged for patients. Nurses should not read in the dining room with the patients.

Some of these rules sound picayune and most of them are quite obvious. Remember, however, that nursing — particularly psychiatric nursing — was a new profession at this time and such rules needed to be made. The authors go on to consider the important relations which the nurses bring to the care of patients and state that "The value of nurses' influence is found practically in that it is only people who represent the sane and outside world to the patient. With regard to particular cases, it seems at times as if nothing had any particular effect upon the patient. But looking upon the cases as a whole, we would find many of them — and indeed all of them — more or less affected by the influences around them. Among these influences, we find the most *common*, *constant*, and *most important* would be that of the nurse who has charge of them. We can very rarely point to a very permanent and immediate effect, either of medicine or surroundings, or of any other agency; but in the influence of nurses we would always have as steadily important a factor that can be found. With such considerations in view, we are trying to train nurses to greater usefulness, to more intelligent work, to be more and to do more. According as you fall in with the advance and intelligent work, you will become more valuable in your work, both to us and to the world. Even if you cannot follow, in particular cases, any difference in the patients due to your behavior or care, *use that care and intelligence*, *anyhow.* Use it until it becomes to you a habitual exercise. Cultivate a spirit that is above the pettiness of worrying. Look at the whole broad field, and if any patient is annoying, see the field of your work as a whole, and the years as a whole as they go by, and not stop to worry about particular annoyances especially after they are over. With the broad field of work forming one large picture before you, these trifling annoyances will be but specks upon the surface. You will realize that you are doing a marked injury to yourself by losing your self-control over trifles, and will mar your work and whole life by any *habit* of so doing."

The authors go on to discuss nursing records which they felt should be very complete, nursing duties during emergencies including dealing with suicidal patients, providing artificial respiration, dealing with patients who have been apparent victims of drowning, dealing with patients having convulsions, as well as tube feeding. They discuss care of hemorrhage, cuts and wounds, poisoning, bed sores, black eyes, fights and sprains. Dr. Sarah Linton Phelps then provides some very interesting instructions on the uses of baths and massage in psychiatric nursing. Recalling that virtually no neuroleptic agent nor any modern psychotherapies were available to these physicians, it seems likely that the type of physical care provided by special types of baths and massage may have been somewhat helpful to the patients. Dr. Sarah Linton Phelps described many different kinds of baths, warm sponge baths, cold sponge baths, cold shower and plunge baths, medicated liquid baths, salt baths, soda baths, sulfur baths, mustard baths, alcohol baths which were said to be particularly useful for "any weak or nervous person," vapor baths, hot air baths, Russian baths, hot foot baths, and cold douches for the head. In addition, one could use Turkish baths and rain baths.

An entire chapter on beds and bed making is provided which is unlikely to be found in any modern textbook of psychiatric nursing. The chapter on making beds even has references and suggestions for further reading. A paragraph in this chapter addresses the importance of tact in making beds.

Another chapter which would not be found in a modern textbook of psychiatric nursing indicates that the role of the nurse was as diffuse in the 1890's as it is today. This chapter is on heating and ventilation and teaches the future nurse how to care for a large heating plant in a psychiatric hospital. There is also a major chapter on the importance of fire prevention in a hospital for the psychiatrically ill which goes into great detail and which again would never be found in a modern textbook of psychiatric nursing — but perhaps should be.

There follows a section on giving hypodermic injections which was a relatively new technique and another on the use of the microscope by the nurse. Nurses were expected to cut and prepare tissues for microscopy and also to be able to do routine examination of blood, urine and some tissues under the microscope. Nurses were also expected to be expert in dealing with typhoid fever and other common communicative diseases of the time. The clinical information which the nurse was expected to have of tuberculosis, typhoid fever and other such illnesses probably is greater than that of most physicians today because of the relative rarity of some of those syndromes.

The authors stress the need for excellent nursing care particularly at the start of hospitalization and say that there are three major approaches the nurse must use when a new patient is admitted. First, "The patient should be received with cheerful and encouraging words." Second, "Much closer observation must be had of a new patient than later. We have a patient who will tell us little or nothing, or else tells us inaccurately; but as he is less able to tell us, by so much the more closely must he be noted and his varying symptoms followed." Third, "It is necessary to study the secretions and excretions of the body, as well as the more obvious behavior." They go on to give a sketch of the nursing examination and the write up of the case history. The nursing history should include an actual history of the reasons for hospitalization followed by a biography of the patient. This is followed by what we would consider to be a mental status examination:

Mental elements

1. Power of reasoning
2. Power of attention
3. Power of memory
4. Power of coherent speech
5. Emotional state
6. Delusions
7. Hallucinations
8. Delusive trains of thought (perverted or exaggerated ideas)
9. General behavior (as to dullness, pecularities, etc.)

Physical elements

1. General physical appearance
2. Symptoms pertaining to
    - Lungs and respiration
    - Systemic and digestion
    - Bowels and action
    - Heart and circulation
    - Muscles and muscular action
    - Bladder and urination
3. Brain and nerves (as headaches, backache, tremors, trembling, stuttering, stammering, delirium, etc.)
4. Temperature — fever, chills, pains, sleep, etc.
5. Secretions and extretions:
    - Movements of bowels — time frequency, quantity, character, color etc.
    - Urine and its examination as to color, quantity, specific gravity, albumin, sugar
    - Sweating — skin moist or dry, oily, scaly, etc.

6. Diet — give quality, quantity, appetite for same, complaints, etc.
7. Treatments, especially the nursing part — baths, massage, occupation, amusements, cleanliness, behavior, medicines, effect of same noted, etc.

Nurses are then instructed in the care of some common complaints of the patients including toothache, removal of foreign bodies in the ear, neuralgia, inflammed eyes, warts, corns, catarrh, herpes, cold sores, and frostbite.

The nursing students are also instructed in nutrition and preparing a diet for sick patient including various special preparations.

The book contains some surprisingly complicated medical information for these nursing students including directions for use of cocaine as a local anesthetic and its ocular use. Such information indicates that the Doctors Phelps themselves had a current knowledge of the practice of medicine and expected the nurses to be similarly informed.

Above all, this book urges the nurse to use professional caution and professional judgment while continuing to provide kind and caring treatment: "It has been said to me by thoughtful ones of former classes that it is impossible to use any moral suasion on some of these people (the patients) — that to say 'please' to them would be ludicrous; to speak to them in a low tone of voice would never meet their active violence; that a strong, stern command was necessary in a large share of those lower ward cases; that to meet their noisy complaining and cursing with an appeal to morals or for quiet would be almost absurd, while to assume that they have delicate, refined feelings or tastes, when one knows positively to the contrary, would be both useless and ludicrous. All this is partly true, and we do not have any desire to deny facts. But while not going to any ludicrous extremes such as we are appealed upon to do by those ignorant of the situation, we can yet approximately more closely than we do these same ideas; that is, for example, while we need not meet each demented, stupid patient with a cheerful 'good morning,' we can yet let the spirit of kindness temper and soften all our speech and behavior toward them, until at the very least no rough speeches or carelessly unkind conduct is left to be noted. Such a speech as 'Shut up your mouth,' which was reported to us at one time, has in it no justification by reason of the curses of the patient."

Thus, an examination of this old textbook of psychiatric nursing gives one a much better perspective on how the field has grown and how the role has expanded but also how the role has changed and been diminished over the years. Such is always the case with the development of any profession.

REFERENCES

1. Phelps, R.M., and Phelps, S.L.: *A Text-Book on Nursing in Bodily and Mental Diseases for Use in Training Schools for Nurses in Hospitals for the Insane*, Rochester State Hospital (1895).

4 The Functional-Organic Continuum

Lloyd A. Wells

For a long period, nursing and all the medical profession have tended to view diseases as functional or organic. In nursing, there has been a move away from this unfortunate oversimplification for many years, but frequently this move has not reached the grass roots. In fact, in spite of nursing's long-held and sophisticated theoretical model of illness, most nurses in practice use an oversimplified type of medical model. For many illnesses, this has been a useful model, although its heuristic value is declining.

If we consider disease as a pathologic process and illness as the experience of that particular pathologic process in a particular patient, then we need to consider not only biological but also psychological and social factors in each illness. This concept, known as the biopsychosocial model, has been introduced and emphasized by George Engel (1). It has a great deal to recommend it, and the purpose of this chapter is to demonstrate the biological factors in some so-called functional illnesses and the functional aspects in some so-called biological illnesses. The goal of the chapter will be to review the concept of "functional" illness, to subdivide it into different types, and finally to examine "fully organic" illness, which has psychological overlay, as well as illnesses which have both a major psychological and organic input.

One problem which has been very common in the past and continues to be problematic is that because of the old model in use there has been a tendency for physicians and nurses to assume that if the criteria for some classical organic disease are not met, the patient's illness must be "functional." Even worse, sophistication regarding the plethora of so-called functional disorders has been lacking so that such a patient has often been labelled "hysterical." As with primarily organic disorders, the primarily functional disorders have specific criteria and cannot be used as a vast dumping ground.

The dichotomy, then, is false; nevertheless, it is helpful to list a group of syndromes which can be considered primarily "functional." These syndromes are listed in Table I.

The first necessary consideration for such a patient is whether in fact this is a true syndrome or represents an undiagnosed organic illness. One cannot stress this necessity sufficiently. Again, one needs positive criteria to make a "functional" diagnosis.

One of the most common falsely positive "functional" diagnoses has reference to the patient with a somatic illness which seems exaggerated. People react idiosyncratically to illness. Thus, a person might seem much more dramatic in reaction to certain symptoms than most patient are. This does not make the illness "functional." One needs to consider whether there are personal or cultural idiosyncratic reactions to a somatic illness before going on to consider which particular "functional" illness we might be dealing with.

Conversion reaction is a very common diagnosis for patients with functional illness. In a conversion reaction, there is no somatic disease, but the patient unconsciously uses somatic complaints as communication. Often, the somatic complaint symbolizes a conflict for the patient. For example, the patient who has a partly repressed wish to hit an authority figure might develop a paralysis of the right arm. Thus, the symptom complaint is symbolic and is a way of communicating. In addition, the patient with a conversion reaction has significant gain from his symptom

TABLE I
THE PATIENT WITH FUNCTIONAL COMPLAINTS

Conversion reaction
Hysteria
Obsessive-compulsive syndromes
Hypochondriasis
Somatic delusion
Acute grief/loss
Drug abuse
Exaggerated somatic illness
Conpensation neurosis
Chronic pain syndrome
Malingering
Doctor dependence
Depression

or symptoms. This gain has classically been considered primary or secondary. Primary gain refers to the relief of anxiety, which the patient gains through the conversion reaction. Secondary gain, classically, has referred to the patient's increased ability to cope with the environment because of the symptom. Thus, the patient with a conversion reaction might very well encounter much less anxiety than the ordinary ill patient and might cope well through his illness. Often one's need for dependence is greatly met through illness in this condition. In addition, the patient with conversion reaction usually has what has been termed *la belle indifference.* This means simply that the patient can tell the nurse or physician about horrendous symptoms with pain, for example, rated at 10 on a scale of 0 to 10, yet while the patient is telling the clinician about the horrible symptom his affect seems bland and indifferent to the symptom. Finally, in a conversion reaction symptoms often occur at a time of stress for the patient. This phenomenon, of course, is by no means restricted to conversion reactions. Nevertheless, it very frequently is correlated with them.

The most common "functional" diagnosis is "hysteria." Hysteria, in the author's view, is a valid conception, but before one can react to this word in the literature one must be aware of the particular use of it intended by the writer. Hysteria is used to describe conversion reactions; it is used to describe phobias and anxiety; it is used to describe psychopathic behavior in women; it is used for patients who malinger; it is used to describe a specific personality disorder; and, perhaps most frequently, it is used as an epithet by people who do not really know what it means.

In fact, "hysteria" has been so misused that many people have suggested abandoning the use of the word entirely. This would be unfortunate because the concept of hysterical personality disorder is very real, and this syndrome affects a great many people. Actually, as Chodoff and Lyons described it, the hysterical personality is of a very vain, dramatizing person who shows a great many affects, often in a labile manner (2). These people are extremely excitable and rather inconsistent and unpredictable. Their emotions are marked by not only rapid changes but also a shallowness which the observer senses. In addition, there is often a sexualization of the normal communication process along with a fear of true sexuality. Perhaps the most important characteristic of this syndrome is the fact that the patients are demanding in an extremely dependent way. Obviously, patients with this type of syndrome are patients who anger health care professionals, and one can easily see why this syndrome has evoked a great deal of hostility and why the name hysteria has become an epithet.

Probably, hypochondriasis is greatly over-diagnosed in that people with any sorts of "functional" symptoms are often labelled hypochondriacal. In fact, the term describes a very specific syndrome in which patients have a great many complaints about their health, usually involving several different systems of the body, and in addition to all these complaints they have an over-perception of physiologic events. One patient, for example, talked at length of how he experienced borborygmi. He apparently was unaware of the fact that this was a normal and universal physiological phenomenon.

Many patients who are ill become dependent on medications. Frequently, a symptom which began as a *bona fide* somatic symptom is unconsciously extended to provide continuation of the medication on which the patient is dependent.

Another type of dependence syndrome can be termed doctor dependence. There are many people who have their dependency needs met through physicians and other health personnel, including nurses. While it is frequently impossible to "cure" such patients, who are usually rather unhappy and very unfortunate people, it is frequently possible to meet some of their needs by providing a little bit of time for them. This can be extremely gratifying to such patients.

Another fairly common form of "functional" illness is that of illness obsession. As with any other obsessive phenomenon, the patient ruminates about having a particular illness, often cancer. The patient actually maintains the intellectual insight that he or she does not have cancer, and in this sense the illness obsession is very different from a delusion. Nevertheless, the obsession causes the patient a great deal of anxiety and often interferes significantly in his life. In this situation, it is of little benefit to reassure the patient that he does not have the illness since he actually already knows this. Treatment of the underlying obsessive personality features is often helpful.

Acute grief or loss can also present as "functional" illness. While it is not difficult to realize that a patient who has just lost a close family member, and who presents with similar symptoms to those which the family member had, is suffering from acute grief, it often becomes a difficult situation when the patient is undergoing a pathologic grief reaction. Often, after many years, the patient has a masked form of grieving. In this situation, the physician or nurse often misses the link between grief and the patient's illness. Often the symptoms which the patient has is a method of linkage to the dead object (3).

Depression can often present as "functional" illness. Some of the major manifestations of depression are decreased energy, decreased concentration, sleep disturbance and diurnal variation, along with a depressed mood. Sometimes many features of depression occur without the patient being aware of a depressed mood or communicating it to others. In this situation, a depressive equivalent is said to occur. In the patient with a depressive equivalent, the depressed affect may be subtle, though it is usually present. There is a sleep disturbance. There may be anorexia and weight loss. The patient's symptoms are usually worse in the morning. The patient has diminished concentration and a decrease in enjoyable activities. The patient often has an obsessive personality to begin with. Often, the losses caused by the illness outweigh the gains, which is quite different from the situation in the patient with a conversion reaction.

There are several forms of atypical depression. The depressive equivalent is one of them. Other people have subtle, mild depressions and may focus more on physical symptoms during those times. Others have chronic states of depression. A great deal of phobic, anxious behavior can be associated with a depressive state. Many patients with anorexia nervosa have many depressive features. In addition, there is a syndrome known as hysteroid dysphoria in which a patient has many signs of a hysterical type of reaction along with vegetative signs of depression. People with narcissistic and borderline personality disorders also may have many features of depressive illness.

Another form of "functional" illness is the somatic delusion. In this situation, the patient has a false fixed belief that something is wrong with him. Unlike the person with an illness obsession, this patient truly believes that there is something wrong with him. Usually the somatic delusion fits into one of two groups. The first group is the paranoid group. Patients with this type of somatic delusion often will mention that their brain has been implanted with tiny electrodes, or some similar paranoid type of idea. The person with this type of delusion may very well have a schizophreniform illness. The second type of somatic delusion is that of worthlessness or nihilism. This patient feels, for example, that his brain is being eaten away by maggots because he is such a bad person. This type of somatic delusion strongly suggests depression, and a trial of treatment for depression is certainly indicated in such a person.

Another type of illness along the biopsychosocial spectrum is that illness which involves both psychological and physical factors in a fairly equal proportion. One such illness is the so-called chronic pain syndrome. In a chronic pain syndrome, a patient usually begins with organic problems, often traumatically caused — for example, industrial accidents, often involving the back or other orthopedic injury. Often, these patients have premorbidly been very hard-working people who have not taken many vacations, who work two or more jobs, and who value themselves primarily as providers. Much of their self-esteem is linked to the fact that they are able to work hard and make money. Often they are people whose needs for dependence — which is a normal phenomenon all of us have — have not adequately been met.

Suddenly, such people find themselves in the so-called sick role, and their dependency needs are met for the first time. Often, the patients become addicted to pain medications, and in spite of frequent surgical and/or medical interventions the pain syndrome persists. The illness becomes a way of life in part because of the gains associated with it.

To deal with a chronic pain syndrome is often a frustrating experience because one must deal with its psychiatric, social and somatic factors. The sick role is so inviting to such patients — though they are not consciously aware of this — that any prime focus on the physical symptoms will often reinforce the syndrome as a whole. Often, the best approach to take with such patients is to concentrate on helping them cope with the pain rather than to attempt to remove it *in toto*. Thus, the best approach is to wean the patient from medications, to institute a program of gradually increasing exercises and activities, and to get the patient back to a situation in which he can return to work and to an active role in the family (4). Clearly, many attitudes need to be changed on the part of the patient with such a syndrome. This, too, is a difficult process because many of these people are not truly amenable to insight oriented psychotherapy in the usual sense.

A similar syndrome is anorexia nervosa. Here, young women, for the most part, become obsessed with the pursuit of being excessively thin. They develop an altered body image, often lose more than a quarter of their body weight, become obsessed with the pursuit of control, sometimes vomit in order to control their caloric intake, and exercise vigorously in order to maintain their low weight. This syndrome is sometimes preceded by signs of hypothalamic dysfunction, including cessation of menstruation and other hormonal abberations. Sometimes — perhaps more frequently — the hormonal imbalances do not occur until the illness is well underway. In any event, the symptom complex seems to be a final common pathway for many physiologic and psychopathologic conditions. Here, an illness has an incredible intermixture of psychological and physiological factors, and it becomes impossible to address the question of "which caused which?" and silly to approach the illness from an exclusively psychological or an exclusively organic point of view.

A third type of illness which we should address is the illness which traditionally has been considered purely somatic. One such illness *par excellence* is cancer. While actual studies of psychological influences on cancer and cancer's influences on the psyche have primarily been made in recent years, people have been aware of some influence of each on the other for many centuries, despite the fact that this never really permeated official medical and nursing dogma. Indeed, Galen wrote that depressed women were more prone to breast cancer than were other women. Sir James Paget believed that the level of happiness influences the development of cancer, and there is an old medical aphroism — which is as untrue as most old medical aphorisms — that "no happy man dies from cancer."

One of the great dangers of looking at cancer as a purely somatic illness is that because it is so threatening an illness, the physician often withdraws from the patient and tends to think of himself merely as treating the disease and not the patient. This certainly has influenced the role of the nurse, and many nurses respond by being particularly solicitous to the needs of the cancer patient, but many others tend to adopt the same attitude that this is a disease entity which happens to be encased in the body of a patient. We can look at the cancer as an illness which exemplifies stress (see Chapter 13). There are external stressors for the cancer patient, including the role of family, work, etc., and there are internal stressors — the illness itself and the psychological reaction to it. The cancer patient's reaction can be autoplastic or alloplastic and often is a mixture of the two.

LeShan has seen many patients with cancer and looked at them from the psychiatric point of view. Although his work is somewhat controversial, he has maintained that the onset of cancer is often associated with loss, the inability to express anger, unresolved grief, or an emotional stance of helplessness/hopelessness. Many clinicians who work with cancer patients share similar views, although one cannot be particularly dogmatic about it. LeShan found that 72% of patients with cancer had suffered the loss of a central relative during a period ranging from 8 years to 8 months prior to the onset of clinical disease, compared to 10% in a control group of people (5).

No matter what the previous personality structure and psychological problems of the cancer patient may have been, once the patient finds out that he has cancer he or she is in a very difficult situation. One has to ask what it is like for the patient to suddenly learn that he has cancer. Patients in this society often view diagnosis of cancer as a form of death sentence, and they frequently react by a certain amount of social withdrawal from their family and friends; this withdrawal is often, unfortunately, mirrored by a similar withdrawal of family and friends from the patient. A sense of social isolation often occurs. The patient has to deal with many losses as a result of all this. It is important for the nurse to delineate grief from depression, which can worsen the prognosis of the cancer patient.

The defenses of cancer patients are well worth examining, just as are the defenses of the psychiatrically ill patient. Some of the primitive defenses which are used by many people include splitting, projection, denial, projective identification and repression. These defenses are discussed in Chapter 4. With the cancer patient one often sees the emergence of some of these primitive defenses at various times in the illness. This does not mean that the patient has always functioned at a primitive level, and the use of these defenses does not necessitate a psychiatric consultation. Many of us use such primitive defenses for brief periods when we are under great stress or threat. The same is obviously the case for cancer patients. The defense mechanism of splitting, however, can be particularly hazardous to the cancer patient because splitting usually occurs for these patients within a hospital setting. As a result of this defense, some members of the staff will perceive the patient as compliant while others will see the patient as extremely hostile, manipulative and a "bad patient." These people, needless to say, will not give the patient the same sort of attention they give to other patients. In addition to the use of primitive defenses, many cancer patients use several other defense mechanisms. Among these are identification with the aggressor, in which the patient often seems to ally himself with the physician, which can be helpful to both; sometimes, however, the patient seems to ally himself with the disease itself and this, of course, can greatly undermine the treatment. Other patients use a great deal of sublimation, and in these patients we see a search for the meaning of their illness and the persepctive this gives them on their life. This defense mechanism may sometimes seem alien to the nurse, but it is a high level defense and often extremely meaningful to the patient. I think that the use of sublimation should rarely be challenged by any health care professional. Another common defense of cancer patients is isolation of affect. In this situation, the patient seems to hear bad news about his illness without very much reaction. Isolation of affect often occurs along with the defense of intellectualization in which the patient seems to react to news of the progression of his illness with an intellectual interest and curiosity.

Central to the cancer patient is the need for control. With all the losses entailed by cancer, the patient often feels very much out of control. One way to help the patient deal with the loss of control is to discuss this issue quite frankly. In addition, one should discuss some of the common concerns shared by many people with cancer. These often are not communicated to the physician or nurse, but they should be and they are certainly worth dealing with.

Many patients also believe that their cancer is something they have caused. Of course, sometimes the patient has indeed contributed to the cancer, as in the case of a heavy cigarette smoker who develops lung cancer. There is need, however, to focus on the patient's role in getting the cancer. One is fearful that chapters and articles such as this, which look at the psychiatric and psychological makeup of a patient prior to development of his cancer, can be misread by patients and misunderstood, and make patients feel even more guilty. A surprisingly small number of cancer patients are overtly guilty about having their illness, but paradoxically some long-term survivors of the illness do develop guilt feelings concerning their survival.

For most patients, the major impact of cancer, aside from the physical threat to the organism, is loss of control, and this causes a refocusing of priorities. The nurse can listen to the patient talk about this potential refocusing and can often be extremely helpful.

In addition to the psychological makeup of the patient prior to development of his illness and the defenses used by patients with the illness, we must focus on actual psychopathology which occurs during the course of the illness. A great many cancer patients become extremely tense and anxious about the illness and this is, of course, understandable. The nurse can be very helpful in dealing with such a patient. Grief, as mentioned, is a normal response to the diagnosis of cancer and can be very helpful to the patient in mobilizing defenses and coping patterns. Depression, on the other hand, is not helpful to the patient and, in fact, can possibly foster the rapid development of the disease. A depressed patient with cancer should be treated vigorously for the depression. Some cancer patients become somewhat paranoid. Usually this is a transient phenomenon and, again, the understanding of the nurse and physician team can be most helpful to such a patient. Suicide is one question which frequently occurs in patients with cancer. Physicians and nurses become extremely concerned when such a patient seems despondent or even talks about ending his or her life. In the vast majority of cases, the talk about suicide is nothing more than a means of perceiving that one remains in control of *something* until the very end of life. With all the losses of cancer, sometimes the patient's perception is that the only phenomenon he can control is the decision to terminate or not terminate his life. The knowledge that the patient can do this is often, paradoxically, very helpful to the patient. At the same time, one must assess the suicide potential of every patient who discusses suicide or who shows other signs of it. Of course, with many patients who have terminal illness and who are in enormous pain, one must wonder how realistic an option suicide might be.

Other examples of serious psychopathology in the cancer patient include psychosis and severe depression. All patients with cancer almost by definition have an adjustment reaction to the syndrome. This is to be expected, and the sensitive nurse can be helpful to the patient in dealing with this syndrome. Often, neurotic defenses are mobilized briefly by the cancer patient. These are best left alone unless they are of long duration and significantly interfere with the patient's life.

The situation is a bit more complex, however. Even though there are many psychogenic causes of the problems which cancer patients encounter, some behavioral abnormalities are incorrectly attributed to psychogenic causes. The patient's reaction to the meaning of his illness are always important, but sometimes behavioral abnormalities are caused by the patient's disturbed physiology, whether it is the cancer itself or the sequelae of the treatment of that cancer. There is fairly good data that when large groups of patients on chemotherapy are compared with other cancer patients not on chemotherapy, neuropsychometric testing shows a slight but significant malfunction in cognitive capacities of the patients on chemotherapy.

Another area in which *psyche* and *soma* interact in this illness is that of tumor anorexia. The reasons for this are unclear, and there has been a significant amount of work on this topic. Work with rats given experimental tumors indicates that the decline in food intake which accompanies the growth of the tumor is accompanied by the development of aversions to the specific diet consumed during the growth of the tumor. An immediate elevation of food consumption occurs in the rats when a novel diet is introduced. Thus, the development of learned aversions to a specific diet during a tumor growth could be a causal factor in the development of tumor anorexia (6).

How can the nurse assist the patient with cancer? One important thing which she can do is to be part of a holistic approach to the entire problem. There is a need to treat the illness, not just the disease. There is a great need to instill and encourage hope, even if this is hope of a limited remission or limited control of pain. It is extremely important to have clear communication with the patient and with the patient's family. In addition, it is helpful if there is one primary nurse who deals with the patient and his family whenever possible.

All one needs to do, then, is to be able to talk, share and accept the feelings of the cancer patient; be alert, be flexible and accept being human. Of course, if one can do all these things one is more than human; one is perfect! However, it seems to me that one can certainly strive to meet these particular goals. There is no rule against being innovative in the nursing care of such patients as long as this innovation is in the direction of increasing the patient's self-esteem, sense of hope, and sense of control.

Perhaps one reason there is so little innovation in terms of bedside management of the seriously ill patient is the fear of peer review. However, our loyalty needs to be to the patient and not exclusively to our peers.

In this disucssion, we have focused on some of the problems that the patient encounters in dealing with a serious illness such as cancer. The health care provider also encounters very serious problems. Frequently, the nurse who works with a seriously ill patient uses similar defenses to the patient, including intellectualization, isolation of affect, identification with the aggressor — in this case the illness — and splitting. The nurse may find herself having "good" patients and "bad" patients, or may perceive other members of the staff as good or gad. When these defenses break down, and they sometimes do, the health care provider may have to deal with depression, extreme anger, or the sense of giving up.

Another concern which all health care providers must have for the patient with any illness, and certainly with a potentially terminal illness, is countertransference. This is the nurse's own real reaction to the patient plus his or her transference reaction to the patient — the way the nurse perceives the patient as similar to important objects in her own life. Countertransference is something that we all tend to shy away from and to feel somewhat guilty about, but it is universal and inevitable, and the important thing is to recognize it. If we do not recognize countertransference, particularly if it is negative countertransference, we often end up giving very negative messages to the pateint under the guise of therapy. It is much easier and kinder to the patient to the patient to recognize the feelings we have within us about that patient and then try to understand those feelings. Frequently, countertransference manifestations include boredom, impatience, a sense of wanting to argue with the patient, feeling very inadequate and discouraged, or inappropriately bland or fearful.

Countertransference is not uniquely a psychiatric phenomenon. It occurs in every encounter between nurse and patient, and indeed it occurs in all our social interactions as well. In dealing with the cancer patient, the normally caring nurses initially responds as a human, empathic person to a troubled, threatened patient who may feel helpless. There is an initial urge toward active help of the patient. If that initial urge is not somehow met by the patient, however, the nurse often feels frustrated and either tries harder or withdraws. Unless one is aware of this sort of cycle, one will have trouble with a great many patients.

In dealing with all the patients discussed in this chapter, it is helpful to keep in mind an old statement of George Bernard Shaw, the playwright: "Diagnosis should mean the finding out of all that is wrong with the patient and not the formal and unctuous pronouncement of a name that obsolves from the necessity of further investigation." In this chapter I have attempted to demonstrate the unity of "functional" and "organic" illnesses and the fact that each has a unique psychological, social and biological framework.

REFERENCES

1. Engel, G.L.: The need for a new medical model: a challenge for biomedicine, Science, *196:*129–136 (1977).

2. Chodoff, P., and Lyons, H.: Hysteria, the hysterical personality and "hysterical" conversion, Am J Psychiat, *114:*734 (1958).

3. Volkan, V.D.: The linking objects of pathological mourners, Arch Gen Psychiat, *27:*215 (1972).

4. Swanson, D.W.; Swenson, W.M.; Maruta, T., *et al.*: Program for managing chronic pain: I. Program description and charactrristics of patients, Mayo Clinic Proc, *51:*401 (1976).

5. LeShan, L.: An emotional life-history pattenr associated with neoplastic disease, Ann NY Acad Sci, *125:*780 (1966).

6. Bernstein, I.L., and Sigmundi, R.A.: Tumor anorexia: a learned food aversion? Science, *209:*416 (1980).

5 An Introduction to Psychoanalytic Theory

Eric K. Milliner

This chapter will consider the practical application of psychoanalytic theory and psychodynamic psychotherapy to psychiatric nursing in the general hospital setting. The topic will be approached with four goals in mind: 1) To compare and contrast the psychodynamic model with the other theoretical approaches in psychiatry; 2) To present a psychoanalytically-oriented model of adult personality organization; 3) To employ that model in understanding clinical psychopathology, and 4) To outline a practical approach to nursing care.

HOW PSYCHOANALYTIC THEORY RELATES TO GENERAL PSYCHIATRY

Psychodynamically-oriented psychotherapy is a modified treatment technique based on psychoanalytic theory and practice. It may be useful for the reader to review the history of Freud's original work and the tradition of psychoanalytic thought which has led to contemporary consideration of Ego Psychology which lie beyond the scope of this present chapter. There are several observations about that historical tradition, however, which merit repeating for our purposes. Specifically, it should be kept in mind that Freud's original training was in neurology; and throughout his professional lifetime he remained rigorously committed to a medical model of mental illness. Specifically, it remained his firm conviction that thought and emotion are mediated through the organically-based, neurophysiologic pathways of the central nervous system, and that at some future date psychopathology would be clearly understood and treated as a physically-based illness. However, in his day, as at the present time, our understanding of the specific neuroanatomic and physiologic pathways is insuffucient to allow organically-based diagnosis and treatment of many psychiatric disorders. Therefore, despite his philosophical commitment to an organic perspective, Freud was willing to accept the usefulness of a hypothetical model which allowed him to observe and understand clinical phenomena in greater detail than could be accomplished from an exclusively organic approach. The usefulness of the model is in the fact that it allows us to conceptualize more meaningfully many clinical phenomena which otherwise would defy logical explanation. In this sense, Freud's work employs metaphorical analogies and concepts in a manner similar to other areas of medicine. For example, nephrologists use the concept of "sodium pump" to explain the energy-requiring transport system which moves ions across the semipermeable membranes in the kidney. In that example, no one believes that there is literally a "pump" mechanism involved, but the illustration usefully conceptualizes a phenomenon which ordinarily we would have difficulty comprehending. Freud's theoretical model (elaborated below) has usefulness in a similar fashion. Nevertheless, it should be re-emphasized that Freud's entire view of psychopathology is thoroughly compatible with a rigorously physiologic, organically-based, medical understanding of central nervous system functioning.

There are several basic tenets which separate psychoanalytic theory from the perspective of other schools of psychiatric thought. For our purposes, we will consider five important areas of emphasis: 1) The existence of a dynamic unconscious; 2) The principle of psychic determinism; 3) The behavioral reflection of repetition compulsion; 4) The existence of transference experiences in everyday life, and 5) The usefulness of transference and countertransference phenomena in understanding clinical psychopathology.

Virtually all psychiatrists would acknowledge that there are aspects of mental life which are not readily accessible to an individual's conscious awareness. To some, this material is considered to be simply "forgotten," and is viewed as irrelevant to current mental functioning. However, for the psychoanalytically-oriented clinician, the "unconscious" is viewed as having a specific, *dynamic* influence in governing the overall course of cognition and emotional experience. This unconscious content and its activity and relevance to the overall patterns of mental functioning is termed the "dynamic unconscious."

This leads us to the second principle; namely "psychic determinism." Clinically, we may often observe that the overall pattern of thought, emotional experience, conscious choices and specific behavior are guided not primarily by deliberate voluntary intentions, but rather by *unconscious* factors outside the individual's recognition. By illustration, one might draw a comparison between the structure of mental life and that of an iceberg, where the conscious portion of the mind is that aspect of the iceberg above the water surface. The bulk of mental life, just like the bottom portion of the iceberg, is truly unconscious, below the surface and behind the scenes. In much the same way that the drift of an iceberg is determined not by the wind that blows on the top of the water, but by the strong water currents and massive content below the surface, so also the drift of one's mental life is determined much more by unconscious factors than by one's deliberate, conscious, voluntary intentions.

Since life for many individuals is filled with unsettled conflict, the unconscious factors which determine future choice may be strongly influenced by unresolved factors from the past. Quite separate from conscious intentions (which are often opposite to the outcome of one's actual behavior) the pattern of choices may serve at an unconscious level to recreate old traumatic situations for the purpose of intended mastery of the previous problems. However, rather than accomplishing a more productive outcome, what often happens is that the old maladaptive set of circumstances is simply recreated, with no new mastery occurring and the previous pattern and outcome is repeated time after time. This repetitive pattern is referred to by the technical term "repetition compulsion." A clinical example comes from the case of a women who is married for the fifth time to a physically abusive, alcoholic husband and who swears after each divorce that she will never get involved with a similar man again. She fails to realize that the pattern is determined unconsciously by unresolved conflicts from childhood and the influence of a father who was a physically abusive alcoholic.

The next theoretical focus of clinical importance which distinguishes psychodynamic psychotherapy from other forms of psychiatric treatment is the role ascribed to the "transference" in interpersonal relationships. By definition, "transference" means the inappropriate displacement (from some time in the past) of old attitudes, expectations, emotions, perceptions and patterns of behavior which are rekindled in current interpersonal relationships when the new set of circumstances provides *unconscious* reminders of the past. Transference is most likely to occur in those situations where emotional relationships are potentially intense and often the most conflicted; and where the current interaction somewhat rekindles feelings about primary early childhood experiences with important care providers and authority figures (i.e., parents and other significant people). Transference phenomena are perfectly normal and occur in a variety of day-to-day situations (for example, with teachers, bosses, supervisors, head nurses, etc; and in any situation where someone is perceived as either a care provider and/or authority). While other schools of psychiatric thought recognize the existence of transference phenomena, only psychoanalytically-oreinted theory and practice focuses upon the transference as a mainstay for understanding and treating patients in psychotherapy. Understandably, nurses and physicians are uniquely suited to mobilize intense transference phenomena among their patients, since in the clinical setting it is the professional person who will be viewed as the most immediate "authority" and "care provider." To the extent that transference exists in the clinical setting, the patient's perception of the care provider will be distorted. Often the professional staff will feel that the patient has "unrealistic" or "unfair" expectations and attitudes. As we will see later, however, psychodynamic theory views the existence of transference as a unique opportunity to understand the emotional subtleties of the patient's pathology. (In contrast to psychiatrists of other persuasions who often view the existence of transference distortions as an unwelcomed, unfortunate annoyance.)

Finally, the phenomena of "countertransference" is to be understood as the staff member's equivalent to the transference experience; whereby at an unconscious level we bring into the clinical situation our own displaced, inappropriate attitudes, expectations and emotional reactions to patients, based *not* on the reality of current interaction but rather as a reflection of our own unresolved, pre-existing conflicts. To the extent that these countertransference feelings exist unrecognized within ourselves, they add to the possibility of distorting our perception of the patient and our clinical role.

All of the above points of emphasis serve to distinguish the focus of psychodynamically-oriented treatment from other disciplines within psychiatry (i.e., from the viewpoint of learning theory psychology, behavioral psychiatry, purely organic theories of mental illness, phenomenologic and existentialist viewpoints, etc.).

THE STRUCTURAL MODEL OF ADULT PERSONALITY FROM A PSYCHODYNAMIC VIEWPOINT

Our next task will be to outline a hypothetical, structural model of the adult personality to assist our understanding of personality organization from a psychoanalytic perspective. By analogy, one might consider psychological structures and their functioning to be similar to the anatomy and physiology of normal adult individuals in the physical sense; recognizing that pathology exists whenever the structure and/or functioning of the organism is somewhat disturbed. Conversely, "normality" may be defined as a structure (either physical or mental) which has matured in an age-appropriate fashion and which functions flexibly and adaptively through interactions with the internal and external environments. It should be emphasized that this section will consider *normal* mental structures and their functioning.

I shall begin by outlining the basic content of each of the three major structural components of the mind, and then return to discuss in more detail the specifics of their functioning and how each interrelates with the other. The three components to which I am referring are the id, ego and superego.

The id may be conceptualized as an innate, inborn dimension of mental experience whose content exists from birth and continues throughout life at predominantly an unconscious level. The "drives" which make up the content of the id are best understood as psychological derivatives of biological instincts. The drives are comprised of two basic components; namely, libidinal (sexual) and aggressive impulses. Each drive component must be understood in much broader definition than what the term might spontaneously bring to mind. Specifically, the libidinal (or so-called "sexual") drive includes much more than just adult genital sexual behavior. Specifically, it encompasses all psychological motivation which would prompt individuals toward dependency, affection, gregariousness, and warmth of close human attachment (a small component of which obviously includes genital sexual activity). However, it should be clear that the sexual drive includes much more than just genital sexual behavior. In a similar fashion, the so-called "aggressive" drive includes much more than hostile, destructive behavior. The term includes all aspects of personal initiative, autonomy, assertiveness, independence, control, and the desire to take a stand on one's own behalf; a small portion of which is actually hostile, destructive and truly aggressive behavior in the conventional sense.

The drives residing within the id constantly generate a psychological pressure for discharge and gratification through behavioral expression in the external world. However, unlike the instinctual behavior of animals which is stereotyped in its expression (leading to pattenrs of behavior which are identical for all members of a given species; as for example, the migratory and nest-building behavior of birds and the territoriality of nonhuman primates), the overt expression of human drives is subject to tremendous variation based on the influence of the two other structural components of the mind which we are about to consider. Thus, even though there may be universal qualities of shared drive derivatives within all individuals, their overt expression in actual behavior shows infinite variety and individuality.

The next structural component of the mind is the ego, which might be envisioned as an executive agent. It serves to moderate the input of the id with the demands arising from the superego/ ego ideal, while coordinating the entire intrapsychic apparatus with the demands of the external environment as well. Thus, before going on to discuss specific ego functions in greater detail, it might be well to consider in brief the nature of the superego and ego ideal.

The superego is perhaps most simply understood as analogous to the "conscience;" that system of internalized values, standards, moral principles and criteria for assessing the appropriateness of thoughts and actions. That internalized system of values and standards is combined quite closely with the "ego ideal." This structure can be defined as the "ideal self-concept" toward which each of us might aspire if our goals and aspirations for successful performance were able to be perfected to their ultimate ideal. Content in that area is often role-specific; in that each of us might have an internalized concept of what it might mean to be the "ideal student," "ideal professional," "ideal spouse," "ideal child," etc. Thus, an intact superego provides an internal regulatory mechanism for assessing the appropriateness of behavior; while a well-integrated ego ideal provides a standard toward which we strive and a source of internal motivation for an ever more successful and perfected performance. We will return to a further consideration of the superego and ego ideal later in the chapter. For now, having defined the content of the id and remembering that it seeks constant and *immediate* gratification of drive–determined impulses, one can easily envision the internal conflicts which could easily arise when id wishes comes into opposition with standards and values put forth by the superego and ego ideal. Thus, one primary challenge for the ego, in its role as the executive agent, is to deal with these potentially conflicted intentions (from the two other components) in such a way as to decrease anxiety and keep the potential conflicts to a minimum.

Ego functions may be summarized under the following categories: 1) Defensive functions; 2) Reality testing; 3) Object representations and object relationships; 4) Autonomous functions, and 5) Synthetic functions.

We shall now consider each of the ego's functions in turn:

1) **Defensive functions:** The defensive functions of the ego occur spontaneously, at an *unconscious* level and are not subject to voluntary control. They operate at two interfaces; namely at the boundary between the id and ego, and also (as we shall discuss later) at the boundary between the ego and the superego. These *normal* phenomena are techniques whereby the ego copes with psychological pressures which would otherwise create consciously unpleasurable emotional states.

Two general categories of emotional unpleasure are considered equal in their ability to trigger defense mechanisms. The first is anxiety: namely, a state of psychological discomfort accompanied by an apprehension that "something bad is going to happen" as an undesirable intrapsychic event in the future. The second, depression, may be defined as a state of discomfort accompanied by the cognitive perception that "something bad has already happened," as an undesirable psychological and emotional experience. These unpleasant psychological experiences *may* or *may not* be related to actual events in the external world. (Historically, early psychoanalytic theory assumed that defense mechanisms operate only at the interface between the ego and id; and postulated that anxiety was unique in its ability to elicit those mechanisms. In that context, the anxiety was referred to as "signal anxiety."

If defense mechanisms are adequate to contain and control the impending internal conflict, then much of the content remains partially or totally unconscious and the entire process occurs at an abstract psychological level. However, if defense mechanisms prove inadequate to cope with the threatened psychological imbalance, symptom formation may occur as an extension of the defensive process. In this instance, the abstract quality of the mental process often gives way to concrete, tangible, observable "symptomatic behavior."

Symptoms function to preserve a degree of psychological balance for the patient (often at the price of many maladaptive influences on life styles and interpersonal relationships) by creating an illusion of control and mastery over a conflict which was unmanageable at a psychologically abstract level. For example, compulsive hand-washing may symbolically capture an ambivalent wish and fear of aggressive impulses, reflecting the conflicted obsessive fantasy that germs and contamination could cause illness or death. The intensity of the originally abstract impulse/fear of doing harm to others may lessen, when the symptom gives the feeling that the conflict is resolved and no harm will come so long as the ritualized routine of hand washing is carefully followed. The cognitive shift from abstraction to tangible, concretely symbolized expressions of psychological issues is what is referred to as the "concrete thinking" of more seriously disturbed patients and/or psychologically unsophisticated individuals.

There are numerous defense mechanisms, all of which may be normal but some of which are more psychologically mature in the sense of arising at later stages of childhood psychosexual development. Several representative defense mechanisms will be considered briefly.

The most universal and most psychologically immature (i.e., present from the earliest stage of childhood development) is "repression." This term applies to the unconscious process whereby the ego massively blocks the conscious emergence of unconscious content, and the impulses arising out of either the id or superego are pushed back toward their source of origin. Repression is automatically and spontaneously involved in every instance in which psychologically conflicted material seeks to become conscious. However, being the most primitive of the defenses, it is also, in a sense, the least satisfactory, for it fails to allow any discharge of the original impulse. Therefore, if the impulse is sufficiently strong, repression will fail and other defense mechanisms will be involved in an effort to allow the subsequent discharge to be better tolerated by the conscious ego.

Early in the course of childhood development, a set of relatively primitive defense mechanisms supplements the original efforts of repression. These include projection, denial and identification with the aggressor. Projection is the mechanism whereby an originally conflicted impulse is redefined as arising from some external source rather than being acknowledged as part of one's own mental life. For example, a small child may verbalize fantasies that his stuffed lion is going to attack his baby brother. In this instance, the child's own aggressive wishes are externalized and attributed to the outside object. "Denial" also allows partial conscious recognition of the conflicted wish, but disguises it through a spontaneous negation of its content. For example, a child may spontaneously assert that, "I don't hate my little brother," thereby affirming the opposite of the original conflicted emotion. Through the unconscious mechanism of "identification with the aggressor," an individual who feels vulnerable may adopt character traits of the adversary he fears. A feeling of power and control is often experienced as their original passivity is transformed into an illusion of active mastery. For example, a young child who has been physically abused may internalize qualities of her parent's personality; becoming intolerant, tyrannical and physically aggressive toward her dolls in play.

At a somewhat more sophisticated level, projection may be coupled with mechanisms of "displacement" and "avoidance;" thereby structuring the basic pattern inherent in phobic symptom formation. For example, a child may initially project his originally conflicted aggressive wish towards a parent of the same sex (a normal phenomena during the competitive stage of Oedipal development). However, in terms of being psychologically at ease, it may be as stressful to be the target of aggression as it was to possess the original aggressive drive. Therefore, especially in instances where there is the wish to preserve a close affectionate relationship with the original target of one's aggression, the originally projected impulse may be subsequently "displaced." By this, we mean that the focus shifts from one external object to another (the second object usually being of far less psychological importance than the first). Then, by avoiding the second "phobic" object, the individual is allowed to preserve his positive affectionate ties with the original person. The classic example of this phenomena was described by Sigmund Freud in his case of "little Hans." He outlines the clinical history of a boy who, in the Oedipal stage of development, displaced his originally projected aggressive drive toward father onto horses; developing the phobic preoccupation that horses would bite him. He thereby, unconsciously, became the target of his own aggression which was initially projected and subsequently displaced. However, at the expense of suffering with his symptom, he was able to preserve his affectionate relationship with his father intact.

Another constellation of defense mechanisms involves undoing, intellectualization, rationalization and isolation of affect. "Undoing" is the behavioral manifestation (either in a mental or motor act) which symbolizes both the original conflicted drive and reparative or corrective action in the opposite direction. Undoing is frequently coupled with mechanisms of intellectualization, rationalization and isolation of affect in the formation of an "obsessive-compulsive neurosis." For example, a woman complained of constant preoccupation with worries that some harm might come to her family if the gas burners of the stove were left on over-night. Therefore, before going to bed each evening she would turn *on* all the gas jets in order that she could then be sure to turn them all *off*. In this way, her behavior manifested her ambivalent feelings toward her family; turning on the jets was followed by the "undoing" of her unconscious aggressive impulse. "Intellectualization" and "rationalization" involve the technique and content of providing a pseudological explanation for behavior which is irrational or motivated by conflicted drives. Isolation of affect (manifest by a clinically pseudo-objective and emotionally dispassionate assessment of one's thoughts or behavior) is a defense mechanism which splits the cognitive content from the expectable emotional experience. An individual using this defense experiences the cognitive content without an experiential awareness of the accompanying emotion, the latter remaining totally unconscious.

Reversal and reaction formation are closely-coupled mechanisms of defense which convert the original impulse into its opposite and lead to prompt action in keeping with the distorted, disguised end result. For example, a middle-aged man lived for 18 months at the bedside of his terminally-ill mother, waiting on her hand and foot. Even when his other siblings offered to share the burden, he adamantly refused their assistance. By history, he was the child who, in earlier years, had had the greatest conflict with his mother. His original aggression was reversed, and a reaction formation ensued whereby the manifest behavior was the exact opposite of the original conflicted impulse (i.e., the impermissible wish to be rid of the mother he had always hated).

Sublimation is the most mature of all defense mechanisms. It is that process whereby the original primitive drive is translated into behavior which allows its expression in activities which are socially approved and often admired. For example, originally conflicted homosexual impulses may be subliminated in contact sports such as football and wrestling.

The above discussion has considered only a few of the defense mechanisms. You may familiarize yourself with others from reading in any standard textbook of psychiatry.

2) **Reality testing:** Reality testing refers to the ego's capacity to assess the interface between internal psychological states and external environmental situations. In this regard, the ego has the ability to distinguish between "fact" and "fantasy." In patients whose psychological adjustment has been severely impaired as psychopathologic processes, this ability of the ego may be severely compromised. For example, the schizophrenic patient may be unable to distinguish between his own internal fantasy world and his sensory perceptions of external reality. Hallucinations, illusions and delusional thinking are clinical reflections of impaired reality testing.

3) **Object representations and object relationships:** Object relations are a dimension of ego function which has both conscious and unconscious aspects. For each individual, experiences with significant people in the external environment are accompanied by an internal, psychological, mental representation of those persons in the mind of the beholder. From a psychoanalytic perspective, it is the internal, mental object representation of "significant others" which is psychologically relevant. Certainly, many times, this dimension may correspond accurately to actual relationships in the external world. However, as one moves along the spectrum from normality towards increasing psychopathology, distortions of internal object representations increase accordingly. Therefore, it is not unusual that a severely psychotic patient may describe family members as having personality characteristics strikingly different from those observed by hospital staff when those people are actually interviewed. The patient's impairment of object representations may account for the disparity, rather than the possibility that relatives might be "on their good behavior" when they meet with the nurse. Clinically, psychopathology is best understood through focusing upon the *internal* object representations, for it is the way in which events and people are *perceived* which is most relevant to the patient's emotional

adjustment. Sometimes the patient's mental depiction of important object relationships may be quite separate from the "facts" or actual historical occurrences.

4) **Autonomous functions:** The autonomous functions of the ego have a degree of cognitive and emotional independence from id and superego pressures. These functions exist quite independently and include the type of mental activities ordinarily categorized as abstract "cortical functions." Specifically, this category of conscious ego function includes such phenomena as the ability to perform formal logical and mathematical tasks; orientation in time and place; and activities such as artistic and musical creativity. All these activities are relatively unencumbered by pressures from either the id or superego. Autonomous functions are generally, therefore, unimpaired by so-called "functional" psychopathology; and, by contrast, are frequently compromised by organic, toxic and/or metabolic derangements of the central nervous system.

5) **Synthetic functions:** The ego's "synthetic functions" are the most generalized, and pertain to the ego's executive function in accomplishing a harmonious, compromised, dynamic balance between the demands of the id, superego, and external world. In this respect, the ego serves as an arbitrator, mediator, and final common pathway for handling the frequently opposing and often intense demands of each of these three other areas.

Having considered both the id and ego, we now return to the final structural components of the personality: the superego and ego ideal. Unlike the id (which is present at birth) and the ego (whose potential is present in infancy and which quickly evolves with the development of verbal cognitive capacities), the superego does not crystalize until approximately the third to fifth year of life. Prior to that time, the child's behavior is initially exclusively (and by gradually lessening degrees, partially) regulated by outside rules and regulations. The child, prior to the development of a superego, will modify this behavior in keeping with external standards, not because of internally-experienced guilt but out of apprehension of shame and punishment imposed by external authorities, especially parents. However, after the superego is internalized through taking into one's self a pattern of standards derived from observations of external "authorities," the child's behavior becomes self-regulating. Thereafter, the superego makes its own demands upon the ego, often in direct opposition to drives arising out of the id. As mentioned above, defense mechanisms may be employed at the interface between the ego and the superego, in order to temper the demands of "conscience" and allow some discharge of the original drive. For example, rationalization may temper superego demands when an individual unconsciously says of his sexual or aggressive wishes, "It's okay; everyone else is doing it."

Coupled with the superego is the so-called "ego ideal." The ego ideal refers to both conscious and unconscious dimensions of an internalized perception of "Who I should ideally be" and "What I should ideally become." The adequacy of an individual's self-esteem rests in large measure upon the internal psychological comparison of one's current self-perception with one's "ego ideal." The adequacy of personal psychological adjustment depends in part upon being able to keep the disparity between these two components to a minimum, or to mobilize resources within the self which makes attainment of the ego ideal seem plausible. When the contrast between the "actual" and "ideal" self-concept becomes too great, anxiety or depression may result (based on apprehensions about future failure, or conclusions in retrospect that one has already failed to "measure up" to one's own internal standards of acceptable performance).

Having considered the three main structural components of the personality, one might summarize by stating that adequacy of normal psychological adjustment depends upon a harmonious balance among these agencies of the mind in keeping with the demands and realities of the external world. Flexibility of internal psychological adaptation in response to the dynamic fluctuations within this system is of utmost importance.

A PSYCHODYNAMIC FORMULATION OF CLINICAL PSYCHOPATHOLOGY

The conceptualization of psychopathology from a psychodynamic viewpoint utilizes an understanding of the structure of personality organization and function as outlined above. From that perspective, psychopathology can arise either because of problems in development (i.e., constitutional, structural abnormalities reflecting aberrancies in developmental maturation which cause lifelong defects in personality) or from maladaptive responses to psychological stress arising from either internal conflicts, environmental circumstances, or both (i.e., illness of recent origin affecting a personality whose structure and functioning was previously relatively normal). The former might be considered analogous to congenital heart disease which results in the compromise of cardiac function in a heart which was never structurally "normal." The latter might be considered analogous to acquired atherosclerotic heart disease (of internal origin) or alcoholic toxic cardiomyopathy (of external origin) as illustrations of disease processes affecting a previously healthy myocardium.

In general, the spectrum of personality function ranging from normality on the one hand to psychosis on the other can be summarized according to these considerations:

1) **"Normality"** requires that the *structural* components of the personality have matured in an age-appropriate fashion, relatively free from the distortions which might result from major emotional traumas or maladaptive patterns of mother-child interaction experienced in early development. The normal individual has an ego possessing a flexible, mature spectrum of adaptive defense mechanisms and the capacity for accurate reality testing even under the most stressful circumstances. Such an individual's object representations and intrapsychic perceptions of the relationships between "self" and important "others" is realistic in content and relatively free from conflicts. The self-concept is equally realistic and free from major narcissistic distortions of grandiosity on the one hand and/or self-denigration on the other. The ego ideal is sufficiently attainable that major feelings of inadequacy in current self-concept are avoided, yet is sufficiently idealized that motivation for self-actualization and productivity is sustained. The superego is neither too punitive nor too lax, appropriately structured between extremes, and thus permits reasonable degrees of id drive gratification on the one hand while protecting the individual from maladaptive, impulsive self-indulgence on the other. As alluded to already, these normal "structures" are accompanied by a flexible, adaptive, reciprocal pattern of dynamic *function*, and potential conflicts are dealt with without major dysphoria, impairment of practical daily function or symptom formation.

In summary, the normal individual is psychologically well equipped to be appropriately assertive without malevolent hostility; to be sexually expressive in sustained and intimate relationships without excessive dependency or primitive pre-genital distortions; and to maintain an adequate sense of self-esteem, a wide spectrum of meaningful interpersonal relationships, and a genuine degree of productivity and enjoyment in his work and play. To a significant extent, such individuals have deinstinctualized some aspects of their motivations, so that energy previously devoted to gratifying conflicted sexual or aggressive impulses can be turned instead to creativity, intellectual growth and richer interpersonal relationships.

2) **"Neurosis"** is that form of psychiatric illness characterized by symptom formation in reaction to intrapsychic conflict. Such individuals typically possess a *structure* of personality which is basically intact. However, adaptive *functioning* is compromised by the influence of unresolved childhood developmental conflicts (termed points of "fixation"). Such "fixations" may reflect any of the psychological issues which are phase specific to the period of psychosexual development when the original "trauma" occurred. For example, individuals who experienced excessive frustration or gratification during the "oral period" (birth to age 18 months) may show neurotic vulnerability to conflicts regarding object loss, "basic trust" and intimacy/dependency in adult interpersonal relationships. For those whose developmental conflicts centered around issues of toilet training during the "anal phase" (varying from age 12-16 months to approximately 3 years), themes of compliance/defiance of authority, control, ambivalence, procrastination and sadomasochistic or aggressive conflicts may predominate in adult symptom formation. Likewise, persons who experienced difficulty during the Oedipal phase (ranging variously from age 2½-3 years up to 4½-6 years) may develop phobic, dissociative, conversion or somatization disorders in adulthood as a reflection of childhood sexualized competitive strivings and fears of punishment. The latter is termed "castration anxiety;" and applies to the fear of reprisal for forbidden competitive sexual wishes in both sexes.

When a previously asymptomatic but neurotically-vulnerable individual encounters a major psychological stress (either "intrapsychically' as through increased conflicted impulses or compromised self-esteem *or* "externally" through difficult environmental circumstances), an unconscious defensive retreat to a point of previous "fixation" is frequently mobilized. The term "regression" is applied to this process of reverting to a more immature, developmentally-primitive pattern of characterologic functioning.

At times, regression alone can prove adaptive and sufficient to alleviate the conflict. However, symptom formation may follow if defense mechanisms alone prove inadequate to control the psychological distress. Neurotic symptoms often portray an ambivalent, impermissible or conflicted impulse in disguised, symbolic fashion; affording a degree of permissive expression for the impermissible wish through the symbolic behavior; and imposing a punishment at the same time as a derivative of unconscious superego retributions. Thus, symptom formation serves an adaptive purpose; meeting some aspects of the demands imposed on the ego by id and superego, while at the same time affording an illusion of control over impulses which would cause anxiety if consciously and directly experienced. Thus, at the expense of living with his symptoms, the neurotic individual has re-established a degree of psychological homeostasis through the process of symptom formation. The intrapsychic purpose of decreasing conflict and preserving a psychological balance is referred to as "the primary gain" of symptom formation.

Once a pattern of symptomatic behavior is established, the patient may experience secondary benefits (psychologically, as well as in practical terms) as a consequence of the "sick role." For example, personal and social expectations that one acts responsibly and works productively may be lessened, and increased passivity, dependency and self-indulgence may be more readily tolerated in themselves by the patients as well as by family and the rest of society. "One can't expect much of someone who is sick" becomes the rationalization for a broad specturm of exemptions and benefits which fall under the heading of "secondary gain." Often the "secondary gain" is clinically more obvious and interpersonally more annoying than the "primary gain" which the symptom accomplishes. At times, deeply entrenched patterns of "secondary gain" (for example, family indulgence or financial benefits through disability) may be a major impediment to therapeutic improvement. However, the core of neurotic illness is the original intrapsychic conflict which gave rise to symptom formation. Any adequate understanding and effective treatment must therefore unravel and modify the "primary gain" through the lessening of conflict which neurotic symptoms represent.

Typically, neurotic individuals recognize their symptoms to be abnormal, and react to an awareness of their illness with emotional distress. They perceive the changes in personality, mood and behavior which accompany their neurosis to be at odds with their usual self-concept (i.e., to be "ego alien") and sometimes express the fear that they are "losing control" or "losing their mind." On the other hand, neurotic symptoms, once they are established, often lessen the pressure of pre-existing psychological conflicts, and some patients, especially those with hysterical personality features and dissociative patterns of defense, will exhibit a bland, superficially detached attitude toward their symptoms (termed *la belle indifference*). Because neurotic symptoms re-establish a degree of psychological balance and lessen the pressure of psychodynamic conflicts, there will always be an involuntary and unconscious reluctance to relinquish symptomatic behaviors until the individual finds an alternative and more adaptive way to keep their conflicts under control. Moreover, dealing with stressful issues is often an emotionally-draining, painful or embarrassing process, and these factors combine to create unavoidable, unconscious, "resistances" to therapeutic improvement for patients with any form of psychopathology.

Neurotic conflicts can potentially arise whenever impermissible drives (for example, dependency, sexual or aggressive wishes) threaten to enter conscious awareness or seek expression in external behavior. Also, conflicts at a conscious or unconscious level may involve the dimension of object relations; the mental perception and experience of one's relationship to other important people and the assessment of whether one's actual self-concept measures up to one's internal standards and ideals (i.e., to superego and ego ideal demands).

Every neurotic conflict has three modes of expression, any or all of which may be *unconscious*. These include: 1) cognitive content; 2) an emotional feeling of "affect," and 3) a psychophysiologic, somatic accompaniment or response. Some patients are aware of all three, and would be able to tell their nurse or physician what it is that upsets them, how that conflict affects thir mood, and how their bodies are responding to the psychological stress. However, it is not infrequent that patients will be unaware of one or more of these dimensions. For example, some individuals suffering from psychophysiologic disorders (such as duodenal ulcer, ulcerative colitis, tension myalgias, some forms of hypertension, etc.) may have *no* recognition of upsetting psychological issues or of the emotions which accompany their unconscious conflicts. All they experience are the somatic consequences of their unrecognized, unresolved tension. The understanding of such patients is sometimes facilitated by paying careful attention to their description of physical symptoms which may give clear indication of psychological conflicts which the patient may not recognize. For example, one patient described her chronic abdominal pain following a hysterectomy as "just like morning sickness," yet had no conscious awareness of feeling threatened by changes in her feminine self-concept or her anger and depression about being deprived of the ability to have additional children.

Other patients may be aware of changes in mood (for example, anxiety or depression) with no recognition of the underlying conflict which is upsetting. Typically, anxiety reflects the prospective assessment that "something bad may happen in the future," while "depression" is an unpleasant affect which accompanies the retrospective assessment that "something bad has already happened." It is important to remember that these dysphoric moods may result as much from *internal mental perceptions* as from actual external events; and that both emotional states may reflect unconscious conflicts regarding forbidden impulses or threats to an individual's self-esteem. Gaining insight and working to resolve those underlying issues through intensive psychotherapy may be equally important and sometimes more useful than psychopharmacologic treatment for such patients.

3) **"Character Disorder"** is the term applied to habitual, repetitive patterns of maladaptive behavior, attitudes and emotions which reflect underlying *structural* deficits in personality development. Such individuals experienced serious disturbances during their early childhood when the components of personality were still in their formative stages. Thus, for the characterologically disturbed individual, it is basically "the person who they are and have always been" which is the problem, rather than that an individual with a previously normal personality has developed a new "illness" in later life. The disturbances in psychological functioning which such patients experience are secondary to the distortions of their personality structure, and such individuals do not perceive their "symptoms" to be any different from "just the way I have always been." That is to say, their maladaptive patterns are identical to their customary self-concept and thus their illness is said to be "ego-syntonic." Many do not seek treatment on their own initiative since they lack recognition that anything is wrong. Others are forced into treatment by the adverse consequences of their attitudes and behavior, often, through the coercion of spouses, employers or the court who will no longer tolerate the patient's pathology. Those characterologically disturbed individuals who seek psychotherapy on their own initiative often complain of pervasive, longstanding anxiety, depression, emptiness,

the inability to sustain intimate relationships, and a chronic sense of meaninglessness and purposelessness in life. Despite having serious maladaptive consequences, the various character pathologies tend to be stable conditions which do not deteriorate into psychosis. Thus, except under extreme psychological stress or the influence of mind-altering drugs, such individuals do not demonstrate a loss of reality testing or formal thought disorder; and the autonomous functions of their ego are generally intact.

A detailed discussion of the numerous forms of character pathology lies beyond the scope of this chapter. In general, however, one might consider each character disorder to represent a developmental arrest at one of the numerous stages of childhood psychosexual development where the various structural components of the mind (i.e., id, ego and superego) are undergoing formative growth.

For example, a Borderline Personality Organization reflects structural deficits within the ego, particularly in the area of self- and object-representations. There is a failure to mature beyond the primitive splitting, over-idealization and over-devaluation which characterize the perceptions of children prior to age 18 months and which is normally resolved through the integration of previously split "good" and "bad" perceptions of "self" and "others" during the separation/individuation process (age 18 to 36 months). Children who fail to accomplish this normal maturation and synthesis will show primitive affects and pathologic distortions in their perception of "self" and important "objects" in adulthood.

Character pathology due to problems in superego development can occur either because that structure is too weak and defective or because it is too punitive, inflexible and overbearing. The failure in childhood to internalize an adequate conscience and capacity for self-regulation results in antisocial personality disorders in adolescence and adulthood. Conversely, too hypertrophied a superego may lead to the development of an avoidant or obsessive-compulsive personality disorder.

All of the personality disorders can be formulated from a psychodynamic perspective by similar assessments of structural deficiencies and/or distortions in id, ego and superego development. Since these are lifelong patterns, character disorders are all extremely difficult to treat and respond definitively only to long-term intensive psychotherapy.

4) **"Psychoses"** are those forms of mental illness characterized by a loss of reality testing and other signs of disorganized ego function. Psychiatric individuals are unable to clearly distinguish their internal subjective perceptions and fantasies from the facts of the external world. They often (but not always) lose the capacity to organize their thoughts in a logical goal-oriented fashion (i.e., will have a "thought disorder") and may show evidence of hallucinations, delusions or illusions in the content of their ideas. Defense mechanisms of the ego have been overwhelmed in a major way and massive regression leads to symptom formation at a very primitive, immature and concrete level of psychological functioning. Object representations are often severely distorted under the influence of primitive instinctual drives which are frequently discharged in essentially unmodified form. Ego boundaries between "self" and "others" frequently blur and the psychotic individual struggles desperately to avoid a loss of identity and a sense of psychological "fusion" or "merger" with the environment. The superego may seem totally lost in some individuals whose sexual and aggressive urges are unleashed in completely unrestrained, impulse-gratifying behaviors. In others, the superego may appear psychotically distorted with severe self-punitive intensity. The mood of psychotic patients may range from profound depression or agitation to euphoria, and their affect is often bizarre and inappropriate to the content of their ideas.

A detailed description of the various psychoses can be found in any standard textbook of psychiatry. Although it is often possible to perceive a spectrum of underlying conflicts in such individuals, the first step in treating any psychotic patient is to employ medication (or at times, electroconvulsive therapy) in an effort to allay the patient's overwhelming anxiety, reconstitute his reality testing, and reintegrate his formal thought organization. Only after the psychosis is under reasonable control can psychotherapy (usually of a supportive nature) be expected to be beneficial. Insight-oriented psychotherapy which interprets primitive defense mechanisms, focuses on early childhood developmental conflicts, and further mobilizes the patient's primitive instinctual drives can occasionally precitipitate a psychotic break or lead to clinical deterioration of those patients who are not receiving adequate psychotropic medication.

PRACTICAL CLINICAL APPLICATIONS

From these basic theoretical and diagnostic considerations, numerous inferences can be drawn and suggestions made which have relevance for a psychodynamic approach to hospital psychiatric nursing.

1) Except for those infrequent cases in which a patient is deliberately malingering, psychiatric patients are incapable of voluntarily changing or controlling their symptoms. The staff should recognize that the patient's illness results from unconscious forces which will not be modified by instructions, coercion, reassurance or pleading; and that symptoms may persist despite the patient's sincere good intentions and best efforts to change. Thus, a non-judgmental and non-punitive attitude is essential if one is to establish a meaningful working alliance with any psychiatric patient. This does not mean that one condones or sanctions the patient's maladaptive behavior, but rather accepts the reality that symptoms are the unavoidable accompaniment of illness for which the patient should not be "blamed" or "punished."

2) Many aspects of the patient's pathology will predictably be re-enacted in relationships with staff and other individuals on the hospital unit. This is due to the general tendency toward "repetition compulsion" and the more specific transference distortion which will be mobilized by the patient's perception of the nurse and physician as an "authority" and "care provider."

At times, patients will respond with the unconscious expectation that staff will treat them as they were treated in childhood by parents and other psychologically-important individuals. In other instances, a psychological role reversal will take place (a reflection of the patient's childhood internalizations and "identification with the aggressor") and patients will adopt their parents' attitudes and behavior in their dealings with the staff. It is as if the childhood "victim" has now become the "victimizer" in adulthood.

Anyone who is going to work effectively with emotionally-disturbed patients must therefore accept the fact that he or she will quite often become the target of the patient's pathology. Not infrequently, staff will feel victimized by the patient's unrealistic distortions, dependency needs and ambivalent sexual and aggressive impulses. At such times, it is essential to avoid reacting impulsively with behavior which could range from counterattacking to defensiveness or retreating entirely from further interactions with the patient. Staff must carefully monitor their own sexual and aggressive impulses, dependency needs and narcissistic strivings so that these reality and/or counter-transference-based motivations are not acted upon at the patient's expense.

If appropriately utilized, the experience of being "victimized" by the patient's pathology and the awareness of one's own emotional reactions will provide the staff person a unique opportunity for understanding the patient's illness. Hopefully the nurse or physician can then elicit the patient's interest and willingness to explore both the current interpersonal experience and the developmental roots of such conflicted or maladaptive patterns.

Often, the insights gained in this fashion will be uniquely beneficial and far exceed the usefulness of information which the patient can consciously remember or voluntarily report in the course of routine history taking. Even those patients who might wish to hide various aspects of their psychological conflicts and maladaptive family relationships quite often reveal those patterns unintentionally through their unconsciously-motivated attitudes and behavior with nurses and other staff.

3) In order to establish a meaningful working alliance with any patient, it is essential to side with the patient's capacity for self-observation and to spark their curiosity and enthusiasm for introspection and greater self-understanding. The uncovering work in psychotherapy might be compared to exploration and discovery in archeology. One digs for a long time in search of a better understanding of the "past" and often may struggle for a long time to piece together small fragments before the identity and significance of one's findings becomes clear. The work proceeds best if one works patiently and carefully, rather than charging in too quickly to seize what may seem obviously important, at the expense of seriously disrupting a delicate balance.

The *timing* of an insight is often just as important as the accuracy of its content if the patient is to be able to utilize the new-found awareness therapeutically. Hasty, premature or poorly formulated attempts to give a patient "insight" runs the risk of intensifying his/her intrapsychic conflicts, or heightening the patient's defenses and undermining the working alliance with the staff.

Short-term hospital units are environments which foster premature efforts to give "insight" and provide "interpretations" since staff and patients alike often inappropriately expect that longstanding, complicated problems can be thoroughly resolved during a short-term hospitalization. Inexperienced staff and junior house officers are particularly vulnerable to the pitfall of trying to do "too much too soon" in an effort to convince others and more especially themselves that they are "doing a good job" and producing "results" with their patients.

More appropriately, any short-term treatment of patients with neurosis or character disorders should have realistically limited goals in mind. A hospitalization of less than three months duration may be considered successful if it has achieved the following goals:

a. If those patients with psychosomatic and psychophysiologic symptoms have received a thorough medical evaluation, and treatable causes of organic disease have been ruled out.
b. If symptomatic treatment (for example, medication, biofeedback, a supportive milieu, etc.) has dealt sufficiently with the preadmission crisis and controlled the patient's dysphoria adequately enough to allow meaningful self-reflection and the establishment of a working alliance with the therapist.
c. If the patient has been re-educated and accepts that his symptoms have a potentially treatable psychological origin.
d. If the patient's curiosity has been stimulated and his motivation for greater self-understanding has been fostered by his interactions with staff and other patients, and
e. If a realistic, longer term treatment plan is developed to allow for ongoing therapy after hospital discharge.

For many patients whose illness requires initial or ongoing treatment with somatic therapies (for example, major tranquilizers, antidepressant medication, and/or electroconvulsive therapy for psychotic patients and individuals with endogenous depressive disorders), the above goals are not to be overlooked and psychotherapy (often of a more supportive nature) is an essential adjunct.

4) In the process of psychological exploration, it is important to maintain a position of "technical neutrality." This refers to the therapist aligning himself/herself with the patient's capacity for self-observation (i.e., with the "observing ego") while being careful to avoid siding directly with either the id or superego. One must bear in mind that psychic conflict can be intensified if the staff unwittingly promotes *either* the discharge of ambivalent

wishes (by giving license to sexual or aggressive drives) *or* the primitive reprisals of conscience for forbidden impulses and personal short comings (by promoting superego and ego ideal demands).

All too frequently, patients feel as though every new insight must be put into immediate practice with behavior which appears to correct their original maladaptive patterns. For example, an individual who has always been passive and compliant with parental demands and exceedingly dependent and suggestible may feel compelled by initial insights (and at times by the unwitting admonitions of the staff) to rebel openly and defiantly in a tirade against his parents. The patient may falsely assume that this form of "assertiveness" represents a meaningful change of his former pattern. More likely, the patient is unconsciously exchanging one authority for another and is now passive, compliant, suggestible and dependent upon the hospital staff and seeking to do what he hopes will please their nurse or physician. The aftermath of such behavior is often regrettable, with the patient's conflicts and self-reproach frequently increased, and occasionally with irreparable damage having been done to relationships which the patient would have wished to keep intact in the long run.

Thus, the sensitive therapist avoids giving license for extracting punishments and instead attempts to assist the patient assess his ambivalence and conflicts thoroughly from all perspectives without "taking sides" with either id or superego.

5) In a similar vein, staff need to be alert to issues of psychological ambivalence and to recognize that the *opposite* of the apparent issue may be just as conflicted as the pattern of thoughts and behavior which is obvious and conscious. Unconscious mechanisms of reversal and reaction formation may disguise the real sources of conflict even from the patient themselves. For example, heterosexual promiscuity may cover deeper homosexual conflicts; pseudo-independence and aggression may hide dependency needs and longings for passivity; solicitous and overly-caring attitudes may cover malicious, unresolved hostilities, etc. One learns from clinical experience that frequently the *real* problems are quite different or at times exactly opposite from the patient's initial, conscious complaints.

6) No matter how intense the ambivalence or how heated the aggressive conflicts, it is important to realize that patients need to preserve their positive perceptions of the important people in their lives intact. This may be more understandable if one remembers

that *all* children are dependent (emotionally and in practical terms) upon their parents. No matter how hostile and emotionally insensitive the worst of parents might be, the children in such families will have a degree of loyalty and positive attachment to their parents even though their intensely negative emotions may be more prominent in their conscious awareness. It is the very fact that these relationships are intensely ambivalent which leaves such individuals torn within themselves. The strongly opposing emotions of love and hate are *equally valid* and equally appropriate to various inconsistent aspects of these children's experience with their parents. Thus, it is not that one group of feelings is "wrong" and the other "right," but rather the truth of the patient's psychological experience is that opposite, conflicting emotions coexist and are directed toward one and the same object.

The task of therapy is *not* to eliminate certain aspects of the patient's emotional experience. For example, it is an inappropriate goal to attempt to "get rid of the patient's dependency" or to "eliminate the patient's hostility." Only if the staff and patient were equally willing to remain selectively blind to some aspects of the patient's experience would such a goal be superficially accomplished, at the possible expense of fostering an impairment of the patient's reality testing.

The truth of the matter is that many individuals grow up with intensely inconsistent emotional experiences and with strongly incompatible yet coexisting opposite emotions toward important people in their lives. Thus, the challenge of therapy is to help the patients:

a. To recognize the existence of their opposite emotions without labeling either component as "bad;"
b. To balance their opposing emotions in keeping with the reality that important people in their past have both good and bad aspects to their personality (some more so than others);
c. To realize that the presence of coexisting, conflicted emotions need *not* destroy the internal perception of those important relationships or seriously damage the patients' concept of themselves as good people.

Frequently, it is early in therapy when the patient gains initial insights regarding the emotional injustices, slights and traumas imposed by parents and other important persons; at this point the patient may be tempted to totally eradicate the influence of those people from his life. It is then that the therapist must work most diligently to avoid sanctioning or promoting the patient's aggressive impulses by seeking to accomplish a balance with feelings in the opposite direction.

One highly useful approach is to assist the patient become more empathic with the experience of those they hate. For example, if a patient can come to realize that parents are well intentioned in caring for the patient to the best of their ability (even though they may be psychologically unsophisticated and emotionally insensitive) the patient will likely be less enraged than if the parents are perceived as ruthless or totally selfish. In other instances, the patient may come to realize that his parents were also "victims" and that the grandparents' or great-grandparents' pathology has been passed on in the family from one generation to the next. If the patient can develop empathy for the parents as "well intentioned and not deliberately insensitive" or "victims themselves who are struggling with unresolved conflicts from their own rotten childhood," then the anger in response to the injustices and traumas sustained at the hands of such parents is often softened and partially resolved.

Helping patients to accomplish empathic understanding requires finding a similarity between the patient's experience and the situation in which the other person (for example, the parent) is involved. The patient is then encouraged to use his own emotional experience as a basis for transiently setting aside his own perspective to view the situation from the vantage point of the other person. Empathy cannot be artificially achieved nor fabricated, and is feasible only if there is an actual emotional similarity between the experiences of the individuals involved.

Helping a patient gain empathic understanding is to be clearly distinguished from "making excuses" or "justifying" the conduct of those with whom the patient is in conflict. Such approaches would not only be perceived as "phoney" and inauthentic, but would also quickly undermine the working alliance with a therapist perceived as having greater allegiance with others than with the patient.

7) Empathy is also a useful tool in the therapist's efforts to understand his/her patients. The same principle applies, namely that the therapist seeks to find some aspect of personal emotional experience which bear sufficient resemblance to the patient's conflict that one can transiently set aside one's own perspective to experience the situation from the patient's point of view. This does not mean to say that the therapist must have had the same

experience as the patient in order to understand him. Rather, from personal past situations one looks to find a set of circumstances wherein the *emotion* might have been similar. It is the similar emotion, rather than the actual content, which provides a bridge for understanding.

For example, a nurse might be caring for a business executive who is experiencing unreasonable anxiety related to fears of failure which the patient recognizes to be irrational. The nurse may be reminded of personal anxiety which seemed overwhelming before a recent in-service examination, even though the nurse knew he/she was well prepared. The issue of "fearing failure" and the emotion of anxiety may be quite similar in each situation, even though the factual, life situation of patient and nurse are entirely different. Empathy is appropriately utilized to help the therapist become *experientially* aware of the patient's dilemma. Becoming more personally attuned to the patient's emotions should help the nurse:

a. To understand the patient's conflicts and suffering more accurately and
b. To develop a more compassionate and devoted commitment to working together with the patient on the patient's problems.

It is important to emphasize, however, that it is *not* helpful to share the personal content of one's own experiences with the patient. Self-disclosure is often an unrecognized self-indulgence on the part of the therapist and even seemingly "innocent" content of one's own past or present experience may unwittingly burden the patient whom you are sincerely attempting to help. For example, one nurse mentioned that she would be absent from the hospital unit on Saturday, and in response to her patient's inquiry explained that she was taking time off to be home for her daughter's birthday party. The nurse returned to the unit the following Monday to find her patient ruminative and despondent. The patient verbalized feeling horribly "responsible" for keeping the nurse away from her home and from being with her children on other days of the week. It gradually became clear that the patient was displacing early childhood feelings about her own mother's lengthy, work-related absences from home, and distorting her perceptions of the nurse through that transference. The patient had struggled for years to resolve feelings of personal guilt when her mother's devotion to work had led to the parents' eventual divorce when the patient was four years old. Thus, feeling that she was "keeping her nurse at work and preventing her from being home" was a burdensome conflict reactivated by the nurse's "innocent" self-disclosure, which fortunately, in this case, was able to be worked through productively. However, in principle it is always best to avoid self-disclosure, and to preserve the personal quality of relationship with one's patients intact. Stated simply, one needs to be "friendly" *without* "becoming friends" with one's patients, since clinical objectivity and therapeutic efficacy often stop where casual social interactions begin.

It is important to pay attention to the emotional connotation and impact of other "trivial issues" which may play a major role in establishing the tone of the relationship between nurse and patient. For example, addressing a patient by his last name conveys a different attitude and expectation than being on a first name basis. Specifically, it implies:

a. That the interaction is professional rather than social;
b. Respect for the patient as an adult; and
c. An expectation that the patient will function in response at an adult responsible level to the best of his ability.

Conversely, calling patients by the first name may unwittingly:

a. Undermine the patient's confidence in the professional attitude of the staff;
b. Be interpreted by some patients as a presumptious and intrusive familiarity on the part of staff;
c. Promote psychological regression and be experienced by some patients as infantalizing or demanding.

Whether one calls patients by their first or last name is perhaps not so important as *thinking* about the connotation of one's actions in advance and knowing one's patients sufficiently well to understand how one's actions will be interpreted. This principle has application in numerous ways.

It may be trivial to be concerned, for example, about the difference in connotation between conducting psychotherapy with hospitalized patients in their hospital room versus holding the same session in a hospital office, until one experiences a homosexually conflicted paranoid patient responding in panic or a hysterical patient starting to make sexual advances. Innumerable examples could be cited to emphasize the point that subtle connotations are at times the most important factors which govern the overall perception of interpersonal relationships, including those between patient and nurse.

8) The psychiatric hospital setting may create unique problems regarding patients' rights to confidentiality. On the one hand, the patient's willingness and capacity for self-disclosure in psychotherapy will be seriously undermined unless confidentiality can be assured. On the other hand, a sharing of information between physicians, nurses and paramedical personnel is a prerequisite for a meaningfully coordinated treatment effort. Therefore, it is essential at the beginning of any hospitalization for the primary therapist to clarify with the patient exactly how information from individual treatment sessions will be recorded and shared with other members of the staff. The patient should be assured that the staff will not share any information with anyone other than members of the treatment team directly involved with the patient's care and even then only to the extent necessary for care plans to be effectively coordinated.

Inevitably, patients will come to know about each other's problems by living together in close proximity and through group therapy and less formal social interactions. However, the staff needs to guard against deliberate or unwitting disclosures of one patient's problems to another. For example, it can be all too easy for staff to use one patient's experience as illustration when talking with another, or for patients to overhear staff discussions of other patient's problems. If breaches in working alliance are to be avoided, such indiscretions by staff need to be carefully prevented.

Inappropriate bemusement, ridicule or sarcasm by staff about patients' problems can be particularly devastating to the treatment effort. Even when such humor occurs "behind closed doors," the staff needs to carefully assess their *own* possible counter-transference hostilities, professional insecurities and personal neurotic conflicts which may be responsible for engaging in such behavior.

The nurse in the psychiatric hospital setting is often in the uniquely frustrating position of spending the most time with the patient while not being perceived by either patient or physician as the "primary therapist." It is difficult to serve an adjunctive role when the nurse may feel more knowledgeable, experienced and/or experientially involved with the patient than the doctor. However, if treatment is to proceed well, there can be only one "primary therapist," and administrative policy often dictates that is it the doctor who is in charge. Optimally, therefore, the nurse should function as a facilitator and advocate of the doctor-patient relationship.

This is accomplished best by providing the patient with emotional support and encouragement to persist in working things through with the doctor. It requires that the nurses restrain their understandable wish to "do the therapy" and to "be involved in the action," and the self-discipline to abstain from promoting too much ventilation of conflicted issues by patients outside their regularly scheduled sessions. It requires considerable abstinence and maturity for a nurse to be able to say to a patient, " I know what you are saying is very important, but perhaps you would benefit more from discussing this with your doctor. Do you think that you can bring it up with him/her during your next treatment session?" If the patient has a resistance to doing so, the nurse may have an excellent opportunity (in the appropriate role of "facilitator of therapy") to help the patient overcome his emotional impediments. This differs significantly from nurses and/or paramedical staff "doing therapy" in terms of helping the patient with the *content* of his underlying conflicts, a job far better undertaken by the primary therapist.

It is important for the nurse to accept, therefore, that all the intimate details of the patient's problems may not, and in many cases should not, be shared with anyone other than the primary therapist. Rather than feeling excluded from "knowing the hidden secrets," the nurse will hopefully appreciate and respect the need for confidentiality which the primary therapist may choose to exercise (or which the patient may request of him/her) in discussing the patient's case, even with other members of the staff.

Finally, the nurse is frequently in contact with friends and family members of the patients under her care. No situation demands greater attention to issues of confidentiality and the patient's right to privacy than the interaction of staff with family. Several guidelines are useful in assuring preservation of a working alliance with your patient:

a. Except for superficial social greetings, any "discussion" of the patient's care with family or friends should occur only with the patient's advance knowledge and permission;
b. There is less risk for misunderstanding if the patient is present during such discussions;
c. It is best for staff to adopt the policy of considering the details of the patients' problems and treatment to be

confidential and to support the patients in deciding for themselves how much or how little of that information to share on their own initiative with family or friends; and

d. It is essential to avoid any behavior which would convey to patients that you are dealing with things "behind their back." For example, telephone calls are best handled by:
    1. Establishing with the caller at the *beginning* whether or not the patient knows of the conversation;
    2. Telling the caller that you will inform the patient of the content of the conversation in its *entirety*; and
    3. Assuring the patient that you will inform him fully of any such conversation of other chance meetings or discussions which might happen to occur without the patient's foreknowledge.

By adopting such policies consistently, many unfortunate conflicts and breakdowns in therapeutic alliance with patients can be avoided.

9) Helping patients to assess interpersonal emotions and conflicts as they occur on the hospital unit is a frequent task for the nursing staff. The process is somewhat easier if the patient is dissatisfied with someone else (whether another patient or staff member), and is considerably more challenging and emotionally threatening if the patient's accusations are toward yourself. However the approach to the issues is the same in both instances. First, one must deal with one's own defensiveness and demonstrate through one's attitude a *genuine willingness* to help the patient assess his perceptions of the situation. If, instead, a staff member responds by counter-attacking, defensively retreating, or conveying a general attitude of indifference by summarily dismissing the patient's complaint as "just part of his illness," a valuable therapeutic opportunity will frequently be lost.

Secondly, one must help the patient assess the possible *validity* of the patient's subjective perceptions and emotions. This can be facilitated by asking the patient to describe in detail, "what things has the other person said or done which give you that impression?" (or if the patient is discussing feelings directed toward yourself, you would ask, "What things have *I* said or done which give you that impression?") The nurse's tone of voice and general attitude in asking such questions will convey whether or not he/she is really open to hearing an honest answer from the patient, and *only* if that is true will this therapeutic effort have any chance of succeeding. The patient's response may in fact point out a factual basis for his perceptions, and if so, the staff member needs to be willing to acknowledge whatever degree of truth there might be in the patient's observations. The willingness on the part of staff to admit to their failures, mistakes and shortcomings is not only essential in preserving a working alliance with the patient, but has important therapeutic implications as well. It allows the patient an opportunity to validate the accuracy or inaccuracy of his reality testing, especially in the area of object representation and perception of interpersonal relationships. Moreover, it is often a "corrective emotional experience" for the patient to interact with a current "authority" and "care provider" who is open to admitting his/her mistakes. This often contrasts sharply with the patient's childhood experience with parents who never admitted any personal faults, and instead left the patient as a child feeling responsible for any and all interpersonal difficulties.

Once the staff member has helped the patient assess the degree of truth in his perception, the therapist can then move to address any degree of distortion which also may be present. However, it is *only after* the therapist has taken an honest look at the possible validity of the patient's allegation that the patient will be receptive to the next step.

For example, if the patient cannot focus specifically on *anything* having been actually "said or done" to give him this impression, it is then useful to inquire with the patient whether he may have been responding to the present situation with attitudes and expectations carried over from past situations (i.e., a transference distortion). Most frequently, one finds a small degree of truth in the patient's perceptions and complaints (which must be acknowledged, as a first step) and a major overpersonalization and disproportionate emotional reaction which is a reflection of the patient's psychopathology. Once the staff acknowledges the former, the patient is often willing to work productively with the therapist to resolve the latter.

For example, a patient may angrily assert that his nurse is "bored and uncaring" and go on to say that the reason is that the patient knows himself to be a worthless, rotten person. In a non-judgmental and genuinely inquisitive fashion, the nurse might respond by asking, "Have I done or said something which gives you that impression?" If the patient were to say, "Yes, you keep yawning and look half asleep and are constantly glancing at your watch," then the nurse would have to honestly assess whether or not that is true and respond accordingly. This would require a much different approach than assuming that every patient's complaint is a "transference distortion" or a reflection of the *patient's* pathology. For example, if it is true that the nurse *is* sleepy, but because of working a double shift the previous day rather than because of "boredom" with the current patient, it would be very useful to clarify those facts and admit to one's own limitations with an apology for not being alert and able to listen in an optimal fashion. Only following that clarification of *reality* can the nurse hopefully proceed to help the patient work through the distortions of having concluded himself to be a "worthless and rotten person" from the experience. One might then discover, for example, that as a child the patient had come to accept personal responsibility and self-reproach for mother having to work two jobs which left her chronically tired and irritable following a divorce for which the patient blamed himself.

I would re-emphasize the importance, however, of assessing and affirming the *reality component* of the patient's perception before attempting to proceed to sort out the neurotic transference distortion. Otherwise, the patient will feel that the staff member "always turns things around against him," the working alliance will be undermined, and an opportunity for therapeutic efforts will be lost.

10) Many psychiatric patients suffer from chronically low self-esteem and are very vulnerable when it comes to taking pride in themselves and in their own accomplishments. Often .they were raised by parents who failed to provide them with feelings that they had value as persons in childhood. Their accomplishments were either ignored or alternatively were seized by parents to be put on display for the parents' own egotistical gain. In either case, the child has little reason to feel personal value or merit as an indiviudal.

How an individual feels about his own self image and the conflicts which may arise from having an unrealistically grandiose *or* an unrealistically devalued self-concept are categorized under the heading of "narcissism." Maladaptive consequences arise if there is an unrealistic assessment by the individual in *either* direction. Maintaining a realistic balance between extremes is essential for normal psychological functioning. Thus, it should be clear that "narcissism" in itself is *not* pathologic if one refers to a healthy "good feeling about one's self." In psychiatric nursing, however, normal narcissistic needs may create a major risk and impediment to the patient's overall improvement.

Staff must bear in mind that the patients are extremely vulnerable and insecure in terms of narcissistic adequacy, and have been deprived of their "narcissistic supplies" through many traumatic experiences in the past. Consequently, patients will fear similar experiences in their relationships with staff; expecting either: a) that their accomplishments will go unrecognized, or b) that their accomplishments will be ripped away and placed on display by nurses, physicians or other staff who acknowledge the patient's accomplishments *only* as a self-serving announcement of the staff's "professional accomplishments."

Frequently, a compliant/defiant pattern can result as the patient struggles on the one hand to "improve" in order to win recognition and approval from staff, while on the other hand the patient may wish to withhold, hide or actually destroy their progress in therapy out of fear and anger that staff will simply "rip it all away" to put on display for themselves.

On the one hand, *every* staff person is doing his work with a degree of self-serving, narcissistic motivation behind the scenes; and that is perfectly normal. On the other hand, to the extent that we "need" the patient to get better in order to feel good about *ourselves*, to that same degree, the patient's capability to improve for himself may be jeopardized. Optimally, a working alliance in any treatment situation is a *mutual* effort, and if a patient resolves his original narcissistic conflicts, it may be possible for both patient and therapist to share credit for the outcome rather than either person perceiving himself as "the winner."

SUGGESTED READING

Bibring, Edward: "Psychoanalysis and the Dynamic Psychotherapies." Journal of the American Psychoanalytic Association. 2:745-770, 1954.

Bird, Brian: *Talking with Patients.* Philadelphia: J.B. Lippincott Co., 1973.

Brenner, Charles: *An Elementary Textbook of Psychoanalysis.* N.Y.: International Universities Press, 1973 (also, Anchor Books, paperback, 1974), especially chapter VIII "Psychopathology" and chapter IX "Psychic Conflict and Normal Mental Functioning."

Cameron, Norman: *Personality Development and Psychopathology.* Boston: Houghton Mifflin Co., 1963, especially chapter 7 through 13.

Chessick, Richard: *The Technique and Practice of Intensive Psychotherapy.* N.Y.: Jason Aronson, 1974.

Greenson, Ralph R.: "Empathy and Its Vicissitudes." International Journal of Psychoanalysis. *41:*418-424, 1960.

Kubie, Lawrence: "The Retreat from Patients." Archives of General Psychiatry. 24:98–106, Feb., 1971.

Nemiah, John: "Chapter 21: Neuroses," in Freedman, Kaplan and Sadock. *Comprehensive Textbook of Psychiatry II.* Baltimore: Williams and Wilkins Co., 1975, Vol. 1, 1198–1278.

Schafer, Roy: "Generative Empathy in the Treatment Situation." Psychoanalytic Quarterly. 28:342–373, 1959.

Watzlawick, Paul: *The Language of Change.* N.Y.: Basic Books, 1978.

6 Emergencies

Lloyd A. Wells

INTRODUCTION

One of the exciting things about any of the mental health professions is that one can be confronted at any time with a situation which is a true emergency. In this chapter, I shall address some common emergencies, including suicide, the assaultive patient, substance-related emergencies and iatrogenic emergencies, as well as some emergencies which one confronts on an out-patient basis. In addition, I shall discuss pseudoemergencies.

SUICIDE

In our historical period, no one is neutral to suicide in the abstract; and dealing with and reacting to a suicidal patient or the suicide of a patient or acquaintance is always an extremely traumatic process. It arouses a great many countertransference affects in all of us. This has not always been the case, and there have been periods in human history when a stoic suicide was considered a good death and was reacted to quite calmly and even proudly by friends of the deceased. Indeed, in parts of the world today suicide is seen as a different type of event than it is viewed in Western society.

The mental health professional faces his or her most important and immediate task in dealing with a suicidal patient. While it is possible to over-react and hospitalize and limit people who may not be truly suicidal because of one's suspicions, it is far more grievous to make an assessment that someone does not need admission or close observation only to have that person commit suicide shortly thereafter.

In this section, I shall attempt to address some of the main thories about the dynamics of suicide, some of the demography of suicide, precipitating factors in suicide, ethical issues which impinge on suicide, legal issues which are also involved, and the process known as the psychological autopsy.

These discussions of suicide begin with a brief mention of Emil Durkheim, the sociologist who suggested that suicide was most often related to an altered and unacceptable relationship between the suicidal patient and his society. Although this theory did not really involve the intrapsychic dynamics of the patient, it is always important to consider the patient's relationship with society and important components of society in explaining the suicide and assessing a potential suicide. While Durkheim's theories are not enough, they are all too often neglected when one considers the purely intrapsychic factors involved in suicide.

Freud discussed the suicidal person's ambivalent struggle with his own aggression and suggested that this was a major component and indeed the determining force of most suicides. Certainly, suicidal people do have an immense struggle with their aggression and its targets. An examination of suicide notes very frequently reveals a great deal of covertly and sometimes overtly hostile thought content. Menninger addresses this ambivalence in his famous dictum that every suicidal person has conflicting wishes to kill, to be killed and to die, and this is generally true.

Adler, Freud's erstwhile disciple, thought of suicide in terms of its interpersonal control, and certainly suicide does serve to control the actions of significant others, at least for a time. In a failed suicide attempt, the interpersonal control aspects often come to the fore, and the suicidal gesture or attempt is taken as an indirect way of asking for alterations in the person's family or social subsystem.

Many suicidal people do have a belief that somehow life will go on after the suicide and indeed will be improved, and the thought disorder which is found in many people who are at the brink of suicide often does not demarcate between death and a continued existence.

Other people who are struggling with the same dynamic of death and rebirth often view suicide as a gamble and as expiation of guilt. These people are likely to attempt suicide by such means as Russian roulette or other methods that could either succeed or fail, with the success or failure of the attempt left to chance or destiny. Such people feel that if the attempt succeeds they will get what they deserve, and if it fails the courage they have shown in going through with the attempt will somehow resolve issues of guilt and aggression. Anyone who has worked with patients admitted to a hospital following a suicide attempt is struck by the fact that some of these patients do come out of their depression extremely rapidly and feel quite good about themselves. Weiss pointed out that dynamics of such patients are quite similar to those seen in the gambler, and he was right (1).

The concept of subintentional death is also worth considering because although many people in our society commit suicide, a vast number are involved in subintentional deaths (2). These are people who usually for very complex motives lead lives which are replete with acute and chronic dangers which could result in their deaths. One can even extend this concept of subintentional death to such destructive lifestyles as seem to be associated with the development of lung cancer (smoking) and myocardial infarction.

Others use their own death as an attempt to find meaning in life and to make some kind of cohesive whole out of their existence. The execution of a type of prisoner is a case in point. Some of these men have lived a psychopathic existence without regard for any meaning except for their own immediate gratification. Although it is certainly possible for many of them to avoid being executed, they virtually seek their own death and dwell on the courage with which they face it. For these men, self-willed execution provides a sense of meaning, accomplishment and cohesiveness.

Joseph Sabbath has written poignantly and with great accuracy about suicidal adolescents (3). I think many of his arguments can be extended to adults as well. He has developed the concept of the "expendable child." Many adolescents (and adults) who commit suicide fall into the categories of feeling that life is futile, feeling unable to cope with life, or wishing others to "drop dead." Usually these are people who are perceived by parents, spouses or other significant family members as somehow expendable. As with the concept of fostering, the message is covertly and usually unconsciously conveyed to such a patient that his death would not be tragic for the family and indeed might serve to meet the needs of the family. Such fostering is frequently found in families of suicidal adolescents and also occurs in the families of adults. In addition, this message is also given covertly and unconsciously to patients on psychiatric units by the staff on those units. It is for this reason that one must monitor one's countertransference reactions to suicidal patients with extreme care, even at the cost of some loss of pride or sense of altruism.

Who is at high risk for suicide? If one were to pick the most probable candidate for suicide one would select a 68-year-old white, obsessive, Protestant physician whose wife died a few months previously and whose license to practice medicine was revoked because of his alcoholism. Indeed, the elderly are most prone to suicide, with higher frequency in males. People who are single, widowed or divorced are at higher risk than married people. Whites and American Indians are apparently more prone to suicide than blacks. People of low social class or falling social class are also more prone to suicide, as are the unemployed or otherwise socially disrupted. Alcoholism and depression particularly increase the risk of suicide.

There has been a great deal of nonsense written about suicide rates in different countries and what they mean. For example, in many statistical presentations Eastern European countries have a very high suicide rate followed by some of the Scandanavian countries. Some South American nations have particularly low suicide rates. People pontificate that communist societies or sexually-liberated societies cause people to kill themselves, but in fact the determination of suicide rates depends entirely upon the expertise of the system of certification of death, and in areas where there is a careful, methodical and unbiased medical examiner, suicide rates are generally considerably higher than in other areas.

There are various assessment scales to determine suicide risk. It is perhaps less important to actively administer a scale than to know the exact questions to be asking, and many of these are included on the scale. One should certainly ask about the presence of suicidal thoughts, and if a moderately depressed patient denies ever having thought about suicide one should be extremely suspicious, because virtually everyone has thought about suicide at one time or another. One should attempt to assess whether there is dissonance between cognitive and affective thinking about suicide because in my view this is one of the best predictors of suicide. If someone is both cognitively and affectively contemplating termination of life, he represents an extremely high suicide risk. One should ask whether thinking about suicide is frightening. One should especially ask about sources of help should the patient become actively suicidal. Many suicidal people live in an increasingly constricted world and are unable to recognize that help might be available for them. One should ask about suicide in the family or among friends, and one should ask about previous suicide attempts on the part of the patient. One should ask whether a suicide plan has been made and what it is. One should inquire about details of the plan and whether any steps have ever been taken to carry it out. One should ask about recent losses and recent social disruptions.

As mentioned, depressed people and alcoholic people have a high suicide rate. In fact, a family psychiatric history does increase the risk of suicide statistically. Schizophrenic patients commit suicide more frequently than is commonly realized, often in response to delusional thinking, particularly delusions of external control. Patients with personality disorders, although they are usually seen as not having intrinsic suffering, do suffer a great deal, and many passive-dependent, obsessive and passive-aggressive people do commit suicide. The history of a past suicide attempt greatly increases the risk of future suicide attempts, at least statistically. Many people who fail at a brief or even a longer attempt at psychotherapy or some other psychiatric/psychological interventin commit suicide. If someone terminates therapy abruptly or unhappily, one should consider carefully whether there is any apparent suicide risk.

Physically ill patients are also at increased risk for suicide, especially patients with chronic, debilitating illnesses, of which the patient in renal failure on dialysis is a good example. Although it was thought for a long time that patients with cancer had a high suicide rate, recent studies suggest that the suicide rate is not much higher than that in the general population except during the period shortly after the diagnosis is made. Prisoners, gifted and creative people, and soldiers, particularly in peacetime, are at increased risk for suicide as well; few groups are spared.

What are some precipitating factors in suicidal attempts? Of course, some common features of the suicidal person have been discussed above. Given someone who fulfills any of these risk factors, an actual attempt or completed suicide often occurs with the additional stress of a major loss. The usual losses one thinks about involve death. Especially if the person who dies is considered in an ambivalent way by the suicide victim, with intense love and intense hate which have never been resolved, the patient is likely to feel suicidal. The loss may be a real one in terms of death or it may be a threatened death. One can anticipate a suicidal attempt by someone who is already at high risk and then encounters the death of an ambivantly held object. It is more difficult to anticipate suicide as an anniversary phenomenon, but it often occurs as such. The original ambivalent conflict can be reactivated by an anniversary of a death, marriage, etc.

The loss can also be by separation, divorce or some other major upheaval. The loss can be a real or perceived loss of health or threat of one's own death. In fact, a common mechanism of coping which is used by many seriously chronically ill people with heart disease or cancer is the perception that they can at least maintain control of the time and circumstances of their own dying. People with such fantasies rarely kill themselves, but they cause a greate deal of worry among their caretakers.

Among major losses is a loss of social position or vocational position, particularly when the person has been somehow disgraced.

There are a great many ethical issues in the treatment of a potentially suicidal patient. Almost all patients who commit suicide are ambivalent about their death almost up until the last. In such a situation the mental health professional should feel comfortable in intervening even with the use of involuntary hospitalization and treatment. If a person comes to a mental health professional's office or facility and talks about killing himself, he is making an indirect plea to be rescued from the consequences of such an act, and the professional should act accordingly by hospitalizing the patient. Consider, however, a different situation: an 80-year-old deaf woman whose eyesight is failing is visiting with her husband in the hospital where he is dying of cancer. His death is expected within two weeks to a month. They have been married for 52 years with a very happy marriage. They never had children. They were estranged from both families because of cultural differences. The 80-year-old woman's major hobby over the years has been reading and watching television, both of which are virtually impossible now because of her eyesight. She has no friends aside from her husband. In a casual conversation with the nurse, the patient mentions how difficult it is for her. The nurse asks what plans she has made for her life following her husband's death. The patient mentions to the nurse that she is quite undecided but that it is possible that after his funeral and after taking care of her affairs she might seriously consider suicide sometime within the next year.

In a situation like this, the nurse is faced with a difficult decision. Many professionals in this situation would hospitalize the patient, but this would deprive her of the change to gain some self-esteem through dealing with her husband's death and being of help to him. It is the author's opinion that in situations such as this where the patient is calm and rational and is planning suicide as a rational, well-considered act, the professional needs to be wary of intervening too abruptly. On the other hand, with any suicide threat the patient should be given as complete an evaluatin as possible by an appropriate professional. There is a very thin line between not intervening in a potential suicide and actually aiding and abetting a suicide, which is illegal as well as unethical.

The legal issues in suicide do need to be clarified. There is an increasing impetus to consider the act of suicide of a patient undergoing any kind of psychotherapeutic treatment as evidence of malpractice. In the next decade it is virtually certain that many psychiatric nurses will be sued because of the suicides and/or attempted suicides of patients under their direct or even indirect care. It seems to me that there is little defense against this type of litigation except for thorough documentation that appropriate measures have been taken and that the professional's best judgment was used throughout. I have referred above to some of the ethical dilemmas in intervention with potentially suicidal patients. Errors in judgment will not be considered illegal, although they may constitute malpractice. However, the act of documenting that a patient is probably suicidal and then not intervening in some way may be taken as evidence of complicity in the suicide and the professional could be charged with a felony.

Dealing with the hospitalized suicidal patient requires a great deal of staff cohesion, the implementation of a uniform treatment plan, the careful monitoring of countertransference reactions and the ability to think quickly and flexibly. These are not characteristics which all people have, but in dealing with the suicidal patient we must all attempt to mobilize whatever strength we do have in these areas to prevent what is often a wasteful, ill-thought-out termination of a human life.

THE ASSAULTIVE PATIENT

Early in their careers, many mental health professionals are inordinately afraid of being attacked by a patient. Much of this fear is countertransferiential and represents a method of dealing with anger toward the patient which seems unacceptable. Later in their careers, many mental health professionals become quite casual about the possibility of being attacked by a patient and do not take even reasonable precautions. It is the intent of this section to discuss very briefly some of the common causes of assaultiveness in patients and to attempt to propose practical methods of preventing such actions and of dealing with them if they do occur.

Enormous tomes have been written about the causes of violence; there is a vast literature on the subject. Several good studies have been done and are underway, but there is little theoretical uniformity in terms of comprehensive understanding of the causes of violence.

I think that it is helpful in this context to consider four major causes of assualtiveness: 1) organic; 2) functional; 3) dyssocial, and 4) "normal."

Organic causes of assaultiveness are many. Many old people with organic brain syndromes and many hospitalized patients with delirium become assaultive, usually for brief periods, because their psychological coping mechanisms have become so constricted that there is no other way for them to express fear or displeasure or sometimes even pain. Undoubtedly the most common organic cause of assaultiveness, however, is intoxication with alcohol or other mind-altering substances.

The intoxicated patient may be violent for long periods, and again because of the state of intoxication such a person has very limited coping devices and very few alternatives to expressing aggression in an alloplastic way. In addition, he may become pathologically jealous or may become transiently delusional, both of which tend to make people more violent. In addition, persons who are using mind-altering substances may hallucinate, which is a frightening phenomenon and which again can cause them to be violent. One of the somewhat alarming features of this type of violence is that it is rarely directed at one person. Anyone near the patient may be subject to assault. This frequently includes physicians, nurses and emergency room personnel.

It should also be emphasized that not only acute intoxications but withdrawal states can be associated with assaultive behavior. These include withdrawal states from barbiturates and minor tranquilizers as well as from the mind-altering substances discussed above.

Many neurologic syndromes can cause assaultive behavior. People with traumatic brain damage can often be assaultive, and many people with congenital abnormalities of the central nervous system are assaultive from time to time. In addition, seizure disorders can be associated with assaultive behavior, particularly temporal lobe seizures and especially the situation of temporal lobe status epilepticus.

The psychiatric disorders associated with assaultiveness include schizophrenia, particularly of the paranoid type but also of the schizo-affective type. Usually, again, the patient is feeling unable to address or deal with his ambivalent, aggressive feelings short of violence. Usually, such patients are delusional and their assaultiveness is an effort at self-defense, in their view. Manic patients can also be violent and their violence is usually of an exuberant type and can be extremely dangerous. People with personality disorders, particularly of the antisocial type and explosive personality disorder, also have a great propensity to do violent acts. The entire syndrome of borderline states is replete with a great deal of anger and enormous feelings of rejection; such people frequently harbor fantasies of violence and homicide and not infrequently act on them.

In this country, and throughout the world, there are social groups and communities where violence is condoned. There continue to be street gangs in urban ghettos where part of the culture of the gang includes violence. While we can deplore this violence, it does not necessarily represent psychopathology in the accepted sense. One of the most difficult lessons for neophyte mental health workers to learn is that a violent patient is not *ipso facto* mentally ill and should not always be hospitalized. There are correctional systems and police departments who can often handle such people with a great deal more efficiency than can the mental health professions.

Finally, we come to the category of "normal" violence. This is violence which can erupt in any of us if we are sufficiently stressed. Many of us — and hopefully this is particularly true in the mental health professions — have a very high threshold for evoking violence, but we do have such a threshold and we are capable of violence. Some of the factors which can cause lower thresholds in people often relate to childhood deprivation. Many people with low violence thresholds were abused children. The debate in psychological circles about the causes of violence goes back many centuries but basically has been between two camps: the first that violence is innate and the second that violence is learned. As with most such controversies, the dichotomy is a false one because violence is both innate and learned.

The work of many contemporary ethologists demonstrates quite conclusively that violence is a phenomenon throughout the primate kingdom. Our evolutionary forebears were violent hominids who killed with their hands and ate their prey, whether human or animal, without much compunction — and they needed to be this way to survive. The roots of violence are polygenetically determined, and we cannot forget this. The roots of violence constitute our aggressive drive, which is necessary for life. Nevertheless, we can learn to channel this drive so that it is not alloplastic and destructive to others. Thus violence is innate but violence is also learned. The child who is beaten frequently and otherwise neglected and abused often does not develop a superego in the accepted sense and does not have any compunction about hurting others.

Another unfortunate child is the child with a severe attention deficit disorder or central processing dysfunction. Many of these children with severe problems have great difficulty in considering alternatives verbally or in thought. Here, too, as with the organically impaired patient, the person reacts to a painful or dangerous provocation with a very limited repertoire of responses, one of which happens to be violence.

In clinical situations, violence can frequently be prevented by astute clinical judgment and clinical practice. One of the major problems clinicians have is that once they have established some sort of working relationship with the patient it is hard to conceive of that patient as being physically assaultive to the clinician, and often the clinician who has most contact with the patient and who knows the patient best will miss subtle, early signs that assaultive behavior is about to occur. That clinician may also feel very aggravated and aggrieved when a clinician on a different shift secludes the patient or takes some other preventive action, but often that clinician who knows the patient less well will make a sounder judgment.

To return to the theme that violence occurs when the patient's options seem minimal to him and when his coping mechanisms preclude virtually any other type of response to stress, we need to be aware of this dynamic. Thus, if one is dealing with a patient who may be violent based on this type of assessment, one should try to give the patient options. One should not respond to the patient with anger or accusation but should make the patient aware that, for example, he may leave the room, he may choose not to answer questions, etc. One should never be inquisitorial with such a patient (or with any other patient)!

Should a patient begin to be assaultive, however, it is necessary to take very firm control of the situation. One should not show fear but should talk rationally to the patient and be very firm and direct. If a patient is actually out of control at least three other staff people should be called whenever possible and the patient should be physically restrained. Before restraining the patient who is out of control, the staff members about to do the act should briefly confer about how to restrain the patient. It is often useful to assign one staff member to each extremity. It is perhaps silly to imply that mental health professionals cannot tell left from right, but on many occasions two people will grasp the same extremity, leaving another extremity free. As the group approaches the patient, the leader of the group should inform the patient (and thereby his or her colleagues) what is being done. There should be no attempt made at this point to negotiate with the patient and action should be carried out swiftly. Again, in dealing with a violent patient, there are enormous countertransferiential issues, and the staff must make very sure not to be punitive or aggressive to the patient.

The occasional patient who has a weapon presents a much graver problem. If the weapon is a knife, it is often possible to buffer the staff with mattresses while attempting to disarm the patient. Whenever possible, security personnel and police officers should be involved in dealing with such a patient.

There are many other inpatient and outpatient emergencies that the nurse will be required to address. Among these are emergencies related to the ingestion of drugs and alcohol or the withdrawal from these agents as well as outpatient emergencies and iatrogenic emergencies. Such discussion, however, is beyond the scope of this chapter.

REFERNECES

1. Weiss, J.M.A.: The gamble with death in attempted suicide, Psychiatry, *20:*17 (1957).

2. Shneidman, E.S.; Farberow, N.L.; Litman, R.E.: *The Psychology of Suicide,* New York: Jason Aronson, Inc., 139-140 (1976).

3. Sabbath, J.C.: The suicidal adolescent - the expendable child, J Am Acad Child Psychiatr, *8:*272 (1969).

PART 2

SYNDROMES

7 Schizophrenia

Lloyd A. Wells

One of the great challenges of psychiatry, psychology, psychiatric nursing, social work and all the other mental health professions is the conundrum and enigma of schizophrenia. This illness, under different names, has been recognized for at least 2,000 years. It continues to be the most intractable of the common mental illnesses, and the amount of damage it does economically, socially, not to mention personally, to its sufferers and their families is enormous. Schizophrenia is an illness of young people which is usually insidious in its start. It is a fascinating illness in that the patient's bizarre views of the world and his bizarre distortions of reality are somewhat predictable and similar to those of other patients. Enough is known about its epidemiology and apparent mode of genetic transmission to suggest that schizophrenia is an illness which fits the medical model better than most other nervous and mental disorders. At the same time, despite fascinating suggestions, experiments and theories, its etiology remains unknown. It is an illness which affects people on biochemical, psychological, and social levels. Its worst effects can be dealt with effectively through medications but there is no definitive cure for this illness.

Given all this, major contributions are necessary from all the mental helath disciplines in an attempt to deal with this most difficult of mental illnesses.

What is schizophrenia? No one can say. Nevertheless, there are certain symptoms and signs of this disease with which any practicing mental health professional should be familiar. Although a great deal has been written about how outmoded the system of Eugen Bleuler is, he gave a classical description of schizophrenia and its primary and secondary symptoms early in this century (1). Many of his observations are extremely important in developing a concept of the phenomenology of this illness.

First, the schizophrenic patient has a disorder of affect. He does not have the labile affect of the hysterical patient or the depressed affect of the person with a severe depression or affective disorder, but has an inappropriate affect which is often flattened or sometimes rather silly. This flattened affect sometimes gives the patient the features of an automaton, and it is because of this affect that one sometimes feels that it is virtually impossible to engage oneself with the schizophrenic person in a human type of contact; this "cold" feeling which comes about when one tries to put one's self in empathic contact with some schizophrenic patients, has been referred to as the "*praecox feeling*" by Rumke (2).

The schizophrenic patient also is ambivalent. While ambivalence is the core of all important human relationships and while we all need to be amvibalent and indeed are ambivalent about all major relationships and meaningful events in our lives, the schizophrenic patient's ambivalence is often a core part of his being and allows him to take opposites into himself. The schizophrenic patient is likely to tell one extremely contradictory things and to feel that these are not contradictory at all. "I am a concert violinist and I am not a violinist," is the type of ambivalent statement one often gets from a schizophrenic patient.

The schizophrenic patient is also autistic. This does not mean that he has infantile autism, which is a separate entity, but that he tends to be directed toward fantasy rather than real relationships. Much of the energy that most of us direct toward others and at relationships with others is directed toward the self by the schizophrenic person.

The associations of the schizophrenic patient are loosened or inappropriate. While everyone has associations to any statement of thought, those of the schizophrenic seem deviant. It is also difficult for the person in conversation with a schizophrenic to follow that patient's associations.

Bleuler referred to the disturbances of affect, ambivalence, association and autism as primary symptoms of schizophrenia. They certainly can be found in schizophrenic patients and whether or not they are of prognostic value, they help the mental health professional gain some grasp of the phenomenology of the illness. In addition, there are many secondary features of schizophrenia. Hallucinations, often of an auditory type, are very common in schizophrenic patients. Often the hallucinations are condemnatory, have to do with partially repressed sexual impulses or are not truly formed, e.g., the patient may hear buzzing noises, music, etc. Many schizophrenic patients are delusional. The believe that they are involved in some special mission or the victims of some special plot. They may believe that events have special reference to them, and this is called referential thinking. They may believe, too, that ordinary events are purposely designed to influence them in one way or the other. These symptoms of schizophrenia are more dramatic than the primary symptoms of schizophrenia, and often one tends to think of schizophrenia in terms of hallucinations, delusions, thought control, referential thinking, etc. Not all schizophrenic patients have such phenomena, however.

Schizophrenia can be subdivided into several types, but it is not the purpose of this book to make such a hair-splitting consignment. Nevertheless, paranoid schizophrenia often presents with more of an affective component; the patient may have some vegetative signs of depression or a family history of depression. The prognosis for this type of schizophrenia is often better than that for other types.

Simple schizophrenia is a debatable concept but it is not debatable that many people with severe disturbances of affect, association, autism and ambivalence but without hallucinations, delusions or any formal disorder in thinking make poor adjustments to society and are often vagrants, hoboes, or marginal social characters. There is certainly a relationship between this syndrome and other types of schizophrenia.

The etiology of schizophrenia remains a mystery. Because of its central importance to the field of psychiatry for such a long period, proposed etiologies for this illness usually reflect some of the major models of thought in psychiatry for whatever time period one is considering. Thus, schizophrenia has been seen as the work of infectious agents and of exogenously produced toxins as well as specific psychological deficits. It has also been seen as a genetically transmitted trait, and there is certainly some evidence that there are genetic components to schizophrenia.

There is no easily observed pattern of genetic transmission of schizophrenia, i.e., it is not a Mendelian dominant or recessive, in all probability. However, there is a much greater chance of finding schizophrenia in the offspring of one or especially two schizophrenic parents. For many years, it was argued forcefully that this did not reflect a true genetic phenomenon but that being raised by schizophrenics would certainly predispose one to develop schizophrenic modes of thought. Several studies of children of one or two schizophrenic parents who were adopted at birth are compatible, however, with the hypothesis that this is a genetic disorder.

The two great trends in psychiatric model building at present are those involving neurotransmitters and post-Freudian dynamic psychiatry. Those who hold neurotransmitter hypotheses look at schizophrenia as a disease which involves faulty metabolism of dopamine, and there is certainly some evidence to suggest that this is a factor. The more psychologically minded view schizophrenia as the result of impaired communication techniques within the family, and there is some good evidence for this hypothesis, as well.

I think the important lesson to learn about the the etiology of schizophrenia and so many other psychiatric disorders is that it is in fact unknown. One can get caught up in beautiful theories, but one must evaluate them critically. The second important lesson is that as with medical illnesses, schizophrenia is a bio-psycho-social phenomenon. It is not either secondary to faulty metabolism of dopamine or the result of abnormal communication. It probably involves a great many factors, including transmission and metabolism of neurotransmitters, communication patterns, many epiphenomena in the brain, and a great deal more. It is impossible to fully understand schizophrenia at this time, but those who attempt to build simplistic models involving just one factor may reduce their anxiety, but they really do not learn a great deal about the phenomenon of schizophrenia.

No one would argue that schizophrenia is a good illness to have. At the same time, it is not one which is without hope of alleviation. In fact, there are some factors which lead to a very good prognosis. If the first schizophrenic episode occurs in a young person who has had a well-integrated personality, who has had friends and who has been able to sustain and cope with relationships with other people, who has succeeded at school or at work and who has a depressive component to his illness, the prognosis is not bleak at all. There is reason to believe that early intervention and vigorous psychopharmacological treatment of schizophrenic syndromes improves the prognosis. Neuroleptic medications have revolutionalized the treatment of schizophrenia and today people who were institutionalized for life because of this illness have an average stay in the hospital of less than two months with the first episode.

The drug treatment of schizophrenia does not cure the illness, but is does control many of the phenomena of schizophrenia, particularly the thought disorder, including hallucinations and delusions. The effective medicines, unfortunately, do have side effects, particularly involving extrapyramidal effects and anticholinergic effects. These, however, can be dealt with through the use of other medications; while these side effects are unpleasant and in some cases, such as tardive dyskinesia, even serious, they seem preferable to a life of severe psychosis.

Because the prognosis is better, the diagnosis of affective disorders is more "popular" with many mental health professionals than is that of schizophrenia. Many patients with schizophrenia have a strong affective component to the syndrome. There is a great tendency and desire to say, therefore, that the patient has an atypical form of depression or a schizo-affective disorder. It must be remembered, however, that schizophrenic patients, particularly early in the course of their chronic illness do become depressed at the knowledge of the deterioration of their personality. Such patients are not schizo-affective patients; they are unhappy schizophrenic patients. It must also be remembered that in many patients the neuroleptic medicines used for schizophrenia are depressant.

The specific roles of the psychiatric nurse in dealing with hospitalized psychotic patients are addressed elsewhere in this book. Some of the nurse's specific roles in helping schizophrenic people include the facilitation of the process of sealing over, in which the patient's thought disorder becomes increasingly less prominent. The nurse needs to assess the patient's mental status and needs to be aware of referential thinking, hallucinatory experiences and delusional systems but at the same time he must not intrude on the patient with these questions. There is a process as the patient recovers from acute schizophrenia in which the patient does gradually seal over some of the crazy thinking. The nurse should allow this healing process to occur without any effort to belabor the patient's psychosis or to prove that it still is there.

Another major function of the nurse in dealing with schizophrenic patients is to present and confirm an orientation to reality. In spite of the patient's psychotic thinking and behavior he is still a real person on a real ward which is part of the real world. The nurse can be extremely influential — indeed the most influential person — in helping the patient function and recognize the reality of that world.

The nurse can minimize and distract the patient from his autistic responses to hallucinations and delusional systems. Even if he or she distracts the patient from such experiences he can also be aware of their occurrence and be sure to report them, giving physicians and other health personnel a very accurate data base, which is so important in the treatment of these patients.

The nurse plays a major role in representing reality to the patient, and the nurse can present observations to the patient of his gradual improvement as well as reinforcement that the medications are helping. This not only bolsters the patient's extremely tenuous self-esteem but also helps to impress on the patient the importance of compliance with a medication regimen.

It is a major role of the nurse with every patient, whether schizophrenic or not, to observe for strengths and interests and to reinforce them. the nurse should discourage the use of certain defenses such as intellectualization and should make note of other defenses and coping mechanisms, not only noting their existence but noting their degree of adaptability for the patient.

Finally, both on the ward and at a time when the patient reintegrates to the environment outside the hospital it is a major role of the nurse to facilitate participation in the community. With the use of medications and a good social support system, even a chronic schizophrenic patient who has had many schizophrenic episodes can function out of the hospital most of the time. One of the great dangers of this illness is that the person will live in the hospital for many years and become institutionalized. The role of the nurse in dealing with the schizophrenic patient can be not only to help the patient deal with the demands of everyday living but also help the patient aim at functioning in society and not just on a ward.

REFERENCES

1. Bleuler, E.: *Dementia Praecox or the Group of Schizophrenias*, New York, International Universities Press, (1950).

2. Rumke, H.C.: The clinical differentiation within the group of the schizophrenias, In *Proceedings of the Second International Congress for Psychiatry*, W.A. Stall, editor, Zurich, Orell Füssli Acta Graphiques, (1959), p. 302.

8 Affective Disorders

Lloyd A. Wells

Depression and other affective states including hypomania, dysphoria, sadness and elation have been with humanity from time immemorial and were well recognized and described by classical medical writers in both Greek and Roman antiquity. These disorders were lumped together during the Middle Ages and during parts of the Renaissance but again became recognized as separate types of entities, some pathological and others normal parts of everyday existence, during the 19th and 20th centuries. Although everyone feels unhappy at frequent intervals, not everyone becomes clinically depressed during his or her life. Within the past few years, it has been increasingly apparent that many of the true depressive disorders have both biological and psychosocial roots and sequelae and it is becoming apparent that many of these particular depressions can be biologically demarcated from one another by certain chemical tests and can be treated with increasingly specific antidepressant medications. This in no way invalidates the old observations that depression is connected with the loss of a love-charged object followed by introjection of the object and subsequent increasingly punitive superego. Depressions which are treated biologically alone often do not respond as well as depressions which are treated eclectically.

Depression is a very important disorder to the psychiatric professional since it is a very common, indeed, perhaps the most common type of psychiatric disorder among the population with up to 25% or more of the population experiencing a depressive episode at some point during their lives.

It is a certainty that although more people are treated for depression than for any other psychiatric disorder, nevertheless the majority of seriously depressed people are never treated. The cost of treating depression is exceeded only by the cost to society, employers, families and indeed even to government and welfare agencies of not treating depression.

In human terms, of course, the cost of not treating depression can be measured most in the number of people each year who do commit suicide. While people commit suicide for many other reasons than depression, depression is clearly one of the major causes of suicide in this country and elsewhere.

With increasing knowledge of the neurochemistry of some kinds of depression, there has been a great deal of frivolous and silly debate about whether depression is psychological or somatic. It seems to me that a far better way to conceptualize depression was provided by Akiskal and McKinney when they wrote of depression as a final common pathway. In such a model, whatever the causes of depression, there are somatic sequelae and etiologic factors just as there are psychologic sequelae and etiologic factors. Patients can become depressed with vegetative signs and depression from many different starting points.

Vegetative signs have been mentioned several times thus far. These include a sleep disturbance, whether terminal insomnia, middle insomnia or initial insomnia, anorexia with weight loss or binge eating with weight gain, lethargy with fatigue, lack of energy, diminished concentration and cognitive abilities and a diurnal variation in which the person feels extremely dysphoric and lacking in energy in the morning but gains more energy with some improvement in affect as the day progresses.

There are, of course, many types of depression. The third edition of the *Diagnostic and Statistical Manual of the American Psychiatric Association* lists the following as affective disorders: major affective disorders which include manic episodes and depressive episodes, bipolar disorders, major depressions; and other specific affective disorders which include cyclothymic disorder, dysthymic disorder; and atypical affective disorders which include atypical bipolar disorder and atypical depression.

The major affective disorders, then, include manic depressive illness and severe depression. The hypomanic patient is familiar to most psychiatric nurses with his impulsivity, lack of inhibition, rapidity and pressure of speech and thought, flight of ideas; and frequently has hallucinosis and other features of psychosis. In addition, depsite his ebullience the manic patient often seems to the mental health professional to be very close to depression and dysphoria and indeed the *hypomanic thinking and behavior may well be a defense against the very deep depression.* The severely depressed person is, of course, familiar to all psychiatric nurses as the cornerstone of nursing practice. In severe depression, one must always evaluate the suicide potential of the patient. One should be aware of vegetative signs of depression. In older patients, one should be aware of the coexistence of melancholia with depression; such patients often feel worthless, have somatic delusions of nihilistic and worthless types and respond quite well to electroconvulsive therapy.

Cyclothymic disorders are characterized by a combination of cyclic depressive and hypomanic features which do not sufficiently combine to cause the clinician to reach the diagnosis of manic depressive illness. Dysthymic disorder is essentially a neurotic depression.

Of course, if a patient appears on any unit who is relatively silent, cries, cannot sleep or eat and attempts suicide, it is not too difficult to tell that the patient is depressed. However, many patients have so-called atypical depressions. There is no agreement as yet in psychiatry about etiology or classification of atypical depressions. What is important for the nurse to do during the initial evaluation of a patient is to watch for subtle signs of depression even if an entire, full-blown clinical picture of depression is not present. Thus, it is extremely helpful to know about the patient's sleep pattern, eating pattern and interactional patterns. Frequently, alexithymic patients — that is, patients who are unable to recognize affective states — are not aware that they are depressed. Indeed, their behavior changes may involve some acting out or other atypical kinds of behavioral changes but they have vegetative signs of depression and frequently respond to treatment with a combined approach to psychotherapy and tricyclic or other antidepressants.

Another entity the clinician must be aware of is masked depression. In a masked depression, patients often have a major behavioral syndrome which keeps the clinician from observing the underlying depressive features. Thus many patients who initially seem to be antisocial or even incipiently psychotic have a depressive illness underlying the other symptoms.

Other atypical depressions include so-called hysteroid dysphoria, which is a combination of dysphoric state with hysteroid personality features.

Some panic-anxiety states may also be related to depression.

Although there are a great many therapeutic approaches to depression the most helpful remedies have been medicines and electroconvulsive therapy. These are discussed elsewhere in this book. This does not mean, however, that the depressed patient can be treated as "just another med/surg patient," put in bed and given some medicine. The depressed patient needs a highly structured therapeutic milieu and the nurse has a major role to play in dealing with the depressed patient.

Standard nursing techniques for depressed patients may be found in any basic textbook of psychiatric nursing. I should, however, like to direct comments to three areas which psychiatric nurses should be particularly cognizant of in dealing with depressed patients.

First, a large number of significantly depressed patients have poor hygiene. The fact that the patients are dirty and smell bad reinforces the low self-esteem that these patients have and thus, although it seems trivial, nursing attention to the patient's hygiene can be extremely important.

Second, there is an overemphasis in many nursing programs on verbal reassurance of the depressed patient. It becomes somewhat trite to both nurse and patient for the nurse to reiterate that the patient is a worthy human being 30 to 40 times each shift. The patient does not believe that he is a worthy human being and no amount of verbalization is going to quickly change that view of himself. Indeed, frequently the frequent reiteration of the patient's worth becomes a mechanistic exercise for the nurse, and her attempt to reassure the patient may actually end up further undermining his self-esteem because he can see that the nurse is just parroting a statement rather than speaking sincerely. Although it is important to attempt to build the patient's self-esteem, it is far more useful to do this through non-verbal techniques such as showing consistent caring for that patient than by constantly repeating how good he is.

Third, there is an overemphasis, in my view, in many psychiatric programs on attempting to mobilize the patient's anger. K. Abraham, one of the early theorists of depression, believed that depression was related to internalized anger turned on the self, and Freud was fundamentally in agreement with this view. We now know, however, that though this dynamic is present in many patients, it is probably not the "cause" of most depressions. As indicated, a great many depressive illnesses have major biological roots and sequelae. Furthermore, even when internalized anger turned on the self is a major component of the patient's depression, dealing with that anger is an extremely intricate process which should best be left to psychotherapy. Often, it is not necessary during the patient's hospitalization to mobilize the anger — this can be done more effectively when the patient is well on his way to recovery from the depressive episode. Many nurses feel duty bound to "mobilize the depressed patient's anger." The patient is invited over and over again to get angry — and frequently he is not angry. Thus, this invitation — which becomes more of an expectation on the part of the nurse — can serve to further alienate the patient from his real affective state: the patient does not feel angry but those around him in a professional capacity insist that he is and that he must be. This is not to say, of course, that the nurse should not invite the patient to vent his feelings, and when the patient is indeed angry she should help him cope with that affect.

Depression is an exciting field for the health care professional in that many changes are being made in our approach to it and we are learning a great deal more about it. Contributions from nurses on specific methods of dealing with hospitalized patients who have various kinds of depression are very much needed and will be appreciated by all health care professionals.

REFERENCES

1. Akiskal, H.S., and McKinney, W.: Depressive disorders: toward a unified hypothesis, Science, *182:*20, (1973).

9 Organic Brain Syndromes

Lloyd A. Wells

Many psychiatric disorders are caused by short-term or chronic and even permanent brain lesions and dysfunction. A major aspect of psychiatric nursing consists of caring for such patients and helping medical and surgical nurses to care for such patients. The brain disorder can often be attributed to specific organic disturbances or can be assumed when other functional disorders are excluded and positive criteria for the diagnosis are present. The actual lesion can be anatomical or metabolic disturbance and can be the result of tumors, alcoholism, deficiency states and degenerative types of illnesses.

The diagnosis is dependent on the entire work-up, consisting of not only mental status examination but many laboratory determinations, physical examination and assessment for functional psychiatric disturbances such as depression and schizophrenia.

In the most recent *Diagnostic and Statistical Manual* of the American Psychiatric Association (1), the organic mental disorders, as they are now termed, are divided into organic mental disorders *per se* and so-called organic brain syndromes. If one is dealing with senile or presenile dementias, the term organic mental disorder is officially used.

While there are differences in findings in the nursing mental status examination of different patients with organic mental disorders, there are certain findings common to most of them. On the mental status examination, the patient will be found to have a disturbance of attention or orientation to person, place or time, an impairment of memory, problems in intellectual functioning including vocabulary, ability to understand, ability to perform calculations and ability to learn new material, impaired judgment and emotional lability, often with a very rapidly shifting type of superficial affect.

The current classification of organic brain disturbance is extremely long and will be listed:

- — Senile dementia of different types including delirious and delusional types and also types which combine senile dementia with depression.
- — Presenile dementia
- — Multi-infarct dementia, usually the result of many small strokes in a hypertensive patient.
- — Substance abuse including alcoholism with delirium tremens, alcohol withdrawal, active intoxication, hallucinosis, barbiturate or sedative-hypnotic induced, opiate-induced, cocaine, amphetamine, phencyclidine, hallucinogens, cannabis, tobacco, caffeine and other substance abuse and syndromes whose etiology is unknown or secondary to an additional medical disorder.

The organic mental disorders are often subdivided into delirium, dementia, amnestic syndrome and organic delusional syndrome. Delirium is a syndrome which usually begins quite suddenly and usually resolves. In delirium, the patient has a clouded sensorium whose level of impairment changes quite rapidly. Confusion is virtually always present and there is impairment of cognitive features in a diffuse sort of way. At times, psychotic features are also present. Often the delirious patient becomes worse at night or when the many props which might remind him of orientation are removed or limited. Memory is frequently impaired. In addition to being confused and sometimes having panic attacks, these patients frequently show considerable dysphoria, anger, euphoria and anxiety. Because of the patient's impaired judgment, he may be dangerous to himself if not to others. Many delirious patients can injure themselves because of their poor judgment or dysphoria. Furthermore, if the cause of the delirium is not ascertrained and treated there can be significant impairment and sometimes death. Delirium is usually caused by some extracranial process and is frequently the result of metabolic disturbance including fluid and electrolyte imbalances, thyrotoxicosis and postsurgical states. Infections can cause delirium as can inflammatory processes, with lupus cerebritis being one of the most frequently found. Poisons can cause delirium as can tumor-related pathology, and certainly one of the prime causes of delirium is related to drug ingestion, specifically alcohol, hallucinogens, sedatives and steroids. In attempting to determine the differential diagnosis of delirium, one must consider a schizophreniform illness and other psychotic disorders, but usually the sudden onset of the delirium and thorough mental status examination will show that one is dealing with a delirium rather than a functional psychiatric illness.

The basic treatment of delirium is the treatment of its cause. In the hospital setting, good nursing care is the *sine qua non* of treatment for the delirious patient. In addition, neuroleptic medications can sometimes be very helpful in providing temporary control, as can restraints. However, the role of support, orientation and availability by the nurse is of great importance in the management of this condition.

Dementia is another form of organic mental disorder, and this is usually considered to be a progressive, irreversible type of loss of cognitive functions because of structural or functional loss of neurons. Dementia is very frequently accompanied by personality changes, and psychotic and depressive features can be superimposed. The demented person loses intellectual abilities to the point that he is severely restricted in social and occupational functioning. He also has serious memory impairment. Abstract thinking is frequently impaired, and the demented patient becomes increasingly concrete. In addition, his judgment, particularly for complex tasks, is usually impaired. Sometimes one finds other disturbances of cognition including language disorder, incomprehension of spoken language, and apraxia. Usually the state of consciousness itself is not clouded as it is in delirium or intoxication.

The demented person becomes withdrawn, often becomes anxious and depressed and generally shows inappropriate behavior, frequently becoming quite exhibitionistic. Paranois is also frequently found in late stages, as is depression. The patient becomes unable to function cohesively in family or work and becomes prone to injury as the result of poor judgment. Differential diagnosis here again includes schizophreniform illness and also includes delirium. One of the most important aspects of the differential diagnosis is of pseudodementia, which is a form of depressive illness found frequently in elderly patients who seem cognitively impaired, but are cognitively impaired in a secondary way because of their depression. Treatment of the underlying depression can often reverse the apparent dementing process, and, therefore, observations the nurse may make of a demented patient which reflect any sign of depression are of the utmost importance and should be highlighted.

While senile dementia is the leading cause of dementia in the world, one must also consider metabolic causes including hypothyroidism and pellagra, other degenerative illnesses including Parkinson's Disease, tumors, vascular impairments of the brain and heavy metal and insecticide poisoning.

Chronic infectious processes such as neurosyphilis can also lead to dementia.

Treatment of dementias must again address the underlying disorder if it can be found, and this is the definitive treatment. The role of the nurse again becomes one of providing support and structure for the patient and reassurance for the family. The nurse must be involved in fairly frequent reassessments of living situations with a view toward restructuring them to provide maximal safety for the patient as well as maximal opportunity for him to function.

Amnestic syndromes are a third type of mental disorder, and in them one finds a severe memory dysfunction but otherwise reasonably normal cognitive functioning. There is no decrease in IQ, and patients with amnestic syndromes can solve problems very well but have no memory except for immediate memory. These patients are unable to learn new information and frequently show confabulation — making up sometimes implausible stories — to fill in their major memory gaps. They usually are unaware of their major memory problem. Chronic alcoholism is probably the main cause of amenstic syndromes, and vitamin deficiencies can also cause them.

Finally, organic delusional syndrome is the fourth type of organic mental disorder currently defined by the *Diagnostic and Statistical Manual* and here one finds delusions occurring without delirium or dementia but caused by an organic factor such as temporal lobe epilepsy, psychotomimetic drug intoxication and Huntington's chorea. Here, the differential diagnosis is between organic delusional syndrome and organic hallucinosis, which is the fifth organic mental disorder classified and is defined as recurrent and persistent hallucinations occurring because of an organic problem and not associated with delirium or dementia. This hallucinosis occurs most commonly in patients who are in the process of heavy drinking but it can also be caused by hallucinogens, electrolyte disturbances and sensory deprivation.

The role of the nurse in the organic mental disorders is usually underemphasized. It cannot be stressed enough that the psychiatric nurse can provide a great deal to these patients directly and indirectly. They frequently are hospitalized in psychiatric units where the nurse can make a direct contribution in dealing with the patient's orientation and structuring of activities of daily living as well as the patient's family. In addition, the nurse can play an educational role with the family and to a limited extent with the patient and can also provide liaison assistance to nurses dealing with such patients on medical and surgical floors where they are also very frequently hospitalized. Finally, the observations of the nurse are of critical importance in terms of assessment of the reversibility of the syndrome and the possibility of a pseudodementia in which the patient is actually suffering from a treatable depression.

REFERENCES

1. DSM-III: *Diagnostic and Statistical Manual of Mental Disorders*, American Psychiatric Association (1980).

10 Neuroses

Lloyd A. Wells

Historically, neuroses and personality disorders have been considered as very discrete entities which are easily separated. In fact, it is quite difficult to separate neurosis from personality disorder, and the distinction is probably an artificial one. While the historical distinction between the two has been in part that neuroses consist of maladaptive intra-psychic responses to stress and anxiety, while personality disorders consist of extra-psychic, environmental actions, in fact one never finds a purely intra-psychic or a purely environmental reaction to anxiety or stress.

The entire concept of neurosis has been so tortured that the diagnosis itself has been removed from the DSM-III. On the other hand, neuroses probably comprise a substantial proportion of the mental illness one will encounter, and it seems a bit of an over-reaction to remove this concept from the nomenclature so prematurely.

In general, the patient who has a neurosis is in very good contact with reality, and in fact his reality testing in some areas may be superior. There is no evidence of a thought disorder, and the neurotic symptom or symptoms is felt as ego-dystonic. In other words, the patient is aware that his symptoms are non-logical, which distresses him greatly.

The problem of neurosis and its origin was very instrumental in the development of psychoanalytic theory. To understand the reason for a neurosis in psychodynamic terms, we need first to consider it as a way of avoiding and hence dealing with anxiety. A neurosis develops because of anxiety. The circumstance which caused the anxiety becomes associated with the neurotic symptom, and then, frequently, similar circumstances will invoke the neurotic symptoms because of symptom generalization.

While fear can be considered as an affective state related to a real, known threat to us, anxiety can more appropriately be considered as a similar affective response to an unknown threat which may have conflict in its origin. The ego mechanisms of defense, which have been discussed, partly protect us from anxiety and keep us from feeling anxious all the time. We all use these defenses very frequently. Sometimes, however, the defense mechanisms work inadequately or the anxiety is so overwhelming that they cannot take care of it. It is at times like these then a maladaptive type of pattern might be established.

In Freud's structural theory of the mind, which one must recall is a model and not an established entity, there were three major components: the id, the ego and the superego. The id consists of instinctual drives concerned with pleasure and aggression. Those drives, in Freud's view, seek gratification. The ego, in Freud's view, is an organizer which controls the drives and both delays and changes their goals. The ego modifies the drives of the id to conform with reality and society. Thus, there is a potential conflict between the id and the ego. The ego develops various, largely unconscious, defensive functions in part to deal with the id drives. Patients develop conflicts between the drives and fears of what will happen if the drives are satisfied. This conflict prevents discharge of the drive. The drives are then dealt with primarily through repression, which keeps them unconscious but powerful forces in the patient. The repressed wishes fight their way back to consciousness as neurotic symptoms — disguised versions of conflict. Thus, the initiation of a neurosis can be considered to have something to do with the conflict between a wish and a fear.

It is important in our conceptualization of neuroses, however, to realize that to understand a neurosis one must understand not only its genesis — indeed, often one never does discover what the basic conflict was all about — but the ways in which the neurotic symptoms, which are observable by others, are perpetuated. These symptoms are usually perpetuated by subtle rewards to the patient from the environment and from within himself. Rewards from within the self include a certain relief of anxiety. Rewards from the environment include, frequently, the chance to regress, to be dependent, to be cared for, to be the focus of attention, and a great many other potential rewards. Thus, the symptoms are subtly and unintentionally reinforced. Changing the way in which those symptoms are reinforced can often change the behaviors.

At this point, we should consider one or two specific types of neurosis to exemplify these general considerations. One good example is the conversion reaction. This presumably arises out of intra-psychic conflict, often centering around the expression of the aggressive drive. The patient is often subliminally afraid of expressing anger at a particular person. As a result of this, a somatic symptom forms as a substitute. For example, the hand with which one might strike a parent whom one views ambivalently becomes paralyzed. There is a symbolic intra-psychic meaning to this symptom. As a result of the symptom, the patient's way of life changes. He is often allowed to become more dependent, often on the ambivalently-perceived important person. He sometimes receives some financial compensation. He often does not have to work anymore. All of these social consequences of the neurotic symptom serve to reinforce the symptom and keep it in place.

Neurotic disorders have puzzled physicians from time immemorial because they are clear cut and occur in the absence of other major psychopathology. It is both troubling and fascinating to the physician or other health professional to observe a person with apparently good ego strength who is nevertheless incapacitated by a seemingly trivial and meaningless symptom. The investigation of neuroses played a major role in the advancement of psychiatric theory at the end of the 19th century and during the first years of this century with such investigators as Freud and Janet focusing their therapeutic and investigative interest on a great deal of neurotic entities.

The role of anxiety in the development of neuroses cannot be overemphasized. There is great debate at the present time in psychiatric circles as to the amount of psychodynamics to be found in a case of anxiety neurosis or panic-anxiety symdrome. There is a reason to believe that some patients have these types of disorders without a great deal of previous psychodynamic problems. When dealing with true neurotic entities, however, the author believes it is most helpful to view them as effects of repression and/or displacement of anxiety just as Freud proposed so many years ago. Rather than deal with the painful affect of anxiety, the patient unconsciously focuses all the anxiety on to one area of his life or psyche.

As can be seen from the chapter by Dr. Milliner, there are many mechanisms of defense against anxiety which are central to the functioning of the human organism. Most neuroses can be viewed as the maladaptive use of one of these mechanisms of defense which successfully represses anxiety and its perception in the patient but which causes more severe problems. Often, such patterns develop in childhood or adolescence and at that time are not maladaptive, but as the human being becomes an adult these patterns become extremely harmful to him. Some of the defenses which are exaggerated in some neurotic entities include displacement, undoing, symbolization and many others.

Let us consider a few examples.

A 21-year-old man develops an intrusive thought that he will misplace his diary and that other people will find it and read of the rather tormented sexual identity he may have. As time goes on, this thought preoccupies the paitnet increasingly, and the anxiety concerning his sexual identity is transferred more and more to the object of the diary. This obsession causes him to limit some of his other activities and certainly curtails his opportunities for friendships and social activities. He may go on to develop some compulsive actions as part of this obsessive syndrome. These might include lengthy rituals to protect the diary from being found. Of course, the patient realizes that such maneuvers are unnecessary and have a magical but unrealistic import. In spite of this intellectual realization, he is unable to stop. Gradually, the obsessive-compulsive neurosis which he develops causes him tremendous difficulties in work, socialization and most other meaningful aspects of life. The anxiety associated with the indeterminate sexual identity has been completely moved over to the obsessive-compulsive syndrome but both objectively and subjectively the patient is far worse off than he was before the syndrome began.

It should be noted that in many cases of obsessive-compulsive neurosis, the patient actually uses the obsessive-compulsive disorder to indirectly and unconsciously express a wish. Thus, a patient who is afraid that she will harm a small defenseless child of hers may actually attempt to protect the child by locking herself away from the child or by asking the child to remove sharp potential weapons from the patient. In fact, the patient increases the chance that the child will indeed be hurt.

Take the case of a 40-year-old woman who is unable to leave her home. Over a period of many years, she had gradually experienced more and more attacks of panicky feelings when in public, particularly in fairly anonymous public places such as markets. She had felt inadequate for most of her married life feeling that she had been unable to please her husband and his family. Her social relationships had been superficial. She felt uncared about but had never learned to express any anger directly. Her husband spent more and more time away from home and the couple was childless. Gradually, the woman began to withdraw increasingly into her own home to the point that she became unable to leave. Attempting even to leave her house created enormous feelings of panic and uncontrollable anxiety. At those times, she would weep inconsolably, speak about death and need to be physically assisted back into her house. As a result of this completely disabling syndrome, the patient's husband had to spend increasing periods at home, needed to engage in some marital counseling with the patient and needed to assume a great many of the household routines. Unconsciously, the patient's anger toward her husband was being mobilized and expressed through the means of this neurosis. Again, however, the price the patient paid in terms of the neurosis was totally out of proportion to the gains she had from it.

This is not always the case with the conversion reaction, which is a different type of neurosis in that the gains often do outweigh the losses. In the conversion reaction, of course, a patient has a physical symptom or series of physical symptoms which have no organic basis but do have great unconscious meaning to the patient. One thinks of the example of a 19-year-old farm boy whose tyrannical father has dominated most of the patient's life. The patient, as he moves through late adolescence, becomes more and more preoccupied with hatred for his father and has a great many aggressive thoughts about him and impulses toward him. After a lengthy fantasy about starting a fist fight with his father, he finds that he cannot move his right arm. In this case, the neurotic conversion symptom, the arm paralysis, actually prevents him from carrying out a conflicted ambivalent wish and protects him from the social and interpersonal repercussions of that wish. At the same time, he receives considerable symptom gain in terms of a relief of his anxiety and also in terms of an increased ability to manipulate the environment. Sick people are viewed more tolerantly than others are. Usually the conversion reaction is self-limited and does not persist for a great many months.

A final type of neurosis which we should consider is the type initially described by Franz Alexander and termed by him the neurotic character (1). Here, a person with a basic neurotic conflict between wish and its expression externalizes that conflict and acts it out in every human relationship rather than developing a different kind of displaced reaction to it which is seen in other neuroses. The person with a neurotic character who, for example, has an intense oedipal rivalry with his father will develop such intense oedipal rivalries with every man he meets or works with.

Most of these patients can correctly be viewed as having personality disorders but the concept of neurotic character within the realm of both neuroses and personality disorders is one that I think has merit.

Neurosis remains an entity of enormous theoretical importance. On a practical level its classification and often enough its treatment will change throughout the years. Nevertheless, one needs to think of and recall neurosis as the maladaptive response of a relatively healthy human being to anxiety. While it begins as an intrapsychic phenomenon, it affects not only the patient but all those around him and becomes an intensely important interpersonal issue as well.

Thus, although classically neurosis reflects a purely intrapsychic process, it is in fact intra-psychic and extra-psychic. Further examples of this fact are delineated in the chapters on personality disorders and functional illness.

REFERENCES

1. Alexander, R.: The neurotic character, Int J Psychoanal, *11*:292, (1930).

RECOMMENDED READING

Laughlin, H.P.: *The Neuroses*, Washington, Butterworths, (1967).

11 Personality Disorders

Lloyd A. Wells

One of the most difficult aspects of psychiatric nursing is in dealing with patients who have personality disorders, in understanding the syndromes they have, in appreciating these syndromes within the context of the biopsychosocial model, and of accepting these people as suffering, worthwhile human beings and not as "bad people." Before one can begin to address the question of personality disorders, one must begin to review the entire concept of personality and its development. Personality can be defined in a great many ways, but one definition which covers many aspects, at least, of what we consider to be personality or character is that it is a largely unconscious, consistent and even stereotyped group of patterns of behavior and thinking which give relatively consistent and also unique responses to stimuli from the external and internal environments; that entire series of defenses, coping mechanisms and reactions which makes each of us uniquely consistent and sometimes consistently unique. Thus, personality consists of a large number of mental operations, many of them unconscious. None of the operations in and of themself is unique, but the constellation of them gives a unique character or personality to the individual.

Personality disorders develop out of problems in the initial development of personality. The locus for many later personality disorders can be found in the developmental tasks and problems in resolving them much earlier in life.

In the stage of infancy, which one can consider in an oversimplified way to occur from birth to about age 18 months, the child has several developmental tasks, but the most important of these are identifying oneself as a separate being and, as Erikson has taught us, developing an ability to trust. Should these two tasks not be fulfilled, the child can have extremely serious lifelong problems and usually does. Sometimes, these tasks cannot be fulfilled because of deprivation and psychological or physical abuse by the caretaking people or, paradoxically, by too much attention from the caretaking person such that the child is not able to experience any kind of independence and thus does not learn about himself as a separate, independent human being. Another major hazard of the infancy stage, particularly during the early part of the second year of life, is to develop a sense of basic trust and then have it shattered by the appearance of a sibling on the scene.

The next major stage to consider is the autonomous stage of toddlerhood, which we can consider to be from about age 18 months to three years. Here, there are perhaps more tasks that must be accomplished than were present at infancy. The child must develop the ability to be physically separate and away from the mother or the caretaking person. The child develops a sense of autonomy and a sense of ability. The child starts to come to terms with reality situations and learn to delay gratification of drives and needs, and as he achieves this ability to delay gratification he or she also has to begin to cope with appropriate means of expressing anger and the whole aggressive drive as well as achieve a measure of toilet training. In this stage, there are certainly many possible hazards, and these include overprotectiveness on the part of the parenting people as well as excessive rigidity on their part.

The next stage psychodynamically is the Oedipal stage, which lasts roughly from age three to five. Here, the child has to master a sense of sexual identity and, more globally, achieve comfort with his sense of position in the family unit. Little boys at this age have a great desire to possess their mother and a concomitant fear of injury and mutilation, usually on the part of the father. This is often resolved by identification with the father. In little girls, the fear of injury and mutilation is also present as they desire to possess the father. In addition, many little girls have a largely culturally determined sense of having been discriminated against at this age.

Latency occurs between age six and eleven, and here there are a great many tasks largely involving an ability to function in society outside the family. This is the age in which the child has to cope with school, with peers, with working as well as with social playing, and the child also has to begin to acquire a great many skills that he or she will need in life. Hazards include anything which is threatening to one's self-esteem, and often at this age physical, emotional and intellectual handicaps cause great problems for the child. Similarly, this is an age at which children need a great deal of secure acceptance on the part of their parents.

Adolescence is the next stage, and because of social norms which are changing so rapidly, I would define adolescence as taking place between roughly age 12 when pre-adolescence begins and age 25 when most people are finishing their schooling and becoming vocationally occupied. In adolescence, one must acquire not only a concept of one's self and mature sexual identity but also vocational and avocational identities. This is an age at which the developing person is very, very interested in the pursuit of meaning — the meaning of his or her life, the meaning of different philosophic systems, and it is often a time of grandiose preoccupation as well as extremely precipitous dysphoric episodes. There is, in this age group, often an attempt to work through previous flicts. The hazards of adolescence include problems with permissiveness versus authoritatianism, problems with discipline, problems with parents and any other authority figures as well as the whole question of dependence versus independence. This is an age at which people want to be independent, but at the same time they are very terrified of being independent.

The next stage is early adulthood which we can consider to be from about age 25 through 45 and here the person has to deal with such tasks as marriage, parenthood, establishing realistic goals for work and hobbies, and shoring up weak defenses. In this age group, there is often a sense of failure as some of the grandiose ideals and plans of adolescence are seen to be non-achievable. In addition, defenses which have operated adaptively for the personality in earlier years might seem a bit extreme or exaggerated in this age group.

One particularly difficult developmental task of early adult life is to reconcile the somewhat grandiose and romanticized versions of major life events such as marriage, childbearing, etc., with the often less glossy realities.

With middle age, there continue to be many important tasks, and these include the pursuit of reasonable goals and hobbies, a sense of ease with one's important companions, particularly spouse and family, the maturation process in which more reasonable and more gratifying goals are found and then achieved, and finally dealing with separation and death from people in the older generation, particularly parents. There are, again, several important hazards in this period including the denial of aging and death, which are so frequently seen in middle-aged people who suddenly have a total change in their lifestyle and begin to rather precipitously change course in terms of marriage, job, family responsibilities and so forth. Often, this type of pattern comes from a faint realization that life is not forever and that losses are many, and a subsequent, rather frantic search for love, often of a rather thinly disguised maternal nature.

Finally, we come to the stage of old age. The old must deal with retirement, economic and social problems, and the pursuit of hobbies. Hazards continue to be a major denial of death and also the embrace of death and dissolution, which is sometimes found underlying a rather nihilistic approach to life. A third defense which many aging people use is that of narcissism in which they become increasingly constricted and preoccupied with themselves.

With this brief review of human development, we can once again turn to the concept of personality disorders. It is my contention that personality disorders arise out of faulty development and an inability to meet certain crucial developmental tasks. Thus, a personality disorder can arise *de novo* during any life phase and not merely in childhood and adolescence.

Perhaps Lucretius had some concept of personality disorder when he wrote many centuries ago that "Each man flies from his own self; yet from that self he has no power of escape. He clings to it in his own despite and loathes it, too, because though he is sick he perceives not the cause of his disease." Lucretius captures some of the major attributes of personality disorders. They are caused by actions of people which in turn alienate all other important human relationships. Though the person often has at least a subliminal awareness of this, he or she finds it excruciatingly difficult to change the pattern.

The history of the concept of personaltiy disorders really begins in more modern times with the writings of James Prichard, a well-known English psychiatrist of the nineteenth century. Prichard introduced the term *moral insanity* and by the introduction of this term greatly increased the scope of psychiatry. He wrote: "The disorder is manifested principally alone in the state of the feelings, temper or habits with some impairment in the power of self-government. It is a madness consisting in a morbid perversion of the natural feelings, affection, inclinations, temper, habits, moral disposition and natural impulses, without any remarkable disorder or defect of the intellect or knowing and reasoning faculties, and particularly without any insane illusion or hallucination" (1). Thus, Prichard was describing an illness which was rather metaphorical. In fact, he is describing a syndrome which is analogous to an illness. He points out that this syndrome — moral insanity — is not a psychosis and has nothing to do with cognitive abilities.

After this introduction of the term moral insanity, there was a proliferation of writing about personality disorders, and several other rather pejorative terms for personality disorders were used. These included moral insanity, moral idiocy, moral oligophrenia, and constitutional ethical abberation. Humane physicians referred to these people as "enemies of society." Eventually, the term "coinstitutional psychopathic inferiority" was coined to describe them. This series of diagnoses by otherwise well-meaning, liberal professionals underscores the fact that people with personality disorders do alienate other people, and they do cause a great many angry feelings. The diagnosis can and is sometimes used as an epithet to describe someone who is simply not nice, not likeable or somehow covertly or overtly hostile.

It is difficult to use the term *personality disorder* without recalling that one of its first uses was to describe runaway slaves during the pre-Civil War period in this country.

It is difficult sometimes to distinguish a personality disorder from a neurosis. The neurosis in fact is less grounded in the patient's entire personality and tends to be more monosymptomatic. The neurotic patient, like the patient with a personality disorder, is regressed psychologically and uses autoplastic methods of dealing with stress, while the personality disorder patient uses primarily alloplastic methods, and the neurotic symptom is egodystonic — the patient is extremely uncomfortable with it — while some of the symptoms of the personality disorder seem to be egosyntomic. Nevertheless, when one actually works with both neurotic and personality disordered patients one realizes that these are oversimplifications, that the neurotic has many alloplastic features while the personality disorder patient is often genuinely, if sometimes quietly, distressed by his symptoms and the way he alienates other people. Neither neurosis nor personality disorder exists in a vacuum — both impact on and partially derive from relationships with others.

One can consider the person with a personality disorder as having a "script" in the parlance of transactional analysis, or a "repetition compulsion" in the parlance of psychoanalysis. The patient has certain expectations, goals, etc. At the same time, his life seems to follow a preset course which is usually somewhat destructive in a repetitive, patterned sort of way. Such patients are genuinely unhappy and feel isolated and lonely. At the same time, because of their unhappiness they are quite mistrustful of others and tend not to share their loneliness, sense of isolation and unhappiness with others. Their reality testing is unimpaired, and at a deep level they are aware of their own inadequacies. Their self-esteem is in fact extremely low although, again, this is not frequently communicated to others. Many of them, in fact, have a major streak of psychic masochism. Despite their adequate reality testing, they do tend to project blame for their problems in social situations, and they refuse to accept, often enough, the consequences of their own acts as due to their own acts. The behavior is repetitious and it is, as mentioned, frequently self-destructive or self-punitive. Changes in the environment are not met with ready adaptation by these patients. They have a great need for closeness with other human beings, but at the same time they are terrified of such closeness and often unconsciously provoke rejection or else themselves reject the person who might become close (2).

One can consider personality disorders as largely autoplastic or alloplastic, although in fact all personality disorders are probably mixed in nature. The autoplastic personaltiy disorders might include obsessive-compulsive disorder while the most notable of the alloplastic disorders would be sociopathy. In all personality disorders, I think that there is a major psychological conflict between the need for love and closeness along with the inability to tolerate it. This conundrum can lead to the fear of being dependent and consequently taken advantage of, and the person can react with a pseudo-independent posture plus feelings of resignation and giving up, which would be autoplastic, or with a great deal of rebellion and, again, pseudo-independence, which would be alloplastic. The person with a personality disorder, unfortunately enough, often ends up relating to the world as if he were a puppet. He presents a "false self" to the world, expecting to be rejected, thus convincing himself that though the false self is rejected, he himself has not really been rejected.

As in any other kind of syndrome, stress can add to the problems of the person with a mild personality disorder and often can precipitate a more severe apparent personality disorder.

Obsessive-compulsive personality disorder is probably one of the most common disorders, and it is one shared by many people in the medical and nursing professions. The classic obsessive-compulsive person is neat, tidy, angry and constrained. Not everyone with obsessive-compulsive symptomatology has an obsessive-compulsive personality disorder. The personality disorder will be discussed in this section. Obsessive-compulsive neurosis is another entity in which a person has classical symptoms with a great deal of ritualistic behavior, expiation for past wrongs, and a great deal of symbolism which are all absent from the personality disorder. Other people who are encountering the initial throes of severe depressive or schizophrenic episodes might develop obsessive-compulsive symptomatology as a defense. This usually leaves soon. In western society, many people make what Neal Krupp called an obsessive-compulsive decision — this is an adaptive use of obsessive defenses so that the person is prompt, accurate, hard-working, with many other characteristics we also often treasure.

In the obsessive-compulsive personality disorder, there is a core conflict which includes the fear of and acceptance of authority with a simultaneous anger at having to be submissive to authority, and usually people with obsessive personality disorders have major difficulties with the entire issue of authority and dependence. This conflict becomes a conflict of the wish to submit versus the wish to defy. Thus, acting on the ambivalent wish to submit to authority, the person is punctual, reliable, conscientious and indeed placid and submissive, but at the same time, acting on the ambivalent wish to defy authority and replace it with himself, the person is rather negligent at times, stubborn, with a certain amount of hostile, dependent and cruel behavior.

Again, when he is under a great deal of stress, a person who has made an obsessive-compulsive decision may in fact encounter the symptoms of the obsessive-compulsive personality disorder as a reaction to stress, particularly the stress of loss, which may be real, fantasized or threatened.

In my experience, most people with obsessive-compulsive personality disorders have had a great deal of core conflict about their ambivalent reaction to a younger sibling. This is always worth asking about.

Such patients are difficult to treat because they have little insight about the maladaptive effects of their personality disorder, and they tend to be covertly hostile and to be repetitive and boring.

Another whole type of personality disorder is hysterical personality disorder, a name which is now being gradually withdrawn from the literature but which has a long and confusing history.

Many meanings have been attributed to the term hysteria, even in modern times, and when one sees this word in any kind of journal or textbook one has to ask what the author means. Hysteria can mean a personality disorder, which is to be described in this section; it can mean conversion reaction; it can be applied sometimes to a combination of phobic and anxious symptomatology; it has frequently been applied to sociopaths who happen to be women; it is often applied to people suspected of malingering or being doctor-dependent; and it can be used as a pejorative term for someone that a health professional does not like.

Hysteria has always been linked with repressed sexuality, and at least from the Middle Ages we have illustrations of people who today would be considered hysterics, considered as witches seducing devils. Even as great a neurologist and as humane a man as Charcot could convince himself that compression of the ovaries with a rather cruel-appearing device was a treatment of choice for this condition.

Wilhelm Reich gave as good a description of hysterical personality disorder as any I have seen, many years ago (3). He pointed out that the hysteric tends to take non-sexual matters and give them a sexual overtone while at the same time the hysteric is sexually frigid and apprehensive. He pointed out that people with hysteria change their behavior unexpectedly, that they are very unpredictable and strongly suggestible. He pointed out that they lack conviction and sometimes seem to either quickly agree with one or quickly disagree with one and disparage one without real grounds to do so. He also pointed out that they sometimes were imaginative and creative. On the other hand, they were prone to lie. He felt that they dramatized a great deal, tended to repress their aggressive drive and acted out in subtle — and sometimes not so subtle — ways, and felt extremely low self-esteem, depending on others for their self-esteem with a nearly compulsive need to be loved and admired. Despite an enormous amount which has been written about hysterical personality disorder since that time, these are still the basic traits that one finds in people with this disorder. Sometimes, in addition, one finds rather extravagant use of language in the description of physical complaints as well as a certain discrepancy between the extent of the illness that the patient describes versus the amount of objective disability. These patients frequently show what is called *la belle indifference*, a term introduced by Charcot which merely means the patient tells about truly horrendous events and occurrences with a very bland sort of affect.

There is a shallowness about these people which is apparent to the observer, and one often feels that they are acting. It is as if one is watching people trying to convey deep feelings on the stage rather than people actually expressing deep feelings. As Chodoff and Lyons have pointed out, hysterical personality patients are demanding in an extremely dependent way, which puts the therapist or helping professional in a very difficult position at times (4).

When one thinks of hysteria, one usually thinks of women. Male hysterics tend to be characterized as effeminate and often are. While some can argue that the vast preponderance of the female sex among those diagnosed as having hysterical personality could reflect some genetic trait, it seems far more likely that this is a cultural phenomenon, that hysterical personaltiy is in fact an unconscious sort of parody of what society has expected woman's role to be over the years (4).

Another personality disorder which is almost totally alloplastic is psychopathy or sociopathy, which is also known as antisocial personality. People with this terrible syndrome tend to be extremely impulsive and derive pleasure from enormous, almost daily change. They seek out excitement. They are very aggressive and are simultaneously unable to control their drives. This obviously leads to great destructiveness. Despite all of this, they feel very little guilt because they have very little conscience, and are really unable to love and be close to other people. Anxiety in people with this syndrome appears largely to be brought about by external situations rather than internal feeling states.

In making the diagnosis of psychopathy, one does need to ask whether it is the core of the personality or whether psychopathy and psychopathic traits actually are symptoms of depression or other underlying psychiatric problems.

In people who have a core type of psychopathy, one notices coldness and lack of compassion and one notices that they treat others more as objects for their own pleasure than as human beings with rights, feelings and attachments.

One needs to consider the possibility, particularly in adolescents, that what appears to be psychopathic behavior is in fact a manifestation of depression, of malingering, of hysteria, of borderline syndromes and of an asocial subculture. If one is brought up in a criminal subculture where everyone breaks the law, one might at first appear to be psychopathic when one is merely conforming to the norms of society. Some psychopathic patients — or at least patients who initially appear to be psychopathic — become overtly psychotic when they are confined, and in these patients the apparent psychopathy may in fact be a defense of sorts against schizophrenia or psychosis.

No one knows the causes of psychopathy, although there have been an enormous number of suggestions. There is slight evidence that there is a genetic component to this syndrome, and certainly it is sometimes familial; it is sometimes possible to trace back the condition for four or more generations. There is some evidence that it is a condition related to learning disabilities. Horowitz has shown suggestive evidence that there is an ethologic component in that many psychopathic people have a much more constricted territoriality than do others (5). Most likely, however, most of the components of psychopathy are psychologic and developmental in their nature. The usual formation of conscience occurs as a result of resolving the Oedipal complex. Classically, it is felt that the young child has love for the mother, whom he wishes to possess, and develops a consequent hatred for the father. The hatred is coupled with fear of mutilation. To deal with this hatred and fear, the child identifies with the father as the aggressor and then proceeds to a more mature from of identification, which leads to the ability to form a concept of one's own identity and to form a conscience. In the psychopathic person, the child is very frequently rejected by the parents, and instead of a normal and unconflicted initial love for the mother there is an ambivalent feeling toward her. Instead of the usual mixture of anger and fear directed toward the father, there is extreme hatred. These feelings of ambivalent love and extreme hatred are transferred to society and the person develops neither a mature identity nor a conscience.

The treatment of psychopathy has a long and unhappy history. Somatic and pharmacologic treatments have been used a great deal and are usually accompanied by initial enthusiasm and later discouragement. Long-term psychotherapy, with the exception of a few therapists such as Schmideberg (6), has met with failure. Therapeutic communities which use a great deal of peer pressure seem to be very popular and may help many people with some forms of psychopathy, but they are also difficult in hard-core psychopaths. Authoritarian approaches are often of more help. Incarceration until the psychopath "burns out," which usually occurs in the 40' or 50's at which time the patient is at least able to live in society, is perhaps the best way of preventing psychopaths from being in society. At the same time, it would certainly be unethical and indeed unconstitutional to preventively detain people. Behavior therapy has been helpful in institutional settings to modify the behaviors of psychopaths. At the same time, it is unlikely that the changes made in a behavior therapy program for psychopathy would be continued once the patient was dismissed from a closed type of setting.

In this chapter, I have attempted to discuss the common features of personality disorders and also to discuss two examples of a rather autoplastic type of personality disorder and one example of an alloplastic type.

REFERENCES

1. Prichard, J.C.: A Treatise on Insanity and Other Disorders Affecting the Mind, Philadelphia, Carey and Hart (1837).

2. Spiegel, J.P.: Personality and antisocial disorders, Psychiat Ann, *6:* 9-17 (1976).

3. Reich, W.: Some circumscribed character forms, In *Character Analysis*, New York, Orgone Institute Press, Inc. (1949).

4. Chodoff, P., and Lyons, H.: Hysteria, the hysterical personality and "hysterical conversion," Am J Psychiat, *114:*734-740 (1958).

5. Horowitz, M., Duff, D.F., and Stratton, L.O.: Body buffer zones, Arch Gen Psychiat, *11:*651 (1964).

6. Schmideberg, M.: The treatment of criminals, Psychoanal Rev, *36:*403-410 (1949).

12 Borderline Syndromes

Lloyd A. Wells

The use of the word "borderline" has increased exponentially in psychiatry over the past 15 years. The diagnosis "borderline" is being proffered to explain the symptoms of a great many patients. Nevertheless, there remains a great deal of confusion about the diagnosis and the concept.

The first problem, I suppose, is the name "borderline." There is an implication that this syndrome borders on something—what? Here there is no agreement. Historically, it was felt that there was a group of syndromes which bordered on psychosis, but many would argue with good arguments that the real border is that of the affective disorders, or that the real border is that of the personality disorders. I think the name is archaic and should be discarded. What name would you prefer?

Some of the problems with the entire concept of the borderline is first that although the term borderline is popular, people don't know what other people mean when they use the term. One psychiatrist's borderline is another's hysteria. There is no descriptive consensus about what symptoms exist in borderline disorders. There are a great deal of ideologic proposals to explain borderline behaviors without any concensus about what those behaviors are. Furthermore, the ideologic proposals are often conflicting. Finally, there are few good modern studies on these syndromes.

The historical antecedents for the borderline disorders can be found in Prichard's work on "moral insanity" in the 19th century (1). In 1925, Reich described a disorder which he called the impulsive character which was marked by impulsivity, ambivalence, over-riding aggression, ego weaknesses, narcissism, superego defects, and immature defenses (2). In many respects, he was talking about the borderline. Zilboorg (3) described a syndrome which he described as ambulatory schizophrenia — clearly he linked this syndrome to schizophrenia. Hoch and Polatin in the late 1940's and early 1950's developed the concept of pseudoneurotic schizophrenia (4). They felt that there was a clinical entity which presented with pan-neurosis, pan-anxiety, pansexuality, and a subtle thought disorder.

I think that one can make a case that there is no single borderline syndrome but that in fact some patients who are labeled borderline are typically schizophrenic while others have a personality disorder. I feel that those patients who are subtly schizophrenic should be diagnosed as having schizophrenia, leaving the borderline to patients with personality disorders. Atypical schizophrenia is probably much more common than we think. There are different forms. One is the form in which the patient has the primary symptoms of schizophrenia without psychosis or with latent psychosis. Another more common form is for a patient to have a very subtle form of schizophrenia with the usual symptoms well guarded. The pseudoneurotic form of schizophrenia described by Hoch and Polatin is a real entity as is pseudopsychopathic schizophrenia in which the patient defends against psychosis by psychopathic traits. (Such patients often become floridly schizophrenic when incarcerated.)

Despite the many disagreements about what constitutes the borderline, many experts would regard the patients described in these two case reports as representative.

Case 1

Samantha was a young woman hospitalized on the open psychiatric ward of a general hospital. At that time, she was a 26-year-old married mother of a 6-year-old daughter. Physical problems had been incapacitating for at least four years. They had commenced with severe headaches and nausea for which she was hospitalized on several occasions. She developed urinary retention. After an affair with her urologist, she was transferred to a psychiatric floor. She became unable to walk. She exhausted the resources of the hospital and was dismissed, but she refused to leave. She was finally escorted to the door. Following this dismissal, she was unable to sleep for three nights, weeping constantly. She went to the office of a psychiatrist whom she had never seen before; she refused to leave his office. He sent her to a colleague who urged her to go for walks with her husband and then arranged for her transfer to a hospital a thousand miles away. There she was initially diagnosed as having depression; the diagnosis was subsequently changed to schizophrenia. She was treated with Thorazine and psychotherapy. Her urinary retention worsened and she was transferred to the urology service of a general hospital. She improved rapidly under the care of a urology resident and moved into his bachelor apartment for about a month. She eventually returned home to her husband and child and found a new psychiatrist. Shortly thereafter, she became blind. She was again hospitalized. It was noted she had mood swings and she was given lithium. Her blindness persisted for more than a year and she was transferred to another hospital.

In addition to these symptoms, the patient had several episodes of auditory hallucinations in which she heard a male voice saying, "It's the end." She never had any doubt that the auditory phenomena were hallucinatory; she was frightened by the voice because she felt it might indicate she was psychotic. She also had frequent hypnagogic illusions.

Samantha was the youngest of three children born to wealthy and successful parents whom she perceived as terribly indulgent, although always on their own terms — if she lived up to their expectations, she was loved and pampered. Her mother had severe separation anxiety when Samantha began school. Samantha reported rather smugly "I was just the one." She competed in beauty contests from age three and won a major national contest at age 18. She was just "the one" again. Her father would remind her before these contests that he would die if she lost. While in college, she became pregnant and married. She perceived her husband as a passive man who would occasionally emerge from his torpidity to rape her — usually at her provocation. She was anorgasmic except for one occasion when she watched the husband of a friend beat her friend. Her life was managed by her mother who also cared for her daughter who was just "the one."

The patient's hospital course was chaotic. On more than one occasion, she obtained and used barbiturates. She had several lengthy obsessive-compulsive rituals which helped to diminish her anxiety. She mentioned that she had actually been able to see for a week or two prior to her hospitalization but had been reluctant to mention that for fear of being considered a malingerer. Almost from the start of her hospitalization, she expressed fear of leaving. The pattern of refusing to leave repeated itself and after her dismissal from the hospital, she and her husband stayed in a motel for two days while she telephoned many physicians pleading with them to arrange for readmission.

Samantha showed evidence of considerable intelligence and creativity. She was an excellent group member, understanding and interpreting unconscious and preconscious conflicts of other patients.

Three-year follow-up by letter suggests her life pattern has not changed.

Case 2

The second patient is Lisa, a 28-year-old divorced mother of one who lives with her child. Her chief complaint when she came for psychotherapy was "My thoughts are scrambled; it feels as if something inside of me has died." Lisa had a childhood in which she felt neglected and depersonalized: "I felt jealous of kids who got grounded; at least their parents cared." She was anhedonic throughout childhood and has repressed most of the usual childhood memories. As a senior in high school, she became involved with a boy and "was someone for the first time in my life." She had sexual intercourse with him on several occasions; she was anorgasmic but found intercourse pleasurable. After six months, the boy moved 1500 miles away. She became extremely anxious and made several suicide gestures within a three-month period. As a result, both arms and both legs are scarred with razor blade markings. She was hospitalized at that time and was diagnosed initially as having an adjustment reaction. She was dismissed after several weeks of supportive psychotherapy. Her behavior continued to escalate and two months later she was admitted to a state hospital where she was diagnosed as being depressed and treated with a long course of electroconvulsive therapy. Following her dismissal, she became involved with alcohol and street drugs. Two years later she became involved with another man whom she described as a rather dull-witted alcoholic, heroin-abusing meatcutter who was sexually and physically abusive to her. After they had lived together for two years they married. When the patient became pregnant, her husband decided to move another woman into the house. He urged the patient to welcome this woman emotionally and sexually. He wanted a true *ménage à trois.* The woman moved in a few days before the birth of Lisa's daughter. When her husband confirmed that this new arrangement was final, she had several homicidal fantansies and a dissociative episode in which she apparently loaded a gun and went out to look for her husband. When he saw her, he became alarmed, thinking that she intended to kill herself. When she realized his misunderstanding, she laughed and threw the gun on the ground. She had her baby, moved away, and divorced her husband. Shortly thereafter, she returned to his house and insisted on coming in to watch the girlfriend, threatening to wreck her husband's car if he did not allow this. About a year after the divorce, she began to live with another man who wanted to marry her and was generally kind and good to her. She found him "unexciting." He is a pleasant, intelligent businessman who cares a great deal about her. She easily concluded that she relates well only to men who misuse her. She felt unhappy and unworthy and ruminated a great deal about her inadequacy as a human being. She had frequent anxiety attacks and became phobic about fires. She had terminal insomnia with frequent nightmares in which she possessed something which others wanted and pursued her for, the identity of which was unknown to her. She found it stressful to contemplate the future. She had no hallucinations or delusions. She occasionally had ideas of reference and was extremely autistic.

The second time that I saw Lisa, she told me that she could not be honest with me because she found herself unwittingly and unwillingly trying to conform to whatever expectations she thought I might have. She felt that this was a pattern with her. Indeed, her sense of identity had always been derived from the most dominant figure around her at a particular time. She felt that the style of her hair or the color of her clothes added to or subtracted from her identity as a human being. In the next session, she associated at great length about her primitive fear of abandonment and the consequent destructive wishes it caused. Her free associations occasionally contained cognitive slips and evidence of a subtle thought disorder. For example, she had a fantasy about her husband signing papers so that her boyfriend could adopt her daughter. This idea had not actually been broached with either man but Lisa concluded by saying, "Looking at him signing that made me angry." For a moment, her fantasy was actualized. I quote a bit of free association for the insight it reveals about many borderline syndromes: "I think my mother might have cancer. She has lost a lot of weight and doesn't look herself. Maybe she does. It bothers me a lot. I am afraid of losing her even though I never had either of them. My mother takes my daughter and lets her do bad things. She thinks my daughter is more hers than mine. It makes me so angry. She says I don't keep her in the right way. I wish to God she had cared for me that way. I wish she had punished me. Inside I am aching for attention and discipline. Then they'll respect me and not walk all over me for the rest of my life. I always tried to measure myself by my sister (who is a doctoral level professional). I felt like a minus because she was so smart. I see myself in her. Gullible, gullible. I see that word in my mind on a big sign. It's gullible's travels, my life. I convince myself that I want what somebody else wants just to try to get along, but I don't. If somebody wants to see a dumb movie I have already seen, I really end up believing that I want to see it again even though I could tell you that I don't. Maybe I feel that no one sees me because I am nobody on the edge of nothing. I want so much for someone to ask me to play. In the dark at night I want mom to come in. It's like panic. I need her. I am so scared to call out to them. When I finally did my small voice was so small that they couldn't hear me. I feel like I'm Edith Ann and I am five years old, a tiny, precocious little girl with a smile on a big rocking chair."

Lisa's rather poetic free associations reinforce the fact that the very best descriptions of borderline conditions are probably found in literature rather than psychiatric works.

While there are certainly variants of many borderline personality disorders, I believe that they have the following features in common:

1. Behavior tends to be alloplastic. In other words, the patient responds to stress not with intrapsychic modifications but with a restructuring of the external environment.
2. The patient leads a life of *stable instability*. This is a term which was coined by Melitta Schmideberg (5) who pointed out that although these patients were incredibly unstable and became chaotically over-involved, when one looked at the instability and chaos, one could see that there was a certain predictability and pattern about them.
3. They have neurotic symptoms from more than one discrete neurosis.
4. Borderline patients are extremely impulsive.
5. There is a great need for an all-encompassing, almost symbiotic love among these patients with a concomitant fear of that love. Relationships which can seem extremely intense can abruptly be transferred from one person to another. Some common stylized relationships in which borderline patients involve themselves are highly infantile

relationships and highly sexualized relationships, particularly sadomasochistic ones. Other patients — perhaps the "as if" group of borderline patients (6) — seem to have given up on relationships and consigned themselves to lonely lives.

6. At some time, and for most patients most of the time, there is a real sense of internal emptiness.
7. Affect in borderline patients is often overwhelmingly angry, but in addition to this over-riding anger there are dysphoria, anhedonia and sometimes frank depression.

Patients with borderline personality disorders tend to use primitive defenses. Among these are splitting, dyadic splitting (7), and projective identification. In the defense of splitting, the patient is unable to incorporate good and bad aspects of the same object, and therefore, splits them in two, seeing a good object and a bad object. Thus, borderline patients tend to see others as good or bad. In projective identification, a patient splits off part of himself and projects it to another person, then uses this attribute to identify with that other person. Both of these defenses are common in young children, and projective identification is used by most mature adults when exposed to novel situations. The defense of dyadic splitting is a sort of combination of the two. The good aspects of one person are considered that person's only aspects, and that person's bad aspects are projected onto another person. Thus, for the borderline person there is often a rescuer and a persecutor. Other primitive defenses frequently used by patients with borderline personality disorders include denial, repression and projection.

Borderline patients can present in either a depressive mode or an aggressive mode and the same patient can go back and forth between a depressive mode and an aggressive mode. Frequently, in the aggressive mode, the patient may seem hypomanic.

Since these patients lead stably unstable lives, it is difficult to determine when they should be hospitalized. Criteria for hospitalization might include severe life crises, suicidal indications, homicidal indications, inordinate despair on the part of the patient, or lapse into psychosis. Many borderline patients do briefly lapse into psychosis, particularly dissociative types of psychoses. They usually reconstitute quickly.

Once in the hospital, there is tremendous danger that the patient will regress and that the stable instability of his life will become unstably unstable in terms of a reintegration into society.

For that reason, it is important to reach a diagnosis rapidly and to arrive at some tangible and limited goals for the hospitalization with the participation of the patient in such goal planning. It is extremely important to stabilize the patient — to show the patient the expectations the hospital unit has. Because of the defense of dyadic splitting, these patients tend to see hospital staff as good or bad. Because of the use of projective identification, which becomes a dyadic and shared defense mechanism, many of the staff tend to become involved in this bad dichotomy. Therefore, it is important to watch for this kind of staff splitting and to stabilize the staff in terms of expecting it and dealing with it.

Many of the problems which occur in the therapy of borderline patients can be attributed to the therapist and the therapist-patient interaction rather than to the patient's unique psychopathology. Borderline patients have a remarkable capacity for eliciting countertransference reactions of great intensity on the part of the staff. These can be extremely positive countertransference reactions or extremely negative ones, and they are highly mutable. Often the countertransference remains unexamined and is allowed to merge with the real relationship with the patient. Dealing with borderline patients is extremely stressful and it is easy to reach a therapeutic and empathic impasse. It is difficult to be empathic when one's instincts are urging fight or flight. It is useful to have a formal or informal supervisory or consultative alliance to keep a check on the defense mechanisms used by the therapist. An examination of such items as the staff member's positive or negative feelings to the patient can be very helpful.

In any event, it is essential that the professional realize his own great capacity for destructiveness in the therapeutic relationship with these patients. They have a great ability to encounter and accurately perceive unconsciously-sent messages; their perceptions are usually accurate and should be listened to openly.

One way to monitor the treatment of borderline patients is through carefully watching the countertransference. It is extremely easy to fulfill the patient's expectations and become a persecutor or a rescuer. Most of these patients, in fact, have many persecutors and rescuers; one more is not necessary. Instead, it is extremely important to be honest with the patient and to be empathic without rescuing. This empathy provides the patient with a good-enough-therapist. Interpretations should be nonjudgmental. There is often more of a need to answer the patient's questions than there is with other types of patients. The therapist must demonstrate nonverbally and sometimes even verbally that he or she will not be destroyed by the patient's hate or by the patient's love. I think that instead of being interpreted, high level defenses should be reinforced. Because borderline patients can change rapidly, the therapist needs to be both alert and flexible. Dangers in treatment include decompensation, acting out, and acting in. The use of neuroleptic agents with patients who have borderline personality disorders often results in depression. The use of tricyclic antidepressants, while there have been few controlled studies, seems to offer some promise of helping modify these patients' anger. If used, tricyclic antidepressants should probably be used in low doses.

Dealing with borderline patients, particularly in the hospital setting, is an extremely interesting, ofttimes frustrating experience. The best guide to dealing with such patients is to maintain one's honesty, flexibility, empathy and alertness.

REFERENCES

1. Prichard, J.C.: *A Treatise on Insanity and Other Disorders Affecting the Mind*, Philadelphia, Carey and Hart (1837).

2. Reich, W.: *The Impulsive Character and Other Writings*, New York, New American Library (1974).

3. Zilboorg, G.: Ambulatory schizophrenia, Psychiatry, *4:*149 (1941).

4. Hoch, Ph H., and Polatin, P.: Pseudoneurotic forms of schizophrenia, Psychiat Quart, *23:*248 (1949).

5. Schmideberg, M.: The borderline patient, In *American Handbook of Psychiatry*, Vol. 1, Arieti, S. (ed.), New York, Basic Books, p. 398 (1959).

6. Deutsch, H.: Some forms of emotional disturbance and their relationship to schizophrenia, Psychoanal, *11:*301 (1942).

7. Wells, L.A.: Family pathology and father-daughter incest: restricted psychopathy, J Clin Psychiat, *42:*197 (1981).

13 Adjustment Reactions

Lloyd A. Wells

For many years, people who are interested in the nomenclature of psychiatric syndromes and the whole field of nosology have struggled with the concept of adjustment reactions, situational reactions, and similar terms. They do not really imply serious psychopathology, and represent more than anything else a reaction which is sometimes an over-reaction to realistic, highly threatening stress.

At this point, a consideration of stress itself is necessary. Everyone is interested in stress because it affects all of us. There are many professionals who study stress, from both a clinical and experimental point of view. In evaluating what they write about stress, it is important to be aware that there are many methodologic difficulties in studying this phenomenon. It is relatively simple to design a controlled experiment which will give meaningful answers to questions in chemistry or physics, but it becomes extremely difficult when we attempt to do experiments on the behavior of human beings. All sorts of ethical issues, problems of experimental design, and government regulations intervene. Even if they did not, it is still impossible to control an experiment adequately when it involves the totality of a person's behavior and lifestyle. Nevertheless, a great deal of work is being done on this topic from its physiologic correlates to its purely psychological side.

I mention these methodologic difficulties in order to alert the reader to an unfortunate phenomenon, which is the proliferation of popular writing about stress. There are a vast number of paperback books which not only tell you what stress is, but teach you how to cope with it and with every imaginable variant of it in a totally successful manner. It only costs $2.00 to purchase one of these books and learn all about it. While some of them offer something, few of them offer very much, and many people are purchasing them in a vain hope to avoid living with stress. We cannot avoid it.

On the other hand, when one picks up actual scientific papers about stress, one can become even more confused. In one paper, I have counted as many as 11 different uses or misuses of the word *stress.* It is always possible to misuse the word in medicine and nursing and it happens very frequently. I am not sure that there is one good definition of stress, but it is certainly stressful in itself to know and experience many different uses of the same word.

Rather than going into a lot of semantics and jargon about what stress is, I am going to assume that the reader has a good idea about it. Either an external or an internal change is perceived as stress, which, therefore, has physiologic and psychologic concomitants. There is, then, a reaction to stress, which can be of several types. One could have a purely autoplastic reaction to stress. *Autoplastic* means that the reaction to the stress is entirely internalized — for example, anxiety, depression, or headache. Or, one could have an entirely alloplastic reaction to stress. This means that one's way of dealing with stress is in the outside environment. If the stress involves the head nurse belittling you, you could hit him or her. This would be alloplastic. Fortunately, this is not usually what most of you do. Perhaps the most frequent reaction to stress is a mixed one, which involves psychological reconstruction along with some action to modify the environment.

The causes of stress — so-called stressors — are also of three types. They can be entirely internalized, either physiologic or psychologic. It is stressful to feel ill. It is stressful to have low self-esteem or to contemplate some great action. Or, the stress can be exogenous. It is stressful to have to deal with difficult fellow workers. It is stressful to be in a bad marriage. It is stressful to be cited for some deficiency of one's work. Most stressors, too, are mixed and have both internal and external components.

These are some of the general types of reaction to stress. Generally, people avoid serious autoplastic or alloplastic responses by a variety of behavioral coping mechanisms. Purely autoplastic responses to stress are fairly rare but do occur. These may be subdivided into psychological and somatic types. Stress can precipitate depression. Of course, depression in the sense of unhappiness related to a real life situation occurs to all of us frequently. Some people, however, develop a much more severe syndrome in which they feel extremely depressed, helpless, hopeless, given-up, giving-up, with thoughts of worthlessness. Suicidal thinking almost always accompanies such a depression, although the person may not act on this thinking. In addition, there are other so-called vegetative signs of depression, which include disturbed sleep — either waking up too early in the morning, in the middle of the night, or not being able to get to sleep in the first place — decreased appetite with weight loss, or conversely, binge eating, diminished energy, concentration, and sometimes recent memory, and diurnal variation — the depressed person may feel worse in the morning than during the rest of the 24-hour period.

Although I am using depression to exemplify a totally psychological, autoplastic reaction to stress, I also use it to show how what starts out as an autoplastic reaction quickly becomes much more. The stress triggers the depression, but the depression then sustains itself through a series of positive feedback-type loops with not only the psychological components to it but also many physiological changes, including changes in the transmitters in the brain and some hormones. This, in turn, perpetuates the psychological changes, and the whole process becomes a very frustrating positive feedback loop. Thus, it goes from the psychological to the physical. In addition, it cannot remain totally autoplastic. The depressed person's behavior changes, and this in turn is perceived and acted on by the people around him.

One's reaction to stress can also be totally somatic, such as sudden diarrhea. The sudden somatic reaction to stress is often an unpleasant but not really pathological physical event, such as increased sweating, feelings of nausea, etc. Sometimes, again, the sudden physiologic response to stress becomes sustained into something more pathological. For example, the sudden increase in blood to the brain, which can be a concomitant of stress, may result in a vascular-type headache which might last for several hours. Of course, sometimes the physiologic response to stress is highly pathological. Sudden bad news can engender a myocardial infarction or a stroke in someone whose circulatory system is already seriously compromised. Again, this purely autoplastic response to stress does have alloplastic components, as you can imagine.

More often, people who have a somatic type of response to stress also have many habits which are related to their state of health. People who respond to stress primarily by noting physical sensations often repress a great many feelings and emotions, particularly angry ones. The well-known so-called Type A personality (1), which seems to be more disposed to heart disease than many other types of personaltiy, is the hard-driving, high-achieving person who pushes himself very hard and might have a certain amount of difficulty when his expectations of others are shown to be too high. At the same time, he may have trouble expressing that difficulty. People like this often tend to internalize anger. At the same time, partly because of their great investment in work, they often tend to ignore preventive medicine; they do not have routine physical examinations, they do not exercise regularly, they may smoke, they may drink a bit too much, they do not watch their diet very carefully, and so forth.

Thus, the person who is already somewhat vulnerable to heart disease, in this case, becomes more vulnerable because of an entire lifestyle. The lifestyle itself is not a result of or reaction to stress. Thus, the stressful event, the person's somatic reaction to it, and the person's lifestyle all interact, in a situation like this, to cause a potentially very harmful event — a heart attack.

In a situation like this, one can attempt to have the person get involved in an exercise program, give up smoking, drinking, eating things that he likes, which is often unsuccessful. Or, one can try to modify the person's personality structure, which is also often unsuccessful. This can be a frustrating situation for both the patient and the nurse. At the very least, a person who falls into this kind of category should see a physician every year or every two years to ascertain whether any serious physical changes are taking place.

Another major type of reaction to stress which fits into both autoplastic and alloplastic categories, and also has both psychological and physical components and sequelae, is to react to stress by substance abuse. The person who reacts to stress by misusing or abusing alcohol or some other drug is very likely to become alcoholic. The drug ends up controlling the person. One of the main defenses of the alcoholic person is to say that he is not alcoholic for some special reason — he does not drink in the morning, he does not pass out, etc. A better definition of alcoholism is that the person's life is adversely affected by his use of alcohol — whether medically, socially, in his marriage, in his work, etc. — and even after this has been pointed out to the person repeatedly, he continues to use alcohol (or the drug) rather than stop its use.

The alcoholic or drug-dependent person almost always is insightless about the nature of this stress reaction. The defense system of such a person becomes progressively impaired so that he honestly refutes the most striking and poignant evidence of his dependence. These people might insist that alcoholics are those who lie in the gutter or restrict their drinking to morning, or pass out daily. They insist on their own definition, and insist that upset family members are neurotic. One of the most important things for a fellow worker or family member of such a person to do is to confront that person openly and directly. Sympathizing or agreeing with his definitions will only reinforce his defense system, which is already one of the major obstacles towards seeking help. It can be very helpful, however, to confront such a person directly, often with other friends, family members, fellow workers, etc., and sometimes to give an ultimatum to the person — often this is the only way he will, however reluctantly, accept any treatment for his illness. Incidentally, the most effective organization ever convened for the treatment of a stress-related disorder is Alcoholics Anonymous, and often it can be tremendously helpful to put an alcoholic person in touch with this organization. Incidentally, about the worst thing one can do with an alcoholic or drug-abusing person is to believe or agree with his defense that the drinking or drug abuse is merely a symptom of some deep psychologic malaise; occasionally, or even often, this is the case, but nothing — psychologic problem, family disturbance, job unhappiness, etc. — can be dealt with until the person stops drinking or abusing drugs. The one exception is in the case of teenage drug abuse or drinking, which often represents a complex matrix of family problems and other individual psychopathology.

Along with physical and mixed types of responses to stress, as have been discussed, the next type of major response is a psychological one.

As mentioned above, a great deal of research is being done on stress, although people mean different things by it, and many of the experiments are more poorly designed than one would hope or expect. One of the most interesting areas of research is that which links the onset of illness with stress situations. Holmes, along with many co-workers, has done a great deal of work on this topic, and he has shown that illness often is a reaction to serious stress (2). Others have pointed out that when one is overwhelmed by a stressful situation, because the stimulus barrier has broken down, one ends up feeling helpless, out of control, and without hope. At such times, there is a good possibility that illness will occur, often of a serious physical nature. Some of the major stresses, as Holmes and Rahe have determined, are shown in Table I. Actually, many of these stresses and a high score on the stress scale often precede such important physical illnesses as heart attacks, strokes, and even cancers.

There have been many studies of the stresses associated with work but, unfortunately, most of these have involved transitional phases, such as leaving school and beginning work or leaving work and retiring. Many other studies focus on the stresses of losing a job. There have been few studies on the decision to change jobs. There have been many studies on stresses experienced on the job, but most of these have been of people in blatantly stressful work, such as air traffic control. It is quite obvious that our vocational identity in the professions is a central life activity and is an important part of our identity, our concept of ourselves as adult people. Acting that role as professionals takes up a large part of our time and energy and it is necessary, usually, so that we can have enough money to hold things together. But the work of a professional has a great deal of significance well beyond any kind of economic gain: it regulates our life activity, offers a social identification, lets us associate with other people, and makes an important life experience available to us. In spite of all of this, I think there is a tendency currently for people to value their work less, and I expect that this is part of a perhaps unfortunate cultural trend.

The question arises of how one can recognize stress. Certainly, most people can recognize a potentially stressful situation if it is environmental. They can anticipate stress. Frequently, if the response to stress is alloplastic, such as leaving work early, hitting the boss, and so forth, people can recognize that it is stress-induced. Sometimes, however, when the response is purely autoplastic, people are unable to realize the presence of stress. This occurs particularly often in situations of chronic stress — unhappiness with work, unhappiness in marriage or other important relationship, etc. Particularly if the coping device becomes one which is relatively insightless it is virtually impossible to recognize what is going on. In the case of totally insightless coping mechanisms, such as drinking or using drugs in order to escape from the stressful situation, it is most unlikely that recognition of the stress and the decision to do something about it will come from within us. Hopefully, spouses and colleagues will notice the change and will point it out to us, the person sometimes quite forcefully.

Of course, sometimes people do recognize autoplastic responses to stress as stress related. Often, the feeling of anxiety or feelings of hopelessness, depression, anger, and so forth follow stress, and are recognized as legitimate reactions to stress.

TABLE 1. *The Social Readjustment Rating Scale*[a]

Life event	Mean value
1. Death of spouse	100
2. Divorce	73
3. Marital separation from mate	65
4. Detention in jail or other institution	63
5. Death of a close family member	63
6. Major personal injury or illness	53
7. Marriage	50
8. Being fired at work	47
9. Marital reconciliation with mate	45
10. Retirement from work	45
11. Major change in the health or behavior of a family member	44
12. Pregnancy	40
13. Sexual difficulties	39
14. Gaining a new family member (e.g., through birth, adoption, oldster moving in, etc.)	39
15. Major business readjustment (e.g., merger, reorganization, bankruptcy, etc.)	39
16. Major change in financial state (e.g., a lot worse off or a lot better off than usual)	38
17. Death of a close friend	37
18. Changing to a different line of work	36
19. Major change in the number of arguments with spouse (e.g., either a lot more or a lot less than usual regarding childrearing, personal habits, etc.)	35
20. Taking on a mortgage greater than $10,000 (e.g., purchasing a home, business, etc.)	31
21. Foreclosure on a mortgage or loan	30
22. Major change in responsibilities at work (e.g., promotion, demotion, lateral transfer)	29
23. Son or daughter leaving home (e.g., marriage, attending college, etc.)	29
24. In-law troubles	29
25. Outstanding personal achievement	28
26. Wife beginning or ceasing work outside the home	26
27. Beginning or ceasing formal schooling	26
28. Major change in living conditions (e.g., building a new home, remodeling, deterioration of home or neighborhood)	25
29. Revision of personal habits (dress, manners, associations, etc.)	24
30. Troubles with the boss	23
31. Major change in working hours or conditions	20
32. Change in residence	20
33. Changing to a new school	20
34. Major change in usual type and/or amount of recreation	19
35. Major change in church activities (e.g., a lot more or a lot less than usual)	19
36. Major change in social activities (e.g., clubs, dancing, movies, visiting, etc.)	18
37. Taking on a mortgage or loan less than $10,000 (e.g., purchasing a car, TV, freezer, etc.)	17
38. Major change in sleeping habits (a lot more or a lot less sleep, or change in part of day when asleep)	16
39. Major change in number of family get-togethers (e.g., a lot more or a lot less than usual)	15
40. Major change in eating habits (a lot more or a lot less food intake, or very different meal hours or surroundings)	15
41. Vacation	13
42. Christmas	12
43. Minor violations of the law (e.g., traffic tickets, jaywalking, disturbing the peace, etc.)	11

Reprinted with permission from *J. Psychosom. Res., 11:*213, 1967.

Once stress is recognized, what can be done about it? If one realizes that he is under stress he then should seek to identify the cause of the stress. Sometimes, this is relatively easy, as when one is dealing with the death of a loved one, a major problem on the job, and so forth, but at other times it is relatively difficult to identify the cause of the stress. If it is possible to identify the cause, the person should then go on to examine the coping mechanisms he is using and whether they are in his own best interests or not. Again, one does not have to be a trained psychoanalyst to do this. I listed some common coping mechanisms, and the reader can undoubtedly think of many more. After examining the coping mechanisms and deciding whether they are adaptive or not, the person should move on to think about specific defenses he is using. Again, it is not necessary to be an analyst; it is necessary only to think about the psychological set the person is in, whether he might be using such fairly primitive mechanisms as projection, projective identification, splitting, and denial. He then needs to make a plan. After he has identified the stress, identified the cause, identified his coping mechanisms and identified his defenses, he needs to make a plan of action. This should entail, first of all, the question of whether the cause of the stress can be removed and whether it should be removed. By this I mean that sometimes people need to experience stress and sometimes the stress is actually protecting them from a far worse situation. Fools rush in where wise men fear to tread. One should always be careful in making major changes even when it seems obvious that the change should be made. People should always consider and try to anticipate the negative aspects of any major change before it is made. This is true even if the positive aspects far outweigh the negative aspects. Next, if the person decides that his coping mechanisms are adaptive, he should ask whether he should leave well enough alone or try to change them. If they are maladaptive, he should try to change them, either by conscious decision or by seeking help in psychotherapy. Again, if his defense mechanisms seem to be either crumbling or excessive for a period of more than a few days, it might be worthwhile to seek professional help, or at least an opinion. On the other hand, there is no need to feel that one is psychiatrically impaired just because of a long stressful reaction. If the reaction is excessive or prolonged, one should not feel ashamed of seeking some psychiatric help. Many people feel that the use of primitive defenses implies significant psychiatric problems. I do not believe this to be the case unless the use of those defenses is prolonged. We all revert to primitive defenses in times of stress, and we should not be unduly alarmed about the fact that we have done so.

Many people find it useful to have some specific techniques for dealing with the stresses of everyday life. Some find various exercise programs helpful; others find it useful to find a method of systematic relaxation. Still others are able to cope better if they devote a certain part of the day to a particular hobby. I think that one cannot make a generalization that any of these techniques is helpful to all people, nor is any of these techniques terribly useful at a time of overwhelming stress where the stimulus barrier is really broken down. While some of these devices may seem a bit gimmicky, they do work for some people. More important, in my view, is keeping channels open with important people in one's life. It is particularly important to be able to discuss some of these stresses with one's spouse, for example. If one has to be defensive with one's spouse about the stresses of life, one merely adds an additional stress. It is tremendously important to be able to speak openly and nondefensively about one' real perception of the world, one's real perception of other people, to one person who in turn shares his or her own view of the world. This is what a close relationship with another person is all about, and it seems to me to be a tremendously useful safety valve for everyone. I am not talking about doing psychotherapy with one's spouse, but about sharing one's real perception of stressful and unhappy encounters and situations. It is not necessary in a situation like this for the spouse or significant other person to feel the need to rescue the person or to be uncritically supportive. Usually, when people are under a great deal of stress, more support or the attempt to rescue does not help very much. But one can be helpful by just listening and reacting honestly.

Some specific syndromes associated with adjustment disorder include marital dysfunction, various types of grief reactions, transition syndromes, and pseudopersonality disorders.

While "pseudopersonality disorders" do not constitute any recognized diagnostic term, it is certainly true that many people with certain somewhat maladaptive defense mechanisms which still do not cause major problems to that person, can have these defenses exaggerated at times of significant stress and this exaggeration of the defenses can seem, for a brief period, to produce behavior which seems similar to that seen in patients with personality disorders. Thus, one can never assume a patient has a personality disorder based on a brief exposure to that patient. Chronicity is necessary before making the diagnosis. Usually, in an acute adjustment disorder which precipitates a pseudopersonality disorder, the maladaptive behavior will diminish as the stress recedes.

So-called transition syndromes can also result in and impact adjustment disorders. Often, these transition syndromes occur at times of major separation and major change. When one leaves home for the first time on an extended basis, when one marries, the appearance of a divorce, the birth or departure of children from home — all of these can cause transitory major problems in living for all concerned. Without question, the major transition syndrome with which we all have to deal is that caused by death.

The role of the nurse in dealing with the dying patient and the dying patient's family is detailed in another chapter. The psychiatric nurse, however, should also be aware of the effects that grief and loss can have over a period of years. Two types of situations are particularly important. One of these is the pathologic grief reaction and the other the anniversary phenomenon.

The usual resolution of the grief process occurs, depending on the circumstances, over the period of a couple of years. In some people, however, mourning is somehow blocked, and the patient remains deeply troubled — though often at an unconscious level — by grief for many years. Often, the person who experiences a pathologic grief reaction is the person in the family who has somehow been stoic during the death and burial ceremonies of the loved object. The usual decathexis from the loved object begins with the whole process of dying and certainly is accelerated by the funeral. Some people, however, deny the death or do not allow their emotions to come in contact with the reality of death. In these people, though they acknowledge intellectually that the loved object is dead, he or she continues to be a major part of their thinking, their dreams, and really their life. Such people often think momentarily that they see the loved person in a crowd. They may forget for a second or two that the loved person is dead and go to telephone them even years after the death. Frequently, patients with pathologic grief reactions present to the medical profession with physical complaints or indeed psychiatric complaints which somehow link them to the lost object. For example, if the lost object died of G.I. disease the patient might present with vague symptoms of G.I. disease. It is very important to reiterate that such presentations are entirely on an unconscious basis and that the patient is not malingering.

Once a pathologic grief reaction has been recognized, it is relatively easy to deal with it. In fact, usually brief dynamically oriented, focused psychotherapy can be very helpful in dealing with pathologic grief over a few sessions. It is often necessary to abreact the actual death of the loved one and to deal with feelings of loss and feelings of rage. While one cannot generalize about pathologic grief reactions, it is frequently true that the person with the pathologic grief reaction and the dead person had an extremely convoluted, ambivalent relationship, which the patient tries to deny.

The anniversary phenomenon is often related to pathologic grief but need not be. In this phenomenon patients become depressed or physically ill around the time of major anniversaries of deaths. Often, they unconsciously assume the identity of the dead person. Rather good research has indicated an uncanny frequency of myocardial infarctions on anniversaries of the myocardial infarctions or deaths of significant others. While the anniversary phenomenon is not necessarily a treatable phenomenon nor is it a manifestation of psychopathology, it is still of interest to find out whether important illnesses of a psychiatric or physical nature occurred on anniversaries to give some insight about the person, to explore for the possibility of pathologic grief reaction and to alert one's self for future anniversary reactions.

REFERENCES

1. Friedman, M.: Type A behavior pattern: some of its pathophysiological components, Bull NY Acad Sci, *53:*593 (1977).

2. Holmes, T.H., and Rahe, R.H.: The social readjustment rating scale, J Psychosom Res, *11:*213 (1967).

14 Chemical Dependency

Raymond Island and Mary Jane Island

The general attitude toward alcohol can probably be best described with an anecdote about a small town politician. When asked what he thought about alcohol, he replied: "When you take the beverage that literally kills thousands, takes food from the family, makes a 'lush' out of an otherwise good mother — I'm against it. But, if you mean the beverage that builds schools and hospitals through the taxes it brings in and creates a more relaxed social gathering — I'm for it!"

When dealing with alcoholism, it is important first to define it. We believe the simplest definition is: When alcohol is causing a problem in any area of a person's life, whether family, marital, professional, legal or medical, and in spite of these problems, he continues to use alcohol, this is alcoholism. Alcoholism is an insightless disease and, most often, the alcoholic is the last person to recognize the problem alcohol is causing in his/her life.

Let us first look at the pattern of the alcoholic's drinking. There is a definite progression in alcoholism. Alcoholism usually begins insidiously, and builds gradually, with increasing dependence on alcohol: the perceived *need* to drink, increased tolerance, a relative inability to stop drinking once underway, and eventually a plethora of alcohol-related problems.

It is important to note that not all alcoholics will suffer all the symptoms listed in the chart. They also may not experience them in the order listed. In the final analysis, the most tell-tale sign of alcoholism is how the alcohol is affecting their lives.

The following are some of the most common symptoms.

Preoccupation: The alcoholic is often preoccupied with the next drink when he should be thinking or talking about other, important things. As the alcoholism progresses, preoccupation becomes more and more frequent.

Increased tolerance: As the drinking continues, the alcoholic needs to drink more to get the desired effect. This is the sign that tolerance is increasing. The alcoholic can drink more than others, yet functions where others would show signs of intoxication drinking the same amount.

Blackouts: This is being unable to remember what he has said or done the previous day or night while drinking. They can range from brief periods, with the person being unable to remember things he said, to a more extended time, with the person perhaps being unable to remember how he got home or where he left his car. During the blackout, the alcoholic is able to function quite well and others are unaware he is in a blackout.

Gulps drinks: Does this to get the quick effect of the alcohol, much as the drug dependent person would "shoot" the drug to get high faster.

Drinks alone: This is not social drinking — this is drinking strictly for the effect of the drug, alcohol.

Uses as a medicine: Again, this is using alcohol for the drug that it is, to sleep or to relieve anxiety, tension or stress. This is abnormal drinking.

Loss of control: This is one of the most obvious symptoms of alcoholism and occurs when the drinker, at times, drinks more than he has planned to or wants to. In the early stages of alcoholism, this may only happen occasionally. As the alcoholism progresses, it occurs more frequently.

Protecting supply: The person always makes sure he has enough alcohol on hand. Many times he keeps a bottle hidden in the basement, in the car or in the office to have it available when he "needs" it.

Morning drinking: This usually happens in the chronic stage of alcoholism. It occurs when the alcoholic "needs" to drink just to feel normal and to be able to function.

Decrease in tolerance: This too happens in the chronic stage. Now the alcoholic is unable to drink as much as he was once able to, and sometimes it takes very little before he is showing signs of intoxication.

Defenses

It is very common for the alcoholic to insist that if the problems or stresses in his life would cease, he would be able to "cut down" on his drinking and then he would not have a drinking problem. The alcoholic unconsciously becomes quite defensive about his drinking. Because alcoholism is an insightless disease, he is usually unaware of the defenses he is using. The following are some of the most frequently used defenses.

Denial: Probably the most common defense used by the alcoholic. He denies that alcohol is causing him problems.

Rationalization: Using excuses and alibies for the drinking.

Protection: Blaming others for the problems in his life and saying they are the "reason" that he drinks.

Hostility: Becoming angry whenever his drinking is discussed — a good defense to keep people away from the subject of his drinking.

Confrontation or Intervention

Because alcoholism is such an insightless disease, many times the only way to break through the alcoholic's defenses is through confrontation. The purpose of confrontation is to enable the alcoholic to look at how his/her drinking is affecting his life and the lives of those around him.

Those who should be involved with the confrontation are persons who have been affected by the alcoholic's actions and are important to the alcoholic. Most often these are family, friends and sometimes, employers. Confrontation of the alcoholic should always be done in a loving and caring manner. The alcoholic should be told how his drinking is changing him and how this is affecting his relationships. He should be told specific times and instances that his drinking has caused problems, not just provided with a statement such as "You drink too much." It is helpful if those doing the confronting write down ahead of time specific instances related to the drinking. Confrontation should never be a time of blaming, but rather a time of discussing honestly what alcohol is doing to the person and his relationships with others.

The purpose of the confrontation is, of course, to help the alcoholic see what alcohol is doing to his/her life and that he needs to stop drinking. Typically if he does realize the need to stop, he tries to convince everyone, including himself, that he can do this on his own — that he doesn't need any help. The important think is to get some kind of commitment from the alcoholic. If he insists that he can do it by himself, then it is vital to add in a "what if" clause — to get him to agree to treatment if he is unable to stay sober on his own. In other words, no drinking — no treatment; drinking means he agrees to accept help or treatment. Treatment can be inpatient, outpatient, individual therapy or Alcoholics

Anonymous (A.A.). Over the years, it has been shown that the most effective long-term treatment for most alcoholics is A.A. However, some people need professional help in an inpatient or outpatient treatment center before they are ready to accept the A.A. program.

The economy of A.A., as we see it, is people coming together in weakness and admitting they need the help of others; in their weakness they find strength. Strong people refuse to accept help from others and, as a result, they crumble. When weak people lean on each other, they become strong together — this is A.A.

When entering any A.A. club room, the sign "By the grace of God" stands out, and we both believe that by the grace of God and the forgiveness of the past, we can have a good today and a bright tomorrow.

PART 3

INTERVENTIONS

15 Relationships with Patients

Denise M. Wells

In the nursing literature, the works of Hildegard Peplau and Gertrude Ujhely form a useful foundation for the extensive superstructure of literature on relationships. In the work of Peplau and Ujhely, the professional relationship is basically divided into three phases: orientation, working phase, and termination (1, 2). Both authors have discussed characteristics of each phase and stress the importance of developing a trusting and non-judgmental relationship with the patient. For further discussion of this basis of nursing relationship theory, verbal and non-verbal communication and techniques, the nurse should read the works of Peplau and Ujhely.

Nursing literature seldom discusses the nurse-patient relationship in perspective — that is, how does the nurse function therapeutically within the scope of a therapeutic team? Should the relationship have more importance or depth than any other relationship the patient has? And what exactly does it mean to have a "contract" with the patient?

Seldom do nursing students work actively in a truly integrated role within the psychiatric team. Much of their observation is discussed predominantly with their clinical instructor or staff liaison and, unfortunately, little time is actually spent with the psychiatrist or other active members of the treatment team. Team meetings are frequently generalized or tend to focus on significant material, sometimes failing to give the student an inclusive picture of the patient. Likewise, the clinical instructor may focus on various aspects of a disease entity to illustrate the specifics of psychopathology. Consequently, many graduate nurses lack a good understanding of what a nurse-patient relationship should entail and how it fits within the spectrum of the psychiatric team.

Much of the nursing literature cites the importance of the nurse facilitating a "corrective emotional experience." This catchy phrase was introduced by Franz Alexander (3), a psychoanalyst and theoretician who discussed how psychotherapy sometimes heals. He talked of the fact that some patients could have a "corrective emotional experience" and improve without necessarily working through the transference neurosis. The nursing literature seems not to use this phrase in the same way that Alexander intended. The nurse cannot consciously manufacture a "corrective emotional experience" although many nurses seem to feel that this is part of their role. A corrective emotional experience may be something entirely unintended and indeed it may have very little to do with the therapy itself. Furthermore, it presumably cures largely because of its unconscious relevance to the patient. Thus, it is not something that can be artificially structured or manufactured by the nurse. This is especially so since most nurses who attempt to manufacture a "corrective emotional experience" are catering to the conscious perception of his needs that the patient may have rather than his unacknowledged and unconscious needs which are far more real and pressing.

Many psychiatric nurses illustrate their role and view it as one of being an insight oriented psychotherapist or a facilitator of reality orientation. With appropriate jargon and lingo, they define, identify and subdivide these roles. Often the verbiage masks unconscious and unacknowledged needs of the nurse. Psychiatric nurses, perhaps more than most nurses, experience notable highs and lows in their professional, patient-oriented life. The roller coaster highs and lows become evident as the nurse finds patients with the willingness or the need to meet the nurse's own needs of curiosity, dependence or intellectualization; however, in time, the low sets in as the patient becomes resistant to change or becomes hostile and frequently illustrates a covert unwillingness to help himself get well. This affects the nurse most often when the nurse has an unconscious need to heal the patient because of the nurse's own need for dependence or omnipotence. Our own vulneratilities encourage our interest as psychiatric nurses. We often possess insufficient insight into our own needs and the ways we manipulate variables in the environment to meet those needs. Thus, the young adolescent who experiences her first psychotic break may bring out the maternal nurturing aspect of the psychiatric nurse who identifies with the patient's alienation and loneliness. Such a nurse ends up temporarily, at least, being a better mother — but is the nurse being a better mother to the child or to the child within herself?

After such an encounter with a patient, the nurse may rest assured that the appropriate approaches have been identified and that significant awareness of feelings has been encountered. These specific treatment modalities and specific components of the nursing care plan, however, are sometimes oversimplified, and they can even cause us to lose sight of the totality of each individual, who is certainly much more than the mere sum of his mechanistic parts. Our obsession with the detailed can preclude our understanding and empathy and can thereby protect us by distancing us from the patient. To truly understand an individual, one must walk in his footsteps (though not in his shoes), and one must experience his sense of hurt or loss.

Given these general *caveats*, how can the nurse-patient relationship evolve to be therapeutic?

Initially the psychiatric nurse should glean essential information about the patient from the history. A discussion with the patient's psychiatrist will set the framework of realistic expectations on the part of the nurse. The psychiatrist may identify his focus in psychotherapy and encourage the psychiatric nurse to offer the patient support and understanding; he or she may also make other requests of the nurse. Such an individualized approach involving the primary physician and the patient cannot help but be an improvement over plugging the patient into a "program" which is not designed to meet his specific needs. For instance, the psychiatrist might wish to focus on an adolescent's acceptance of rejection by his family and might encourage the nurse to allow the patient to express his anger. Frequently, what happens is that the nurse is unaware of the content of psychotherapy sessions and becomes frustrated and overwhelmed by the patient's anger. Soon, although the nurse may overtly encourage the patient to express anger, he or she is also setting unrealistic covert limits on the patient to curb his anger and to express it only "appropriately." If the adolescent is unable to deal with his anger in the hospital in a therapeutic setting, where will he come to terms with his rejection?

At other times, the nurse may focus on a patient's anxiety and help the patient to look at coping mechanisms. In some cases, structuring an anxious patient may enable the patient to deal more effectively with continuing insight oriented psychotherapy.

The major theme of which one should be aware in developing a nurse–patient relationship is the ability to correlate the nursing focus or direction with that of the remainder of the therapeutic team. This role does not belittle the psychiatric nurse's abilities but rather challenges the psychiatric nurse to allow the patient the opportunity to use the relationship to work through his feelings, knowing that a nurse-patient relationship affords him a relationship of unconditional acceptance. Is it not far more helpful and professional to accept a realistic role as part of the treatment team doing specifics for the patient which may not be grandiose but which may be far more effective than enacting a nursing fantasy of omnipotent, excellent and indeed perfect care for the patient? Unconditional acceptance or unconditional positive regard does not imply, as many nurses think it does, the approval of all of the patient's maladaptive behavior. It means merely that the nurse is willing to accept the patient in an empathetic way as a real human being in spite of whatever maladaptive behaviors there may be. The nurse does not need to approve the behavior to care about the patient.

This does not preclude the psychiatric nurse from being attentive to the patient's resistance in the form of anger with his therapist and manipulation of the nurse-patient relationship in ploys — which may or may not be conscious — to divide and conquer the staff. Acceptance of the patient's anger, however — *without* a covert cooperation with the patient's ploys — will facilitate his psychotherapy and allow him the chance to develop better adult interpersonal relationships.

Accordingly, nurses may use the nurse-patient relationship to facilitate better observation of parataxic distortions which may provide behavioral data about the nature of the transference relationship with the psychotherapist. Every bit of information in this area can facilitate a better awareness of this person's psychodynamics and the way they fit into a particular disease entity.

Does the patient seek out the nurse as a mother or father figure, someone he can test for approval? Is it difficult for the patient to relate in a woman-woman, woman-man or man-man relationship? Is the patient exhibiting exorbitant demands or is the patient testing to see what happens when the nurse gets angry with him? The direction of a great many nurses is to plot out some chart directing them to use the same specific approaches for all patients with a particular disease entity: for example, verbalize anger, encourage better self-esteem, etc. — and yet there is often no realization that other messages are nonverbally communicated to the patient.

It is essential for the nurse to work closely with other members of the treatment team to coordinate treatment efforts and modalities. If such coordination does not occur, the themes of nurse-patient relationship, doctor-patient relationship, other professional-patient relationship may all be similar, and yet the covert agendas inherent in those relationships may be worlds apart. The nurse may be subtly and unconsciously competitive to gain information from the patient that is unknown to the other professionals. He or she may also seek control by subtly and again unconsciously fostering acting out or regressive behavior. It is difficult for any professional to be in a setting where his needs are not met. If the patient does not meet the needs of the nurse, the nurse should trust his or her colleagues for praise, respect and acceptance. And yet, if one cannot offer a completely cured patient as an end result, what does the nurse accomplish professionally? If the psychiatric nurse can illustrate his or her competencies by contrasting the progress the patient has made with him or her, or the patient's acceptance of her or her, *versus* the progress the patient has made with the psychiatrist, or the patient's acceptance of other members of the treatment team — perhaps then she will be recognized. Of course, it is rare for this fantasy to be completely conscious but it is present in a great many nurses and other professionals. It can be extremely destructive.

The best analogy to the patient-nurse relationship is perhaps found in the family constellation and the role of a traditional mother. The best nurturing role would be one in unison with a paternal role making use of the expanded contact to better understand the individual with unconditional acceptance. Only in this sense will the healthy individual later mature to be capable of separation and individuation from the staff. However, as is frequently the case, different variables come into play in this triangle. We professionals — as do parents — get caught up in rescue fantasies, ploys to divide and conquer, covert fostering of the patient's dependence or regression, or simple meeting of our own egotistical needs — and all this within the guise of a helping relationship!

Little confrontation from fellow nurses will occur if one keeps the focus on the incompetent psychiatrist or social worker or other member of the treatment team. And yet, insecurity prevails within nursing ranks as more concrete guarantees are demanded for identifying and solidifying relationships. For example, for some nurses the initiation of a relationship with a formal contract identifying the nurse's commitment and availability and the patient's obligations in return, seems to supersede any ethical, professional need to share critical information obtained from the patient with other members of the treatment team. The contract can actually serve to prevent the nurse from functioning as a member of the treatment team. The contract as such seems an unnecessary legalism in helping psychiatrically ill patients. Do we sue them if they do not live up to their side of the bargain? The game of pseudoconfidentiality engendered by contracts with patients puts the nurse in the precarious situation of agreeing sometimes to keep information from other members of the treatment team despite the fact that the nurse may not have the necessary theory or experience to evaluate the patient's condition.

One may not qualify all psychiatric nurses on the same continuum. Many who have worked closely with other professionals over the years have assimilated a sound theoretical basis and have had extensive supervised psychotherapeutic encounters. Many are excellent group psychotherapists as well as individual psychotherapists. In many cases, insititutional credentialing would facilitate upward mobility of competent nurses to act as primary psychotherapists and in other highly individualized roles; however, nursing is becoming more concerned wiht its own evolution and frequently overlooks other professionals who have something substantive to offer. Today's training programs for the most part leave wide gaps of ignorance and entitlement. One must sometimes question the audacity of the nurse's intricate involvement in the web of another's life in so important a role with so little real training. Whose needs are being met?

A discussion of nurse-patient relationships would be incomplete without a discussion of recent developments. Theoretical bases have been expanded to include psychosocial transactional systems, kinesics, general systems theory, and other related disciplines. Such a framework provides great breadth. Often, however, the integration of all these different disciplines in the training of an individual nurse tends to be extremely superficial. An analogous situation seems to be the case of many modern mothers who studiously prepare for raising children; and yet, in an abandonment of maternal instincts and a desperate grasp for "the right way" and the "expert way" to bring up a child, such mothers unconsciously structure a superficial relationship based primarily on projective identification with their child. Have psychiatric nurses become so well defended that the actual explicit and implicit communications from the patient have been lost or misinterpreted *vis-a-vis* a theoretical framework which does not lend itself to actual caring and empathy? An increasing intellectual framework for the discipline of nursing relationships can never be allowed to mask the emergence and use of the nurse's "third ear" and her real ability to care for patients in a professional but truly empathic way rather than as a mere job or as a means of meeting his or her own dependency needs.

As nursing develops more of a theoretical framework and as the nursing literature becomes increasingly complex, there are an increasing number of papers delineating appropriate approaches in the treatment of various illnesses and syndromes, discussing the withdrawn, the manipulative, or the hostile patient, for example. Infrequently does the literature delve into the more complex messages that psychiatric nurses convey to patients. In discussing this more abstract reality, we must begin to focus on the verbal and nonverbal messages that nurses communicate. Frequently, the nurse's scope becomes so narrowed that he or she tends to refuse to acknowledge dependency or narcissistic needs, viewing them as inappropriate in some dependent patients primarily because of his or her own difficulty with similar needs. Nurses can fail to comprehend that we all must be dependent to some degree, or the mere reality of any relationship would be non-existent. Yet, I have frequently seen professional nurses communicate hostile messages to patients and their families whose dependencies overwhelmed them. This is not to say that a patient's dependency should be fostered, but rather that a degree of dependence is a basic need for us all.

Many professional nurses have areas of conflict when dealing with some adolescents. It is very difficult to retain one's perspective or even one's self-esteem in a situation where one's control is constantly being tested; however, for the nurse to use a strictly authoritarian role to emphasize who is adult and who is child is mere role playing.

The principal thrust should be one of ascertaining the type of milieu we as professionals provide for the patients we try to help. Do we use our patients in a type of projective identification hoping to increase our own self-esteem? Are we able to work with other professionals to provide a healthy environment without our own covert agendas being played out using the patients as pawns?

Hypothetically, one could draw analogies in asking how different are the psychodynamics that psychopathological families illustrate from the dynamics of the psychiatric team and its milieu. The focus for many nurses in the future will be not to try to secure a job description for which we are not qualified, but rather truly to help patients we treat and to provide and sustain a therapeutic atmosphere in the units themselves. How nurturing is our role? Our constancy, predictability, time commitment and unconditional positive acceptance in a milieu which we structure sets us off from other professionals and provide a highly therapeutic experience to patients if those qualities are conveyed without hidden agendas or strings attached. So often, though, the tone, attitude and covert messages of nurses nonverbally communicated contradict the overt messages. When the patient exhibits inconsistent improvement, particularly in his behavior, do we accept the complexity of the dynamics for this behavior or are we intolerant and unaccepting because the patient has not met our expectations? How different is the nurse in this situation from the disapproving, rejecting parent? Although much of the nursing literature steers clear of discussions of transference and countertransference roles, it is apparent that these dynamics are very prevalent in any ward milieu.

Nurses have always been uncomfortable in discussing that nurturing role. One immediately associates nurturing with mothering and thereby with infantilizing. Nevertheless, nurturing may be defined as providing an emotional environment of nonjudgmental acceptance with consistent focus on meeting the other person's needs and helping the other person to meet his own needs. As society becomes increasingly narcissistic and evolves to a point where families provide less and less in the way of physical nurturance, how many patients will be in need of nonjudgmental acceptance of nurturing and being nurtured?

Acceptance and implementation of a discrete, limited, but unique role for the nurse in the hospital setting, particularly involving nurse–patient relationships, can provide better care for patients and far more professional gratification for nurses than the trend toward role playing other professional disciplines.

REFERENCES

1. Sills, G.M.: Hildegard Peplau: Leader, practitioner, academician, scholar and theorist, Perspectives in Psychiat Care, *16:*122 (1978).

2. Ujhely, G.: *Determinants of the Nurse-Patient Relationship*, New York, Springer, (1968).

3. Alexander, F., and Ross, H.: *Dynamic Psychiatry*, Chicago, University of Chicago Press (1952).

16 Psychotherapy

Lloyd A. Wells

Psychotherapy imposes great demands on the patient and the therapist. Every kind of psychotherapy has a body of knowledge which can be taught but also an art and technique which depends in great measure on personal qualities of the therapist and indeed of the patient. The therapist who models the art of therapy on another therapist often minimizes his own therapeutic impact because that particular art may not be useful for someone of his own personality and gifts.

In this chapter, we shall examine some different types of psychotherapy which can be used by trained psychiatric nurses and which should be understood by all psychiatric nurses. We shall then describe a bit about the therapeutic process which impacts on all therapies, all therapists and all patients engaged in therapy.

There are clearly many types of individual psychotherapy, some of which will be described in this book. Some of the major types include behavioral treatment, client centered psychotherapy, so-called counseling, supportive psychotherapy and the various insight-oriented psychotherapies which can also be subdivided into short-term dynamic psychotherapies and long-term dynamic psychotherapies.

Behavioral therapies are different in many ways from the more dynamically oriented therapies. Some of these differences will be detailed in the chapter on behavioral treatment. It should be remembered, however, that even in this highly structured type of therapy, not based on a developmental or psychodynamic model, there remains a relationship between a therapist and a patient. The effects of this relationship itself on clinical change must be kept in mind at all times.

Counseling is frequently within the purview of the psychiatric nurse, particularly in an outpatient setting. Many patients come to a health professional not because of any serious psychiatric disorder but because of social breakdown. Often, the nurse can be extremely helpful by detailing available resources. Similarly, he or she can provide didactic types of information regarding child rearing, sexuality, meeting psychosocial needs of the elderly parent, etc.

Supportive psychotherapy is an extremely complex area. Many professionals feel that insight-oriented psychotherapy is far more important than supportive psychotherapy, but in fact many patients are able to reconstitute and to manage quite well in spite of mildly maladaptive coping mechanisms if they are provided with a bit of support. It is important to make sure that the support does not become rescuing, however.

Insight-oriented psychotherapy or psychodynamically based psychotherapy is increasingly being used by some well trained nurses. This chapter is not sufficient to train anyone to be a dynamic psychotherapist but is an attempt to describe the use of insight oriented psychotherapy and some of its pitfalls and problems.

One of the goals of insight-oriented psychotherapy is to increase the patient's capacity to make conscious choices which are not determined by previous psychopathology. Many patients who have personality disorders, neuroses and adjustment disorders and many depressed patients tend to see their options as extremely limited and often see their choices as being forced between two bad or impossible options. One goal of insight oriented therapy then is to increase the patient's capacity to see options — more than two — and then to choose freely.

Through the use of dream interpretation, free association and some other projective techniques the therapist is enabled to gain some insight into unconscious processes and conflicts of the patient. For the most part, the therapist does not give answers but reflects data back to the patient consistently asking the patient to provide more interpretation and more background. This type of psychotherapy usually is not focused on one specific problem but on the patient's emotional reactions from earliest childhood on, problems in his relationships with parents, peers and spouse, and transference phenomenon. While transference is usually considered to be the distorted view of the therapist by the patient, an extension of this concept which is very useful is that most patients with personality disorders and neuroses react to all the major figures in their life as if they were the early mother or father. This is often very disguised in its form but it is present. Its interpretation to the patient and the patient's working through of the transference situation can be the major factor leading to an increase in the capacity to make free choices.

Not every patient is a good candidate for dynamic psychotherapy. Many patients should be excluded in the groups of severe affective disorder, psychosis and severe alloplastic personality disorders. Similarly, some poeple who are extremely obsessive but who are not particularly emotionally impaired often wish to begin therapy as a sort of hobby. Such a patient can be difficult and often rejects whatever the therapist attempts to offer. Therapy with such a patient can be satisfactory in terms of outcome but is often very difficult and frustrating for both patient and therapist. In selecting a patient, some attention should also be paid to the emotional reaction of the therapist to the patient. If the therapist has an instant dislike for the patient, this usually indicates a major countertransference problem on the part of the therapist. The natural reaction of many such therapists is to accept the patient and to begin treatment with a feeling of guilt and lack of control. Obviously, in spite of the fact that it is the therapist's countertransference rather than the patient's personality which provides the negative reaction, working with a patient for whom one has no regard can be extremely self-defeating and can be very destructive to the patient. Question should be extended, however, in the case of a patient to whom one has immediately an immensely and unreasonably positive reaction. This again is countertransference and will get in the way of successful treatment.

Before accepting a patient for insight-oriented psychotherapy, the therapist should also concern himself with other possible contraindications. Is the patient intelligent enough to understand? Does the patient have the potential for severe acting out? Does he show the potential for psychotic decompensation? How much potential is there for severe regression?

The initial interview is often most important in evaluating the potential of the patient for psychotherapy. The actual content of that first interview becomes less important, of course, as therapy progresses but the old view held by many analysts that history taking *per se* was contraindicated for psychoanalytic patients is certainly fallacious. The interview data from that first interview is extremely important because it often hints at the whole process the therapy will undergo if it is undertaken. It hints at the tone of the therapy and the style of the therapy. In that first interview, the therapist and the patient should come to some agreement about the patient's problems as they present, the therapist should attempt to reach a working diagnosis and should attempt to establish a certain amount of rapport between himself and the patient. It is important in this first interview to develop an idea about the patient's motivation and the patient's therapeutic potential. After the first interview, or occasionally after two or three interviews, the therapist should be able to propose a formulation of the patient's case. The formulation at this stage of evaluation and treatment can never be as precise and detailed as one would like. Rather, it is a proposed rough sketch of the patient's psychopathology as well as a rough prediction of the proposed therapeutic undertaking.

The formulation should include the patient's primary symptoms and problems, hypotheses about the relationship of those primary symptoms and problems to important events in the patient's intrapsychic and interpersonal life, an assessment of the patient's motivation, liabilities and assets, a view of the patient's types of human relationships, a consideration of possible contraindications to psychotherapy and an understanding and admission of the therapists's initial reaction to the patient. Once interview data have been gathered and the formulation has been made, and once a decision has been made to embark on psychotherapy, it is necessary to discuss the goals of therapy with the patient and to say something about the process. All too often, a neophyte therapist offers therapy to a patient who eagerly accepts. The ground rules for the therapy are never adequately discussed and when common vicissitudes of therapy occur the patient becomes quite frightened and thinks that his case is extremely unusual and often hopeless. It is extremely helpful to any patient embarking on psychotherapy to be told about common problems in early therapy. The patient should be told it is often hard to speak freely and to free-associate, that there will be times when nothing comes to mind, that there will be other times when the patient has a great many thoughts and feelings but feels that it would be wrong or shameful to discuss them. The patient should also be told that there will be times when he tends to exaggerate or censor his thoughts and feelings in order to please the therapist or make the therapist angry. The patient should be told that these events occur frequently, commonly, and are to be expected.

One of the therapist's first goals in early psychotherapy should be the establishment of rapport with the patient. Rapport does not mean rescuing. It seems to me it is a twofold process requiring the need to be real and what has been termed unconditional positive acceptance. The need to be real does not imply sharing all one's reactions to the patient with the patient or sharing all one's own psychopathology and social pathology with the patient. Rather, it means that one should never lie to the patient and that one should allow oneself to acknowledge his own feelings in reacting to the patient. Unconditional positive acceptance similarly does not mean condoning whatever acting out or other alloplastic techniques the patient may be employing. Rather, it is acceptance of the observing ego of the patient, the part of the patient which wishes to get well, and caring for the entire patient.

Early in psychotherapy, in addition to educating the patient, it is important to ask questions in order to get a history. These questions should preferably be open ended because closed questions tend to control the patient. Especially in an insight type of psychotherapy in which the therapist hopes for free association on the part of the patient, it is silly to ask a whole barrage of questions with yes or no answers because they tend to set the tone for future therapy. Another helpful technique is the use of comments by the therapist which can encourage the patient to speak further but do not control him or require him to speak further. Such statements as "I guess I'm thinking that you might be . . ." can allow the patient to expand an answer. One should always avoid so-called school teacher questions which are questions to which the therapist thinks he knows the answer. Frequent use of such questions can tend to browbeat the patient. Similarly, questions whose answer would apparently and obviously be too threatening for the patient to reveal should be avoided in early therapy. Verbal and nonverbal cues from the therapist are extremely important. Verbal cues such as the use of "umph-humph" can encourage the patient to go on. Nonverbal cues such as nodding, apparent interest on the part of the therapist and apparent disinterest, boredom or napping obviously have effects on the patient. Note taking must be left to the prerogative of the individual therapist and possibly his supervisor but can often be used as a counter-resistance by the therapist and a means of isolating himself from the patient. It can be helpful instead of taking notes to train oneself to report the entire hour in detail immediately following the hour either by dictating or writing.

Early in the psychotherapy of almost any patient with a personality disorder or neurosis, evidence of a harsh superego — at least in some areas — will be apparent. It can frequently be helpful to interpret the harshness of the superego to the patient at this time. This can help the patient and therapist ally themselves early against "it" — a part of the patient which is causing him distress — and can greatly promote the therapeutic alliance and transference. In many cases the therapist's more moderate superego can become a goal for the patient. The patient is also often comforted by the realization that the therapist judges him less harshly than his own superego does.

Early in psychotherapy, too, issues of dependence will become very important. The patient will wish to contact the therapist, will wish for his advice, etc. A transference cannot occur meanfully unless the patient's dependency needs are met to some extent. It should be manifestly clear to the patient that he is allowed to talk about dependency needs and in emergent situations to become dependent on the therapist. Therapists who actively remove themselves from dependence never become involved in a truly psychotherapeutic relationship with the patient.

Whatever their intellectual insight about therapy might be, most patients at some level come to therapy hoping for love. When instead of love they get insight, they become frustrated. The therapist must always be attuned to the ways in which the patient is asking for love. Although the therapist cannot provide the kind of close maternal holding love or the kind of oedipal love that many patients desire, the therapist can provide a mature sort of caring. This must be made abundantly clear to the patient. The patient's need for love and caring from the therapist should be discussed with the patient.

Early in the psychotherapy, resistance will emerge. A common mistake of neophytes is not to identify the resistance for fear of alienating the patient. Resistances tend to be of three sorts: resistance to insight, resistance to change and resistance to an examination of personality structure. Some specific resistances which occur in early psychotherapy include shifting from one symptom to another, being too intellectually inhibited to talk freely to the therapist, obsessing to the point that it becomes a defense against self-examination, reporting only superficial details, repressing and suppressing important material as well as resistance to the transference. Acting in or acting out in which transferential conflict is dealt with nonverbally by action either in or out of the office is also a form of resistance. Settling into psychotherapy — as a way of life rather than as a way to seek choices — is also a resistance. One of the most difficult resistances with which to deal particularly for the neophyte is "insight" as a resistance. Here, the patient offers a new insight about his psychodynamics once or twice each week. It takes some time for the therapist to realize that these "insights" are superficial, fragmentary, and a defensive against true emotional insight.

It is never easy to deal with resistance but the therapist's task can be made easier if he educates the patient to recognize resistance with him. As part of the initial education of the patient, resistance should be discussed and named. If the patient anticipates its occurrence, it will be less frightening and less mysterious. Similarly, if the resistance can be named and then viewed and interpreted by the therapist not as something bad that the patient is doing but rather something that "it" is doing to the patient to keep him from making progress in this therapy — which is, of course, always threatening — the patient can examine the resistance without feeling guilty. It is also necessary throughout psychotherapy to be prepared to repeat interpretations about resistance, sometimes endlessly, it is not infrequent for a resistance to occur during an hour, to be interpreted, to be seemingly overcome, and then to have it occur again in virtually the same form a few hours or several weeks later. Reference has been made to the term *counter-resistance.* Counter-resistance is a form of counter-transference which occurs in the therapist and can be as devastating to the course of the therapy as the resistance of the patient. In counter-resistance, the therapist unconsciously minimizes or exaggerates the patient's degree of psychopathology and the success of his treatment. Counter-resistance can work to prolong or shorten therapy and it can work to prevent improvement on the part of the patient; indeed in some unfortunate situations it can even serve to encourage the patient to get worse. In order to monitor counter-resistance, the therapist must be aware of all counter-transference — or as much of it as he can be aware of. As mentioned elsewhere in this volume, counter-transference is a combination of the therapist's real reaction to a patient and his transferential reaction to the patient — the reaction which is based not on the patient's reality but on the important objects in the therapist's life whose emotional intensity is somehow stirred up by the particular patient. While it was felt for many years that counter-transference was somehow bad and that a well analyzed therapist would not have any, it seems to the author that counter-transference is a universal phenomenon and an inevitable one. What remains to be done, then, is for the therapist to acknowledge counter-transference and to try to find it and understand it in each therapeutic contact he has with a patient. In this way, counter-transference can be used to mobilize more understanding of the patient. If counter-transference is denied or somehow blamed on the patient, a therapeutic impasse will occur.

Many therapists get angry with patients who do not get better, particularly if many of their patients are in this category. Therapists get angry and bored by obsessive patients dwelling on minor incidents at great length. Recognition of one's personal idiosyncratic reactions to patients allows one to predict types of patients one will have difficult counter-transference reactions to.

Some very common manifestations of counter-transference which would lead one to examine one's reaction to the patient for counter-transference issues are great boredom in the face of material which should not be boring, flights into fantasy, arguments with the patient, feelings of great discouragement with the patient, an inability to pay attention to the patient, an inappropriate attempt to be kind to the patient and an inappropriate fear of the patient's capacity for self-destructiveness or violence as well as a bland reaction to material which should make one very worried about the patient's capacity for self-destructive behavior or violence.

In addition, there are three patterns of counter-transference which can torpedo any attempt for successful therapy. These are the patterns of rescuing, enabling and fostering. In a rescue counter-transference manifestation, the therapist repetitively removes a patient from the consequences of the patient's actions. This is usually caused by an oversolicitude for the patient which is actually often a reaction formation. Rescuing not only keeps the patient from examining the consequences of his actions but also leads the patient to feel less responsible for his own life. It actualizes the ubiquitous fantasy that the therapist will intervene magically for the patient. Often, the therapist is acting out of guilt and out of some eroticized feelings toward the patient. Over a lengthy psychotherapy, the rescue operation will actually lead to the patient's becoming worse.

Enabling is a more covert type of counter-transference reaction than is rescuing. Enabling therapists give covert though not overt permission for a continuation of a harmful pattern which the patient has. The patient, for example, who, in spite of good economic circumstances, has not paid his bill for a matter of several months and without any comment from the therapist, is receiving a message that it is alright not to pay the bill. The patient who comes for his therapy hour complaining that there are not any bars open because it is election day and is told by the therapist about the private club two blocks away, is involved in an enabling reaction. The therapist does not directly give him something to drink but he makes it possible for the patient to carry out an otherwise impossible act.

Fostering is a third and very common form of countertransference manifestation. Fostering is the unconscious and covert encouragment for a harmful act. Often, a therapist will be quite fascinated by the patient's methods of acting out and by his questions, and by his apparent interest gives the patient the idea that these methods are of particular interest to the therapist. There may be a continuation of them or they may increase in intensity, duration, and provocativeness in order to hold the therapist's attention. This great attention and selected attention on the part of the therapist gives the patient a clear message that this is what the therapist wants to hear about.

Patients have strengths as well as weaknesses and sometimes their weaknesses are characterologically related to their strengths. It is the duty of the therapist to focus on the patient's mature abilities as well as his regressive problems. There is no rule against being innovative in psychotherapy though many of us refuse to be because of our concerns about peer reaction. Finally, psychotherapy is heady stuff. It is fun to construct beautiful, precise psychodynamic formulations. One should, at the same time, keep in mind other alternatives and always look for simpler explanations.

SUGGESTED READING

Bruch, H.: *Learning Psychotherapy.* Harvard U. Press, 1974.

Buckley, P., Karasu, T.B., Charles, E., and Stein, S.P.: Theory and Practice in Psychotherapy: Some Contradictions in Expressed Belief and Reported Practices. J Nerv Ment Dis, *167:*218, 1979.

Hill, L.: On Being Rather than Doing in Psychotherapy. Int J Group Psychother, *8:*115, 1958.

Lewis, J.M.: The Inward Eye: Monitoring the Process of Psychotherapy, JCE Psychiat, *40:*17, 1979.

Saul, L.: *Psychodynamically-Based Psychotherapy.* Science House, 1972.

Szalita, A.B.: Some Thoughts on Empathy, Psychiat, *39:*142, 1976.

17 Psychopharmacology

J. Ramon de la Fuente

Drugs have become a most important tool in the management of many psychiatric conditions. In this chapter, I will attempt to present succinctly some of the foundations for the clinical use of the most common psychotropic drugs: antipsychotics, antidepressnats, lithium carbonate and antianxiety agents will be reviewed on the basis of their mechanisms of action, pharmacokinetics, therapeutic effects, unwanted effects and average dosages. While other drugs such as CNS stimulants (amphetamines and others), beta adrenergic blockers (propranolol and others), anticonvulsants (carbamazepine and others), and other chemical compounds including some hormone preparations do have a place in the treatment of some psychiatric disorders, they will not be discussed here. Readers interested in those drugs, can find excellent reviews in several of the major textbooks of psychiatric therapeutics (1, 3).

Many psychotropic drugs have been discovered by serendipity, their pharmacological activity involves brain mechanisms that are not fully understood and much research is currently being done in the field. This makes it a complex subject where some knowledge about brain organization and behavior, and particularly about brain neurotransmission, is needed to understand why we use these drugs, and perhaps most important, what happens when we use them.

Clinical psychopharmacology is a young subject, dating from the introduction of the antipsychotic medication chlorpromazine in the early 1950's. At about the same time, it was observed that iproniazid, a monamine oxidase inhibitor (MAOI) used to treat tuberculosis, had a euphoriant effect in some patients. Lithium salts were first used in the treatment of psychotic excitement in 1949; however, mainly because of fear of toxicity, its use was very slow to develop in the United States. Benzodiazepines (chlordiazepoxide and others) were introduced in the early 1960's and rapidly replaced the older tranquilizers (barbiturates and others).

Its widespread use, misuse, and abuse have become the subject of much discussion by both the medical and lay communities. All things together, throughout these 30 years, psychotropic drugs have proved as valuable in the laboratory as in the clinic. They have provided powerful means of analyzing brain physiology and animal behavior, as well as some basis for elucidating the actions of other drugs. But overall, psychopharmacology has contributed enormously to the awareness that psychiatric disease has biological components. Whether psychotropic drugs can modify basic disease processes rather than symptoms, remains largely to be established, but nevertheless research in the field has been fruitful so far, and is likely to be even more in the years to come.

ANTIPSYCHOTIC DRUGS

The term antipsychotic refers to the clinical action of these drugs, also called major tranquilizers, antischizophrenic agents and neuroleptics. Neuroleptic means "that which takes the neuron" (4) and refers basically to the side effects rather than the therapeutic actions, and because they are not really tranquilizers nor are they specific antischizophrenic drugs, the term antipsychotic appears most appropriate.

Table I shows the various chemical groups of antipsychotic agents, their generic names, trade names and conversion factors for dosage in relation to chlorpromazine, the prototype drug. On the basis of their side chain, the phenothiazines can be divided into three subclasses: the aliphatic compounds, the piperidine compounds and the piperazine group. All the chemical groups of antipsychotic agents listed in Table I have the common property of blocking dopaminergic receptors.

While these drugs are useful outside psychiatry for the treatment of vomiting and vertigo, for instance, or to potentiate the analgesics, their main indications are:

1. To calm down disturbed patients whatever the underlying pathology, but most commonly those with acute psychosis, schizophrenia, mania or organic mental disorder;

2. As maintenance therapy to prevent acute relapses in chronic schizophrenia;

3. As maintenance therapy to suppress psychotic exacerbations, mostly in chronic paranoid patients; and

TABLE I
GENERIC NAMES, TRADE NAMES
AND ESTIMATED DOSAGE RATIO OF ANTIPSYCHOTICS
IN RELATION TO CHLORPROMAZINE

Generic Name	*Trade Name*	*Conversion Factor*
Phenothiazines		
Aliphatic		
Chlorpromazine	Thorazine	1:1
Promazine	Sparine	1:1
Triflupromazine	Vesprin	1:4
Piperazines		
Acetophenazine	Tindal	1:5
Butaperazine	Repoise	1:10
Carphenazine	Proketazine	1:4
Fluphenazine*	Prolixin	1:50
Perphenazine	Trilafon	1:10
Prochloperazine	Compazine	1:6
Thiproperazine	Dartal	1:10
Trifluoperazine	Stelazine	1:20
Piperidines		
Mezoridazine	Serentil	1:2
Piperacetazine	Quide	1:10
Thioridazine	Mellaril	1:1
Thioxanthenes		
Aliphatic		
Chlorprothixene	Taractan	1:2
Piperazine		
Thiothixene	Navane	1:25
Dibenzazepines		
Loxapine	Loxitane	1:6
Clozapine	Leponex**	1:2
Butyrophenones		
Haloperidol	Haldol	1:50
Droperidol	Inapsine	1:50
Diphenylbutyl-piperidines		
Pimozide	Orap**	1:200
Penfluridol*	Semap**	1:50
Dihydroindolones		
Molindone	Moban	1:10
Rauwolfia alkaloids		
Reserpine	Serpasil	1:50

*Long-lasting effects
**Not commercially available in the U.S.

4. In low doses, to control anxiety and agitation in selected patients, although it must be emphasized that these are not primarily antianxiety drugs.

Mechanisms of Action

What was once thought to be a relatively simple question — how do antipsychotic drugs exert their therapeutic action? — has become an increasingly complex one. While these agents produce a plethora of pharmacological effects, interference with dopaminergic transmission is a most likely mechanism ascribable to their clinical efficacy.

The dopamine-receptor-hypothesis was first suggested twenty years ago (5). It stated that these drugs specifically attach to dopamine receptors in the nervous system, and it is consistent with the dopamine hypothesis of schizophrenia, as they ameliorate the clinical course of the illness. Evidence to support these receptor-blockade hypotheses is largely based on clinical observations: their ability to induce an extrapyramidal syndrome that mimics naturally-occurring Parkinson's disease; their ability to induce a neuroendocrine syndrome featured by galactorrhea, amenorrhea and occasionally impotence; and their ability to alleviate the schizophrenic-like symptoms induced by dopaminergic agonists such as amphetamines.

Laboratory studies have been somewhat more controversial in terms of how antipsychotics interfere with dopamine tramsmission, and which particular pharmacological effect best correlates with clinical efficacy. However, since dopamine receptor binding was demonstrated in brain membranes, evidence supports the hypothesis that these drugs do act by blocking post-synaptic dopamine receptors. In fact, it has been possible to measure the ability of a wide range of antipsychotic drugs to displace radioactive labelled haloperidol from these membranes, and to determine the affinity of binding of each drug to the dopamine receptor. Further, a significant correlation has been found between clinical and pharmacological potencies of these drugs, and their ability to displace radioactive haloperidol from post-synaptic receptors (6).

No drug has a single effect, and in the case of antipsychotics, the varying incidences of side-effects suggest that other mechanisms of action are involved as well. It has been well documented that these drugs can block other central nervous system receptors in addition to dopamine receptors, such a muscarinic acetycholine receptors, histamine H-1 and H-2 receptors, alpha-adrenergic receptors and serotonin receptors. Their interactions at these receptor sites largely determine their clinically unwanted effects that will be discussed below, but they are too nonspecific to explain the therapeutic action of these agents (7). Table II shows the estimates for the affinities of some antipsychotic drugs to brain receptors.

Pharmokinetics

Chlorpromazine and butaperazine are the most extensively studied antipsychotics in terms of their kinetics. The former, probably because it has been the prototypic drug for many years, and the latter because of its simpler metabolism, which was thought to represent a significant advantage for these studies. Too many factors, but mainly individual variabilities and differences in the techniques employed, not to mention the study designs, have made it difficult to interpret the meaning of the contradictory findings that have been reported. Chlorpromazine, for instance, is absorbed erratically and incompletely when taken orally; goes through a large first-pass effect due to metabolism in the liver and possibly in the gut, its systemic bioavailability has been estimated

TABLE II
ANTIPSYCHOTIC AFFINITES* FOR BRAIN RECEPTORS
Estimates calculated from data of various authors (7, 13, 15) should be considered as approximations

Drug	*Dopamine*	*Serotinin*	*Muscarinic Acetylcholine*	*Alpha adrenergic*	*Histamine H-1*	*Histamine H-2*
Chlorpromazine	++	+++	++	+++	++	++
Clozapine	+	++	+++	++	+++	+
Fluphenazine	+++	++	+++	++	++	++
Haloperidol	+++	+	+	++	+	++
Penfluridol	++	+	–	+	+	–
Perphenazine	–	–	++	+++	++	–
Pimozide	+++	++	–	++	+	–
Thioridazine	++	+++	+++	+++	++	+++
Thiothixene	+++	++	–	++	++	–
Thifluoperazine	++	++	+	+	+	–

* + = least; ++ = intermediate, +++ = most

to be about 25%, it is highly protein-bound (approximately 98%), and its metabolism is complicated and virtually complete. About 160 metabolites have been postulated but few have been identified and fewer tested for pharmacological activity. Its plasma disappearance is bimodal, with a distributive half life of about two hours and elimination half life of about 16 to 30 hours. The drug can be metabolized fast or slowly which is genetically determined, and metabolic tolerance can be developed since patients can induce enzymes to metabolize the drug faster after a few weeks of treatment. With such kinetic behavior, one can understand why attempts to correlate plasma concentrations with clinical response have not been very successful. There is not a good consistent correlation between dose and plasma levels, although blood levels between 150 and 300 mg/ml or higher have been found to be associated with clinical improvement (8).

Although it is reassuring to know that plasma concentrations of chlorpromazine are highly correlated to levels in the cerebrospinal fluid, central effects can be caused by an active metabolite, and unrelated to the levels of the compound. The main problem with chlorpromazine is that the weight of the presumed "therapeutic window" is not known, and although there might be an inverted-U relationship between plasma levels and clinical response, the upper and lower limits of such a window remain to be determined.

Pharmacoclinical response correlations in patients treated with butaperazine, a not very commonly used drug but technically easier to work with, have been better documented. Evidence for a U-shaped dose-response curve with this agent comes from studies where the drug has been administered on a constant-dose schedule to acutely symptomatic schizophrenics, and measuring plasma and red blood cells concentrations. Red blood cells levels may be a better correlate of clinical response than plasma levels. The assumption is that for drugs to reach the receptor side in the brain, they must pass the blood-brain barrier, and the distribution of the drug across the blood cell membrane mimics the passage through the blood-brain barrier (9).

Studies on haloperidol (10), show that this drug also has a rapid distribution phase, and an elimination half life of 12-22 hours. Peak blood levels have been observed 20 minutes after intramuscular injection but its systemic bioavailability remains unknown. Its metabolism appears to be simpler than that of the phenothiazines, and its metabolites are inactive. It possibly crosses the placenta. The weakness of its affinity to muscarinic-cholinergic and alpha-adrenergic receptors have made it a good drug to use parenterally in elderly, agitated patients.

Data available regarding other antipsychotics are scanty and not enough experience has accumulated as yet to draw conclusions.

Antipsychotics can accelerate the metabolism of other drugs, and reciprocally their own metabolism can be increased. Barbiturates, several anti-parkinsonian drugs and even cigarette smoking have been implicated in inducing liver enzymes, resulting in a decline in plasma concentrations of various antipsychotic drugs. By contrast, some drugs can increase plasma concentrations of antipsychotics by competing for the liver enzymes. The tricyclic antidepressants, imipramine, amitriptyline and nortriptyline, all compete in this way with chlorpromazine and might potentiate its actions. These combinations are not generally recommended because they can lead to drug toxicity.

Therapeutic Effects

The most common indications for use of these drugs in psychiatry is to reduce severe agitation, psychomotor excitement or disturbed behavior from whatever cause. Symptomatic tranquilization is indicated in patients with schizophrenia, particularly when restlessness, excitement, paranoid delusions and destructive behavior are present; in affective disorders, particularly when manic or hypomanic episodes are to be controlled, or when agitated and paranoid features are predominating; in the acute psychoses, including most of those that are substance-induced, and in some cases of delirium or other organic mental disorders; in the chronic symptomatic psychosis where restlessness, confusion, or violent outbursts are the target symptoms, and finally, in a few selected cases of patients with neurotic or personality disorders where low doses can be of much help.

It is important to emphasize that the above list of indications to use these drugs for tranquilizing purposes, reflects mostly a symptomatic approach, irrespective from the specific diagnosis. While its main indication is to treat schizophrenia, it should be pointed out that more than 25 years of experience with these drugs has demonstrated that they do not "cure" schizophrenia. Rather, the drugs curb the progress of the condition by cutting short the acute, initial attack and subsequent episodes, and by delaying relapse when the drugs are taken as maintenance therapy. Nevertheless, experience shows that in patients with paranoid schizophrenia, symptom suppression with these drugs is often complete as long as medication continues (11).

About twenty years ago (12), the National Institute of Mental Health carried out a study of 463 newly admitted, acutely schizophrenic patients each of whom was treated with one of three phenothiazines in flexible dosages or with a placebo. About 75% of the patients given active drug were much improved after six weeks as compared with only 25% of those given placebo. Several areas of psychopathology were rated significantly more improved by drug than by placebo. These included: ineffective social participation, confusion, poor standards of self-care, agitation, slowed speech, incoherent speech, irritability, indifference to environment, hostility, hallucinations, ideas of persecution, and disorientation.

From many other studies of this sort, it seems that the most helpful single therapeutic step in managing acutely ill schizophrenic patients is the administration of adequate, but not excessive, doses of antipsychotic medication. However, this must be combined with a supportive environment, sympathetic nursing and appropriate social measures.

Maintenance therapy refers to the long-term drug treatment of schizophrenic patients who are in remission or partial remission. Several controlled studies have shown that patients taking antipsychotic medication are much less likely to relapse than those maintained on placebo. However, the main problem has been that of drug compliance. Most patients relapse because they stop taking their medication regularly although there are some who do relapse and then cease medication. Life events also seem important and tend to cluster in the previous weeks before relapse. Drug maintenance therapy often seems relatively ineffective in preventing such event-related relapses.

The chronic schizophrenic does benefit from antipsychotic treatment although less than the acute patient. Hallucinations, delusions, anxiety, and restlessness are particularly amenable to amelioration by drugs, and there is general agreement that use of antipsychotics facilitates patient participation in social rehabilitation programs.

Unwanted Effects

Throughout the years, a long list of side-effects of antipsychotic medications has been accumulated. Most of them, however, are fairly minor. Some of them present rather acutely, while others are a consequence of its long-term use; some are mediated by dopamine receptor blockade, while others relate to blockade of other neurotransmitter receptors.

The most common and sometimes the most troublesome are the neurologic side-effects of antipsychotic drugs (13). The earliest effect is acute dystonia, which is particularly likely to occur in males and in children, and is most common as an effect of butyrophenones and aliphatic phenotiazenes. It is featured by torticollis, tongue protrusion, facial grimacing, opisthotonos, and oculogyric crisis. The main problem with this syndrome is to recognize it and not to ascribe it to a seizure disorder, tetany, or hysteria. Sometimes a single dose of the drug is sufficient to induce the condition, which usually responds promptly to the parenteral administration of an anticholinergic agent. Akathisia (motor restlessness, fidgeting, pacing, and a drive to move about) is another common early motor symptom complex. It should not be mistaken for increasing anxiety or agitation, nor should it be treated by increasing the dose of an antipsychotic drug. Antiparkinsonian agents may have a beneficial effect, as may antianxiety drugs with muscle-relaxing properties such as diazepam. Sometimes the dose of the antipsychotic drug needs to be reduced. Akinesia is another side effect on which walking and fine-movement control are affected. More severely impaired patients show coarse tremor, excessive salivation, stooped posture and festinant gait, all of which are signs of drug-induced parkinsonism. The onset of the extrapyramidal syndrome is usually within the first month of treatment and there appears to be some sort of tolerance as the signs usually fade away over 2 or 3 months with a decreasing requirement for anticholinergic medication. Antipsychotic agents with higher milligram potency induce parkinsonism with greater frequency than less potent agents. Akinetic mutism, catatonic reactions and the so-called neuroleptic malignant syndrome are less common and usually associated to relatively high doses of potent antipsychotics.

Drugs for the treatment of parkinsonism should not be used routinely with antipsychotic medication. There is no clear-cut evidence for any prophylactic effect; instead, they may cause unpleasant anticholinergic side-effects, increase risk of delirium (especially in elderly patients), decrease gastrointestinal absorption of other drugs, and even habituation and abuse may also occur. Sound practice requires an attempt to withdraw these drugs a few weeks after the onset of an extrapyramidal reaction.

Tardive dyskinesia is a late-developing extrapyramidal syndrome that has led to reappraisal of the value of uninterrupted and indefinitely prolonged antipsychotic therapy. The syndrome consists of involuntary or semivoluntary movements of a choreiform nature, sometimes with a dystonic component. These classically affect the tongue, facial and neck muscles, and often also the extremities and muscles that control posture and sometimes those used in breathing. Early signs of tardive dyskinesia are movements of the tongue or extremities. Oral-lingual-masticatory movements are common, especially in the elderly; it is common to find abnormalities of posture and involuntary movements of the fingers in younger patients. The movements of tardive dyskinesia usually become worse if the antipsychotic agent is withdrawn, and can be suppressed temporarily by readministering an antipsychotic agent. It has been suggested that this syndrome might represent a functional level of hyperactivity of central dopamine mechanisms, possibly arising in compensation for prolonged blockade of dopaminergic-synapse transmission by an antipsychotic drug. The syndrome may be irreversible or persist for many months even after withdrawal of the antipsychotic, and although painless, it is usually embarrassing and distressing, especially in relatively well-functioning outpatients. The incidence of the syndrome has varied widely among several epidemiological studies but has averaged at about 10-15% of patients maintained on antipsychotic medication for several years. The treatment of tardive dyskinesia is highly unsatisfactory, so the best way to deal with this potential problem, is to avoid the condition by reserving long-term antipsychotic medication for those who really need it. Regular review of dosage and treatment regimen is essential.

Other unwanted effects of antipsychotic medication include hyperprolactinemia, that can be associated with amenorrhea and galactorrhea in women and with gynecomastia and loss of libido in men. Antipsychotics may cause some EKG changes such as prolonged ventricular repolarization. Arrhythmias have been reported, and one has to be cautious in patients with heart disease. Another long-term side-effect of chlorpromazine and other phenothiazines is the accumulation of the drug and its metabolites on pigments in the cornea, lens and skin. This leads to a purple-gray decolorization, especially in sunny climates but vision is not usually impaired, in contrast to the retinal degeneration that can follow high doses (more than 800 mg day) of thioridazine.

Postural hypotension and reflex tachycardia are related to the alpha-adrenergic blocking effects of these drugs. Dry mouth, blurred vision, urinary hesitancy, and constipation are related to their anticholinergic effects. Sedation, drowsiness, and probably weight gain are likely to reflect their antihistaminic properties. Among the rarest adverse reactions are cholestatic jaundice and agranulocytosis.

Choice of the Drug and Dosage

No substantial evidence exists that the various antipsychotic drugs differ significantly in effectiveness. However, clinicians often see patients that respond to one drug and not to another.

A significant difference among antipsychotic drugs are their unwanted effects and as mentioned above, these may result from interactions at various neurotransmitter receptor sites (7). Thus the high affinity for muscarinic acetylcholine receptors of the aliphatic and piperidine phenothiazines makes anticholinergic effects to be common with these drugs, and minor or negligible with other compounds such as haloperidol or trifluoperazine. A similar situation is observed in regard to their sedating, as mesoridazine and thioridazine tend to keep the patient less alert than haloperidol or molindone. But really what is the only major alternative regarding antipsychotic drugs is the use of long-acting injectable preparations (14).

Long-acting injectable antipsychotics can help individual patients who have responded poorly to all medications, particularly those who are drug defaulters and those who metabolize the drug rapidly. Fluphenazine is available to be given by injection into the gluteal muscles once every 2 to 4 weeks. By using this route of administration, the drug can be absorbed into the systemic ciruclation avoiding the first-pass metabolism in the liver. This provides some rationale for the effectiveness of these drugs in relatively low dosage. The use of them can be optimized if attended by the institution of a specially organized clinic with adequate social support in the community.

Thus, the dosage requirements will vary according to several factors. To attain an adequate effect in a critical patient, an intramuscular dose of 100 mg of chlorpromazine or its equivalents is usually necessary. However, as unwanted effects may be troublesome after such a loading dose, or in less urgent circumstances, a build-up of oral medication is preferable. The dose is usually titrated for the individual patient to obtain the optimal response which is the maximum therapeutic effect with minimal side-effects. The dosage will vary widely from patient to patient and caution should be stressed with elderly patients. In patients over 60 years of age, half of the ordinary adult dose should be given initially until one can become well acquainted with the patient's individual tolerance.

In schizophrenia, moderate dosage, say 400 mg of chlorpromazine a day or its equivalent, is usually more effective than lower doses. However, it is doubtful whether the routine use of high doses (more than 600 mg of chlorpromazine a day or its equivalent) offers any real benefits, although there are patients that will respond only to higher doses. Kinetic properties of most phenothiazines allow for a once-a-day schedule, and furthermore, some of them given as one dose at night, often exert useful hypnotic effects.

ANTIDEPRESSANT DRUGS

Antidepressants can be roughly divided into two major groups. The monamine reuptake inhibitors, namely the tricyclic antidepressants and related compounds, and the monamine oxidase inhibitors (MAOI's). Both were discovered by accident, and their modes of action still pose many questions. The classical biogenic amine hypothesis of affective disorders (16) stems directly from studies on the acute pharmacological effects elicited by a number of clinically effective antidepressants. However, at times, the amine hypothesis has been so vigorously promoted that its basis in psychopharmacology has seemed forgotten.

Work with antidepressant drugs as tools for pharmacologic research and as therapeutic agents has generated continuous excitement since the early days of their discovery. First came the observation of mood elevation in patients with tuberculosis treated with isoniazid (a MAOI) in the 1950's. In the 1960's it was found that the so-called tertiary amines (imipramine and amitriptyline) could be converted *in vivo* to secondary amines (desipramine and nortriptyline). Then came the findings that such conversion could alter the affinity and potency with regard to inhibition of serotonin and norepinephrine reuptake, and finally, the more recent findings about the action of antidepressant drugs on noradrenergic-receptor functions and their regulator control of specific biological responses.

At a practical level, there have been two main problems: the incomplete response to antidepressant therapy and the discrepancy in the time course between biochemical and pharmacological effects and their clinical therapeutic action. In controlled trials, about one-third of depressed patients show a satisfactory response to placebo, and another third respond to the drug. Why the remaining third do not respond is still unclear, although some explanatory hypotheses have been suggested. Some of them stress that the problem has been the cause of the depressive illness, which remains largely contentious, with both dimensional and dichotomous models being put forward. This has made it very difficult to interpret the results of some drug trials.

Another serious clinical problem has been the many troublesome side-effects of these drugs. All this has led to the introduction of newer compounds: tetracyclic, bicyclic and monocyclic antidepressants have been developed and marketed in some countries with claims that they are more effective and have fewer side-effects or more rapid action. However, some skepticism should be kept on regarding these claims as there are no hard data to document them.

At the present time, monoamine reuptake inhibitors still are the standard therapy for depressed patients, whereas MAOI's seem to be most applicable in patients with what has been called atypical depression. The so-called new second generation antidepressants can provide improved therapy for some patients although none has consistently shown greater efficacy than older agents. Table III shows the various chemical groups of antidepressant drugs, their generic names, trade names, and usual daily dosage.

Tricyclic and Related Compounds

Mechanism of Action

In general, it is accepted that the therapeutic effects of these drugs are related to their activity in blocking reuptake into the

TABLE III
GENERIC NAMES, TRADE NAMES AND USUAL DOSAGE OF ANTIDEPRESSANT DRUGS

	Generic Name	Trade Name	Dose/Day/mg
Tricyclic Antidepressants	Iminodibenzyls		
	Imipramine	Tofranil	75-300
	Desipramine	Norpramin	75-300
	Trimipramine	Surmontil	50-300
	* Clomipramine	Anafranil	75-200
	Dibenzocycloheptenes		
	Amitriptyline	Elavil	75-300
	Nortriptyline	Aventyl	50-200
	Protriptyline	Vivactil	20-60
	* Butriptyline	Evadyne	150-300
	Other tricyclis		
	Doxepin	Sinequan	50-300
	* Dothiepin	Prothiaden	25-150
	* Opipramol	Insidon	150-300
	Tetracyclics		
	Maprotiline	Ludiomil	75-300
	* Mianserin	Bolvidon	20-120
	Mao Inhibitors		
	Isocarboxazid	Marplan	10-30
	Phenelzine	Nardil	30-75
	Tranylcypromine	Parnate	10-30
	Second Generation Antidepressants		
	* Nomifensine (Tetrahydroisoquinolone)	Merital	50-200
	Amoxapine (Dibenzoxazepine)	Asendin	100-300
	Trazodone (Triazolpyridine)	Desyrel	50-400
	* Iprindole (Triheterocyclic)	Prondol	45-180
	* Viloxazine (Bicyclic)	Vivalan	150-300

* Not commercially available in the United States

presynaptic vesicles of norepinephrine, serotonin and possibly dopamine. These active uptake pumps are located in the cell membranes, and its inhibition increases the amount of neurotransmitter at the receptor site.

While some selectivity on monamine reuptake inhibition exists, most of the agents are mixed reuptake inhibitors. The tertiary amines tend to inhibit serotonin uptake more than norepinephrine uptake, while the secondary amine derivatives tend to do the reverse. Nevertheless, inhibition of uptake mechanisms is not a necessary property for antidepressant efficacy. There are drugs that are potent antidepressants and poor uptake inhibitors, and drugs that are powerful uptake inhibitors but useless as antidepressants. Table IV shows the relative potencies of antidepressants in inhibiting monoamines reuptake.

Most of these drugs are also potent antagonists of muscarinic acetylcholine receptors, histamine receptors, alpha-adrenergic receptors and serotonin receptors. In general, these functions are not thought to be responsible for clinical antidepressant activity, as a large number of drugs lacking antidepressant properties, are also potent antagonists for these receptors. However, the powerful anticholinergic properties of some of them have led to the speculation about the role of central atropine-like action in the antidepressant effects, and an acetylcholine-related depression has been proposed. Their sedative effects have been related to the antihistamine properties, and the postural hypotension they may induce, to their affinity for alpha-adrenergic receptors in the brain. Table V shows the estimated affinities of some antidepressants for brain receptors.

Recently, it has been shown that these drugs cause, upon chronic administration, a down regulation of central noradrenergic receptor function, and although the exact mechanisms whereby these agents can modify the sensitivity and density of these receptor sites is not known, depression can now be conceptualized as a receptor-related disease (21).

TABLE IV
ANTIDEPRESSANT POTENCIES*
FOR INHIBITING NE AND 5-HT REUPTAKE

Estimates calculated from data of various authors (19, 20) should be considered as approximations

Drug	*Norepinephrine (NE)*	*Serotonin (5-HT)*
Amitriptyline	+	+++
Clomipramine	++	+++
Desipramine	+++	+
Imipramine	++	++
Maprotiline	++	+
Nomifensine	+++	+
Nortriptyline	++	+

* + = least, ++ = intermediate, +++ = most

TABLE V
ANTIDEPRESSANT AFFINITIES* FOR BRAIN RECEPTORS
Estimates calculated from data of various authors (17, 18) should be considered as approximations

	Histamine		*α-adrenergic*		*Muscarinic*	*Serotonin*	
Drug	*H-1*	*H-2*	*α-1*	*α-2*	*acetylcholine*	*HT-1*	*HT-2*
Amitryptiline	+++	+++	+++	+++	+++	++	+++
Desipramine	+	+	+	+	+	+	+
Doxepin	+++	++	+++	+++	+++	++	+++
Imipramine	++	++	++	++	++	+	+
Nortriptyline	++	++	++	++	+	+++	++
Protriptyline	++	+	+	+	++	+	+

* + = least, ++ = intermediate, +++ = most

Pharmacokinetics

Antidepressants are rapidly absorbed and extensively metabolized. However, blood levels following single oral doses will vary considerably among individuals. This variation is probably related to first-pass metabolism through the gut and liver which has shown a marked genetic influence. Protein binding is usually high, more than 90%, so the concentration at synaptic receptors is presumed to be low. The half-lives of these compounds in general, suggest that a once a day dosage after the steady state has been reached is sufficient and it might lead to better compliance (22).

While recent technological developments have made it possible for virtually any clinical laboratory to establish techniques for measuring plasma concentrations of these drugs, the relationship of blood levels to clinical response is quite contentious. Evidence of a curvilinear relationship between clinical response and plasma concentrations has been presented for the secondary amines and protriptyline whereas claims have been made for a straight-line relationship between clinical responses and high concentrations of tertiary amines. However, recent studies have failed to confirm such a relationship for either amitriptyline or imipramine. Furthermore, an effect of that nature would be difficult to explain because treatment with tertiary amines is essentially treatment with a mixture of the parent drugs and deaminated derivatives. In summary, correlations between antidepressant plasma levels and clinical response are not very solid, and while monitoring plasma levels can be useful in some cases for the psychopharmacological management of patients with affective disorders, its routine use cannot be justified at the present time (23).

Toxic effects are observed when antidepressants are used with other drugs of similar actions such as antihistaminics or anticholinergics. Barbiturates and alcohol enhance hepatic enzyme induction, and can reduce plasma concentrations of antidepressants. Conversely, phenothiazines and antidepressants may mutually compete so that the plasma concentrations of both are increased. Reversal of action of some antihypertensives such as guanethidine and clonidine has been noted, and drugs that bind to proteins such as aspirin may also alter the clinical effect of antidepressants. While some of the dangers of interaction between monamine reuptake inhibitors and monamine oxidase inhibitors may have been overemphasized, this combination should be avoided except for very specific and well controlled cases as will be discussed below.

Therapeutic Effects

Anxiety and insomnia, two of the most common symptoms of depression tend to be relieved within the first few days of treatment although fully normal sleep patterns may not resume until several weeks of treatment. Increased energy and less concern with somatic symptoms usually develop during the second or third week of treatment. Lifting of the depressed mood, either recognized by the patient or his family might be one of the last symptoms to be relieved, often not being evident until the fourth week of treatment. The same is true of disturbed sexual function. The expected course of response should be explained to patients so that they do not become discouraged with treatment and stop it too soon. Some patients initially feel much worse on these drugs, especially the more sedative ones.

Refractory patients should be carefully re-evaluated. Frequently, it can be due to misdiagnosis, subtherapeutic dosage, noncompliance, or a biochemical basis for the depression not being touched by the drug used. Attempts have been made to identify patients who are likely to respond more specifically to certain antidepressants. Urinary measurements of norepinephrine metabolite 3-methoxy-4-hydroxiphenylgloycol (MHPG) and some neuroendocrine tests have been studied on these effects with promising results (24, 25).

Unwanted Effects

The wide range of pharmacological actions of these agents, are reflected by a host of side-effects. These unwanted effects are quite common at the initiation of therapy but usually lessen as treatment is continued; by and large, they are not serious but they can be uncomfortable. Anticholinergic effects due to blockade of muscarinic-acetylcholine receptors include dry mouth, blurred vision, constipation that might lead to paralytic ileus, urinary retention, exacerbation of narrow-angle glaucoma, confusion that occasionally can develop into delirium, and speech blockage. The antihistaminic effects are mainly sedation, that can actually be used to advantage, and weight gain which might be mediated by hitamine H-1 receptor antagonism. Some of the cardiovascular reactions can be due to alpha-adrenergic blockade such as postural hypotension, but there are also some direct effects on the heart such as intraventricular conduction delay and flattened T waves. Patients with pre-existing heart disease are particularly suspectible and one should be cautious. A recent myocardial infarct is considered in general as a contraindication but fortunately, these drugs are seldom needed at this time in any case. Sudden deaths have been reported in association with amitriptyline but further surveys are needed before firm conclusions can be drawn.

Allergic reactions such as skin rashes and mild cholestatic jaundice have been reported. Agranulocytosis is very rare. A fine tremor in the upper extremities and ataxia can occur particularly with bipolar illness although it is difficult to be sure that this is not a spontaneous switch. Finally, some teratogenic effects have been suggested, but no excess of fetal abnormalities has been proved to be associated with maternal use of the drugs in therapeutic doses.

Choice of the Drug and the Usual Dosage

Few clinical differences have been found among monamine reuptake inhibitors. However, it has been proposed that the secondary amines which act preferentially on noradrenergic systems should be more effective in increasing psychomotor activity and drive, whereas tertiary amines which preferentially block serotonin reuptake have a greater effect on mood. Nevertheless, it must be remembered that the tertiary amines are metabolized to secondary amines so that the former have a comprehensive profile of action lacking in the latter.

The side-effects which vary widely among these agents should be considered preferentially when making the choice of the drug to use. Not only the anticholinergic effects but the cardiotoxic and sedative properties, and its potential for interacting with concomitantly administered drugs such as antihypertensive agents and sympathomimetic compounds should also be considered. The risk of suicidal overdosage may suggest the use of toxic drugs, perhaps a tetracyclic. As for the speed of action, there seems little to choose among these agents. New second generation antidepressants are always a good choice for patients who have been resistant to conventional antidepressants.

Because many patients will be seen during a recurrent depression, it is valuable to obtain a complete history about previous responses to drug treatment. The proper choice of drug for a particular patient may then become clearer. Lacking such history, one should inquire about family members who may have been treated for depression; the assumption is that etiologic type of depression may run true in close family members. Caution should be taken when prescribing antidepressants to elderly patients. Side-effects are often more troublesome, particularly hypotensive episodes. Once nightly dosage is preferred by some patients, but others prefer divided doses throughout the day.

Doses of antidepressants have largely been determined empirically. The usual range of dosage is listed in Table III. The desired effect, is weighted against the undesired effects. It is usually advisable to start medication at a fairly low dosage and to increase it gradually over a number of days to therapeutically effective levels. If there is no or only minimal response to treatment at the end of three weeks, increase to the maximal dose or a change of medication is in order. Once the patient responds to the antidepressant, the dosage should be reduced to a maintenance level which is usually about half of the dosage needed for the acute treatment. Patients should be kept on maintenance treatment for about 6 to 9 months. Some patients have been on maintenance treatment for years with apparently good control of their illness and no long-term adverse effects. If the depressive episode was the patient's first and if it responded quickly and satisfactorily to drug therapy, one would be tempted to gradually withdraw treatment during a period of a few months. If relapse does not occur, then drug treatment could be completely withdrawn. However, relatives should be instructed in how to detect early signs of relapse since the patient himself may be a poor judge of that.

Monamine Oxidase Inhibitors

Thanks to recent work, MAOI's are currently having a resurgence, but have never recovered their initial popularity, and have been generally eclipsed by the monamine reuptake inhibitors. However, the MAOI's have always had their devotees who claim that there is a limited but valuable place for these drugs in the treatment of some depressed patients. Symptoms that seem to respond most to treatment with MAOI's are: irritability, hypochrondriasis, and severe anxiety. Further, these agents have proved to be especially effective in the treatment of phobic anxiety, particularly of agrophobia. Another area of usefulness might be in the hypersomnic, anhedonic, depressed patient.

Mechanisms of Action

Monamine oxidase (MAO) is an enzyme that exists in a number of forms with various substrate and inhibitor specificities, and various mechanisms of distribution in body tissue. MAO type–A oxidatively deaminates serotonin and norepinephrine but not phenylethylamine, whereas type–B has reverse specificity. Conventional MAOI's inhibit both unselectively, but drugs have been developed that can inhibit selectively each type of the enzyne. (Clorgyline for type–A, and deprenil for type–B.)

Inhibition of MAO leads to the build-up in the tissues including the brain, of many aromatic amines normally present in only minute amounts. This includes the monamines active in neurotransmission and other amines such as tyramine. Brain MAO is obviously difficult to study in human beings and much has been inferred from indirect methods, such as urinary amine excretion and MAO activity in accessible tissues such as blood platelets. Since MAO concentrations in most tissues are excessive, fairly extensive inhibition is required before amine disposition is altered. Something of the order of 80% inhibition has been found necessary in various experiments before brain monamines alter in concentration (26).

As with other antidepressants, there is a gap between the time course of inhibition and clinical response. MAO inhibition, at least as monitored by blood platelets, is fairly rapid, often within a few doses of the MAOI drug, yet clinical response might be delayed for 2 to 4 weeks or even longer.

Pharmacokinetics

MAOI's are divided into two chemical groups: the hydrazines (phenelzine and isocarboxazid) and the nonhydrazines (tranylcypromine). Thus, their pharmacokinetics are varied. Isocarboxazide, for instance, is rapidly absorbed and is metabolized by hydrolysis and then is excreted in the urine. Phenelzine has been more extensively studied and it is possibly the most widely used MAOI because it has less inhibitory activity in the liver and more in the brain, thus being less hepatotoxic. A major route of its metabolism is acetylation by hepatic acetyltransferase. The rate of acetylation is genetically determined, and is bimodally distributed in the population; persons are either slow or fast acetylators. Slow acetylators seem to develop more unwanted effects with phenelzine than do fast acetylators. Also, the rate but not the eventual degree of MAO inhibition and clinical response, appears marginally greater in the slow acetylators. Tranylcypromine, the amphetamine-like MAOI is rapidly absorbed and almost entirely metabolized and eliminated within 24 hours.

Therapeutic Effects

MAOI's appear most useful in only certain types of depressed patients, usually referred to as patients with anxious depression, secondary depression or atypical depression. These patients usually show phobic signs and hysterical features (hysteroid dysphoria), have had a poor response to other antidepressants, and in general tolerate MAO inhibitors well.

While phobic, hypochondrical, hysterical, depressed patients particularly seem to benefit from MAOI's, it should be pointed out that patients with classical "endogenous" depression may also respond. In fact, they are used for this purpose fairly routinely by many psychiatrists outside the USA (27).

Unwanted Effects

Autonomic effects include orthostatic hypotension, dry mouth, constipation, impotence, delayed ejaculation and dizziness. However, only the hypotension is of practical significance, particularly in the elderly. CNS effects include drowsiness, restlessness, and insomnia. Seizures may be precipitated in susceptible patients. Other less common effects are hepatocellular jaundice, headaches, ankle edema, blood dyscrasias and skin reactions.

The best known untoward effects are the dietary interactions. While many foods have been recorded as being implicated, serious reactions are unlikely if patients avoid meat and yeast extracts, red wine and mature cheese. Their reaction is characterized clinically by a severe and sudden headache usually occipital in site, vomiting, chest pain, hyperpyrexia and restlessness. It usually subsides within a few hours but complications and death may supervene. Therefore, careful precautions are mandatory when prescribing MAOI's.

The mechanism of their interaction mainly involves tyramine but tyrosine, L-dopa, histamine, dopamine and phenylethylamine have also been implicated. Tyramine is formed by the decarboxylation of the amino acid tyrosine and is present in many fermented foods. Normally, it is deaminated by MAO in the gut wall and liver, and it is thus detoxified and prevented from entering the systemic circulation. When MAO inhibition is induced, tyramine is no longer detoxified and enters the circulation. Then it is taken up into noradrenergic nerve endings. These already contain surfeit of noradrenaline consequent on the MAO inhibition. The tyramine releases large quantities of noradrenaline, which constricts blood vessels in muscle by an alpha-adrenergic reaction, producing hypertension. The treatment of hypertensive crisis is to block the alpha-adrenergic receptors by parental administration of phenotolamine. Chlorpromazine which also blocks the alpha-adrenergic receptors can also be used i.m. The blood pressure must be monitored and the drug dose repeated as necessary.

Drug interactions are important. Any indirectly acting sympathomimetic medication can cause a hypertensive reaction, the mechanism being that described for tyramine. Agents such as amphetamine and phenylephrine which is a common constituent of cough medicines and nasal decongestants should be avoided. Alcohol, barbiturates, opiates and insulin can also be involved in dangerous interactions because the MAOI's also inhibit a wide range of enzymes that are required in the breakdown of many drugs.

Because food and drug interactions are so common, patients should carry a reminder card, alerting medical attendants in case treatment is required for an accident or another illness. If a patient taking MAOI's requires an operation, anesthetists must be warned. Detailed tables of food and drug interactions with MAOI's are readily available (28).

Choice of the Drug and Dosage

As with most psychoactive drugs, clinical usage is more dependent on side-effects than on main effects. Phenelzine is said to be the safest of the MAOI's and should be chosen by those with limited experience in the use of these drugs. Tranylcypromine sometimes is effective when the others have failed, but it is more likely to be associated with unwanted effects.

As a rule, use of these drugs in children should be avoided as their safety and efficacy in this age group are not well established. In the elderly MAOI's are sometimes effective when tricyclic medication has failed. In general, these medications are not recommended for use in physically ill patients because of interactions with other drugs.

Usual dosages are listed in Table III. They should always be initiated at a small dose, and then titrated according to clinical response and tolerance of side-effects. Doses should be divided through the day, since a single larger dose at night is not recommended.

Combined Pharmacotherapy for Depression

One of the most controversial topics in psychopharmacology has been the combined use of monoamine reuptake inhibitors and monomine oxidase inhibitors. Although this combination has been considered hazardous, reviews in recent years have suggested that if it is prescribed cautiously untoward reactions are rare. The safest combination appears to be that of amitriptyline and isocarboxazid, although phenelzine and tranylcypromine have also been used safely. The tricyclic must be given first, and the MAOI added gradually. Guidelines for the safe use of this regimen have been published elsewhere (29).

The pharmacology of the toxic interaction is that of excessive central and peripheral concentrations of monamines. The reported untoward reactions have been featured by hyperthermia, restlessness, agitation, hypertension and later hypotention, convulsions, coma and death. While this combination may be justified in some refractory-depressed patients, no clear benefit has been consistently documented. Thus, it should be restricted to carefully selected patients. Instructions must be followed to the letter, and informed consent from the patient must be obtained.

LITHIUM CARBONATE

In the late 1940's, an Australian researcher injected urine from manic patients into guinea pigs and found it to be toxic, the main agent of toxicity being urea. Uric acid seemed to increase the toxicity and in these experiments, lithium urate was chosen as a highly soluble salt. Unexpectedly the guinea pigs were protected from urea toxicity and became "tranquilized." The responsible agent was identified as lithium. In later experiments, lithium quieted some manic patients to whom it was administered. However, because of its known toxicity, it was not approved to the U.S. for treatment of acute mania until 1970. Lithium was then claimed to be also a prophylactic, preventing not only manic attacks but also depressive episodes.

Lithium is a cation, which substitutes other body fluid cations such as sodium and potassium but unlike these, lithium is fairly equally distributed between extracellular and intracellular body compartments. It is first transported into cells mainly by diffusion and moved out slowly by the sodium pump. Not surprisingly, a wide range of neurophysiological and neurochemical processes are modified by lithium. However, it is unlikely that any one action of lithium could be singled out as the mechanism for its clinical effect.

Lithium alters many neurotransmitter functions, diminishing the release of many of them and accelerating the reuptake of others. In the cell, lithium interferes with energy processes, acting on cyclic AMP production. Together with electrolyte and neurotransmitter changes, a very complex set of actions is attributable to lithium. However, its mode of action remains uncertain.

Pharmacokinetics

Lithium taken by mouth is rapidly absorbed from the gut. Because it peaks serum levels in 1-3 hours, sustained-release preparations have been introduced. These vary in their bioavailability and each preparation must be judged on the absorption course by the manufacturer.

Distribution into body tissues is a little delayed, at nonuniform rates and different gradients. In humans, serum concentrations decline with a biphasic course, rapidly during the first 6 hours and then at a slower elimination rate during the ensuing 24 hours. Lithium is not protein bound; it is excreted almost entirely by the kidneys, less than half of an administered dose being cleared in 24 hours. Lithium excretion by the kidney is linked to sodium balance so that if sodium intake is lowered, lithium excretion is reduced and toxicity can appear (30).

Because of the low therapeutic index of lithium, toxic concentrations can be reached easily. It is essential clinical practice to monitor serum lithium concentrations at appropriate intervals. Monitoring it is particularly important when treatment is initiated or dose regimen changed. Samples obtained weekly during the first month of treatment and thereafter at intervals of 2 to 3 months are recommended depending on the reliability of the patient and the variability of previous concentrations. The blood samples must be taken at the same time of the day each time, the optimal time being approximately 12 hours after the last dose. Concentrations between .6 and 1.4 mEq/liter are usually considered therapeutic. However, concentrations between 1.0 and 1.4 mEq/liter are suggested during the acute phase, and between 0.6 and 1.0 mEq/liter during the maintenance phase. Red blood cell concentration and saliva concentration may also provide adequate estimates, but they are currently reserved for research purposes. At any rate, lithium estimates must not be used as a blind substitute for clinical observation.

Clinical Use

Lithium is used routinely to treat manic and hypomanic patients and to prevent attacks in patients with recurrent affective illness. These attacks comprise both manic and depressive episodes in bipolar patients, episodes of mania in recurrent manic patients, and depressive attacks in unipolar patients. The role of lithium in the acute treatment of depressive episodes is a controversial issue.

Other conditions in which lithium treatment has been claimed effective such as schizoaffective disorders, chronic alcoholism, cluster headaches, etc. remain controversial as no conclusive evidence exists for its therapeutic effects. Other uses of lithium currently being studied include behavioral disorders in children and adolescents, pain disorders, leukopenia, tardive dyskinesia, thyrotoxicosis, Felty's syndrome, and others.

The therapeutic effects of lithium are not often apparent for at least a week. This is particularly relevant when treating manic patients where antipsychotic drugs almost always have to be used concurrently at the beginning of treatment. The delay on lithium action reflects its pharmacokinetic behavior with a slow build-up to therapeutic concentrations. Attempts to hasten the onset of action by pushing the lithium dosage rapidly need careful monitoring to avoid toxicity and, in general, are not recommended. Combinations of antipsychotics and lithium are not uncommon. Adverse reactions to the combination of haloperodol and lithium have been reported in some cases, but such interaction, if anything, seems exceptional.

Improvement of depressed patients with lithium is not always complete. Combining lithium and tricyclic therapy is frequently more effective than the use of lithium alone for reducing the intensity of depressive episodes in most patients. In the acute phase of depression, lithium alone might work, but not as effectively as antidepressants. In general, this combination carries no clinical problems.

Continued treatment with lithium has been shown to reduce the relapse rate of patients with bipolar affective disorders. Whether prophylaxis with lithium is more effective in bipolar than in unipolar patients remains controversial. While trials comparing lithium with tricyclic antidepressants as maintenance therapy for patients with recurrent depressions suggest that both are effective, lithium seems most suitable in those with a long history of affective episodes. Any patient who has had 2 or more distinct manic and/or depressive episodes should be evaluated and considered a candidate for lithium treatment. Some clinicians initiate lithium therapy very readily but others are more reluctant and may first try maintenance with a tricyclic antidepressant, especially in unipolar patients. If a patient treated with lithium does not show an adequate response within the first year of treatment, the drug should be discontinued as there is no reason to expose the patient to the risks of lithium treatment without due benefit.

Maintenance therapy does not necessarily mean complete prophylaxis. For some patients, attacks are only attentuated to the point at which they can be managed on an outpatient basis, but very close supervision is needed to keep them off recurrent hospitalizations.

Unwanted Effects

Most of the side-effects of lithium are harmless and reversible, the most common being nausea and a fine hand tremor, drowsiness and fatigue, especially during initial treatment. To minimize the tremor, which can be somewhat embarrassing, addition of a small dose of beta-adrenergic antagonist such as propranolol is usually sufficient.

Ataxia, dysarthria, difficulty in concentration and mild confusion and disorientation are the commonest early signs of incipient toxicity. Other features include muscle twitching and fasciculations of limb and face, as well as nystagmus and visual disturbances. Severe toxicity is accompanied by seizures, delirium, and eventually coma and death. Muscular flaccidity, hyperreflexia and irreversible brain damage have also been reported.

Endocrine effects feature edema, weight gain, and hypothyroidism with or without goiter. Lithium-induced goiters are usually diffuse and not large enough to be really noticeable. The incidence of this complication is low. Patients with pre-existing thyroid function at the lower limits of normal are more at risk than those with average or increased thyroid function. The hypothyroidism which may be confused with a retarded depression is usually reversible either by stopping lithium treatment or with use of thyroid preparations or replacement therapy. It is not necessarily a contraindication for lithium therapy, and if a patient is thought to be at high risk of recurrence of mania and/or depression, replacement therapy is wiser than discontinuing use of lithium. Lithium affects thyroid function at several sites. The main effect is to inhibit the release of thyroid hormones which leads to an increasing TSH secretion, compensatory augmentation of thyroid function, and sometimes goiter. If the compensation is insufficient, hypothyroidism ensues (32).

Kidney effects are by far the most preoccupying (33). Polyuria and polydypsia can occur in up to 40% of patients using lithium salts, but these symptoms do not always bother the patients who may not even mention them. The primary mechanism of the polyuria seems to be an inhibitory effect of the adenyl cyclase in the kidney which is normally sensitive to antidiuretic hormone. The syndrome is almost always reversible so that lowering the dose is indicated. Disturbing reports of long-term nephrotoxicity have appeared in the literature. Focal fibrosis and other morphologic changes have been reported. While it is possible that eventual renal damage may occur even with therapeutic levels of lithium, most reported cases have been associated with other symptoms of toxicity.

EKG changes and heart arrhythmias may occur rarely with lithium treatment at therapeutic concentrations, and more commonly at toxic levels. Acneiform eruptions and other skin reactions have also been reported. Lithium possesses teratogenic properties and major cardiovascular anomalies (Ebstein's anomaly) have been reported. Lithium passes the placenta readily and also passes into the milk. As with most drugs, it should be avoided during pregnancy and while taking it, breast feeding should be discouraged.

Dosage and Treatment Schedules

Before starting lithium therapy, a complete physical examination should be performed, with particular attention to kidney and thyroid function. Cardiac disease requires cautious appraisal but is not an absolute contraindication. Indicated pretreatment laboratory tests include CBC, urinalysis, creatinine level, serum electrolytes, thyroid function tests and EKG. The baseline values are important in assessment of both short and long-term side-effects.

Initial dosage will depend on the severity of the illness and the age and body surface of the patient. Individual dosage requirements may be predicted from a single oral dose (31). In general, the average dosage is approximately 900 to 1200 mg per day, but it must be individualized.

ANTIANXIETY AGENTS

The terms used to describe these drugs have changed in the last several years. It seems appropriate to call them antianxiety agents as the term implies a specificity against anxiety although they are frequently called minor tranquilizers. The distinction between the terms antianxiety and hypnotic is also somewhat artificial, inasmuch as most antianxiety agents in higher dosage given at night have sleep-inducing actions, and many hypnotics in lower divided doses given during the day are useful to treat anxiety. However, one should bear in mind that benzodiazepines, which are by far the most commonly used drugs to treat anxiety and induce sleep, fall into different classes depending on their duration of action which is a function of both, the length of their elimination half lives and the formation of active metabolites. This section will be devoted primarily to these agents.

Most benzodiazepines are used as daytime tranquilizers but at least two of them (temazepam and flurazepam) have been promoted as hypnotics and another one (clonazepam) has been marketed as an anticonvulsant. The many benzodiazepines available in clinical practice present us with some problems. Each one of them has been promoted as having its unique properties and advantages. What is clear from pharmacological studies is that they all have antianxiety effects, hypnotic properties, muscle-relaxant activity and anticonvulsive effects when given in appropriate doses.

Clinical comparisons have consistently shown no advantages of using one benozodiazepine or another. However, many studies have not used adequate doses nor equivalent patient populations when testing for clinical differences between these drugs. In general, when using benzodiazepines one must prescribe a dosage that is able to produce the described clinical effects in a particular patient; if with an adequate dosage there is little improvement after two or three weeks, it would seem that other treatment modalities should be considered, and finally, it should be remembered that the level of improvement reached after 4 to 6 weeks is most likely the maximum improvement attainable. Some of these issues have been addressed in detail elsewhere (34).

Mechanisms of Action

Despite various proposed sites and mechanisms of action of benzodiazepines, for the most part, the evidence is contradictory and inconclusive. It is unlikely that a single neural action could explain all of the clinical effects of these drugs.

Attention to elucidate the brain mechanisms associated with therapeutic actions of benzodiazepines has been focused on neurotransmitters (35). Although there is evidence that these agents may affect levels and turnover rates of dopamine, norepinephrine and serotonin, a most persuasive possibility is that these drugs may mimic or enhance the synaptic actions of the inhibitory amino acid neurotransmitter gamma-aminobutyric acid (GABA).

High affinity binding sites for GABA and benzodiazepines at synaptic membrane fractions have both been demonstrated and further, the muscle relaxant potency of benzodiazepines seems to parallel their affinity for their receptor sites. An interaction between these two different receptors has been recently suggested. GABA and GABA-agonists seem to increase the affinity of binding sites for benzodiazepines, an effect that is blocked by

GABA-antagonists, which themselves lower the affinity of the drug receptor sites. Such interactions are interesting since a naturally-occurring protein that inhibits GABA affinity in rat brain membrane fractions has been purified. This "endogenous inhibitor" of GABA receptor is also able to inhibit the binding of benzodiazepines, and conversely, benzodiazepines seem able to displace the endogenous inhibitor and convert the GABA-binding properties of the membrane to their high-affinity state. However, the benzodiazepine and GABA-binding sites do not show a parallel distribution among brain regions and clarification of the relationship of these highly specific mechanisms is awaited.

At a physiologic level, benzodiazepines depress activity in the reticular limbic system while leaving the cerebral cortex relatively unaffected. Following parenteal administration, consciousness disturbances are particularly profound.

Pharmacokinetics

Kinetic studies for benzodiazepines have taught us a great deal about clinical actions, potential benefits, and adverse effects. One way of looking at kinetic behavior of these drugs is by their biotransformation pathways. Essentially, there are two kinds of benzodiazepines: those that are transformed by oxidative pathways which occur slowly and give the drugs, at least in chemical terms, a long duration of action, and those that are transformed by conjugative pathways which occur rapidly and give the drugs a short duration of action. It should also be noted that many of the metabolites produced by oxidative transformation are active, whereas the metabolic products of conjugative transformation are pharmacologically inactive.

Drugs metabolized by oxidation tend to accumulate more because their rate of elimination is slow, whereas drugs metabolized by conjugation tend to accumulate less because they are eliminated faster. The steady state is reached faster by the conjugayed drugs, but if a single dose is missed, blood levels will decline rapidly.

It should be emphasized that factors other than elimination half-lives are operative during single dose administrations. What largely determines the duration of action of a single dose is not so much the elimination half-life as it is the volume of distribution. After distribution is complete, the elimination phase becomes dominant. But the volume of distribution largely determines the duration of action after a single dose. This becomes clinically important because drugs with fastest gastrointestinal absorption rates, such as diazepam and clorazepate, are the ones that reach the blood faster after single doses. They have, therefore, the most rapid and profound onset of activity after a single dose. However, the duration of their action may be short because of its large volume of distribution.

Table VI shows the generic names, trade names, and kinetic properties of benzodiazepines. In considering these, it is essential that not only the kinetics of the parent compound, but also of their active metabolites are taken into account. It is the total of the parent drug plus active metabolites that contributes to the overall clinical effect. This is particularly important during chronic administration when occasionally, metabolite levels are higher than those of parent drugs. The presence of active metabolites is also very important for determining their classification as short-acting or long-acting agents. Once a compound forms considerable amounts of an active metabolite with a relatively long elimination of half-life, it should be regarded as potentially long-acting,

TABLE VI
GENERIC NAMES, TRADE NAMES AND PHARMACOKINETIC PEOPERTIES (34, 36) OF BENZODIAZEPINES

Generic Name	*Trade Name*	*Estimated Half-Life*	*Active Metabolites*	*Biotransformation Pathway*
Chlordiazepoxide	Librium	8-28	+	Oxidation
*Clobazam	Rubanyl	18-42	+	Oxidation
Clonazepam	Clonopin	19-42	–	Reduction
Clorazepate	Tranxene	30-200	+	Oxidation
Diazepam	Valium	26-52	+	Oxidation
*Flunitrazepam	Rohypnol	10-31	+	Oxidation-Reduction
Flurazepam	Dalmane	47-100	+	Oxidation
Lorazepam	Ativan	10-20	–	Conjugation
*Nitrazepam	Mogadon	20-48	–	Reduction
Oxazepam	Serax	5-10	–	Conjugation
Prazepam	Centrax	30-200	+	Oxidation
Temazepam	Restoril	8-20	–	Conjugation
*Triazolam	Halcion	4-10	+	Oxidation

*Not commercially available in the United States

despite the fact that the compound itself might be eliminated quite rapidly.

A great variation between individual kinetic parameters has been noted with these drugs. Such large variability may be attributed to interindividual differences in drug metabolizing capacity (determined by genetic factors, environmental factors, age, sex, diet, etc.) and in drug distribution (determined by body constitution, protein binding, etc.). Therefore, one should bear in mind that an individual patient under treatment may show a pharmacokinetic behavior towards a certain benzodiazepine which is at the extremes of the range and rather far away from the average. These might require substantial dosage adjustments in order to obtain optimal responses. In addition to its clinical implications, pharmacokinetic differences among these drugs are also important for the development of tolerance and abstinence (37).

Clinical Use

The benzodiazepines are the drug treatment of choice in the management of anxiety, insomnia, and stress-related conditions. None of the currently available compounds have any clinical significant advantages over the others. Nevertheless, as mentioned above, some rational choice can be made to attempt to fit the patient's symptom patterns to the pharmacokinetics of the various drugs. Patients complaining of persistent high level of anxiety should benefit from long-acting drugs whereas patients with fluctuating anxiety might benefit from shorter-acting compounds.

For hypnotic purposes, pharmacokinetic considerations are also pertinent. Ideally, hypnotics should induce sleep rapidly and their effects should not persist the next day. Flurazepam, for instance, is inappropriately long-acting unless a persistent anxiolytic effect is welcomed the next day. Lorazepam and temazepam seem most appropriate for pure hypnotic purposes. Lorazepam and diazepam can also be used for relaxation procedures, for preoperative medication, and for sedation during minor operations.

The benzodiazepines have been widely used in management of the alcohol-withdrawal syndrome. Because cross-tolerance exists, large doses are often needed to suppress the withdrawal symptoms. Similarly, benzodiazepines can substitute for alcohol in the chronic alcoholic, especially in those who resort to drink to quell their anxiety symptoms. Caution is needed or else the alcoholic may be converted into a chronic benzodiazepine user. Diazepam has also been used in the treatment of spacticity and tetanus. It helps relieve muscle tension in spastic patients but does so less successfully in patients with upper motor-neuron lesions. The use of diazepam and other benzodiazepines to control seizure activity is well established. However, sedation may limit its use in convulsive disorders.

Doses and Dosage Schedules

Establishing the dosage of a benzodiazepine for a given patient is largely an empirical process. A reasonable approach is to start the drug at the end of the day so that enforced sleepiness can be appreciated. Long-acting drugs can be given in single daily dosage in the evening so that advantage is taken of the hypnotic effects (anxious patients usually complain of initial insomnia anyway), and a mild sedation compatible with unimpaired activities is attained during the day.

However, some patients will request (and it can be acceptable) flexible dosage schedules, but one has to be careful for not reinforcing drug-taking behavior. Usually, doses during the day should be about one-fourth the nighttime dose.

Rapidity of the desired effect and duration of activity are good criteria to determine which of the many available benzodiazepines should be used for a particular patient. A careful evaluation of the presenting signs and symptoms of anxiety and of possible associated problems (medical and nonmedical) becomes mandatory before prescription.

Doses vary, but they should very rarely exceed 30 mg of diazepam a day, which is roughly equivalent to 60 mg of prazepam or chlordiazepoxide, 45 mg of clorazepate, 75 mg of oxazepam of 6 mg of lorazepam (38).

Patients should expect that treatment will be of limited duration and drugs used only when symptoms are discomforting or disabling.

The chronic anxious patient will usually do very well with small doses. Attempts should be made periodically to withdraw the drug. However, some patients will need to be maintained on medication for long periods of time. Provided they receive adequate follow-up, physical dependence should not be a major concern, although psychological dependence is likely to occur.

Unwanted Effects

At high doses, tiredness, drowsiness and a profound feeling of detachment are common. Headache, dizziness, ataxia, confusion and disorientation are less common but may affect the elderly in particular. Marked potentiation of the effects of alcohol occurs. Others far less common unwelcome effects include weight gain, skin rashes, menstrual irregularities and impairment of sexual function.

An increasing hostility is frequently reported by patients starting a course of treatment with benzodiazepine. The clinical significance of this phenomenon is unclear. Adjustment of dosage up or down usually attenuates the impulses.

Dependence, both psychological and physical, can occur with benzodiazepines. Abrupt discontinuation may result in a withdrawal syndrome, featured by anxiety, agitation, restlessness, insomnia, tension and even seizures. This is more likely to occur with the short-acting drugs for reasons of their kinetics (39). Psychological dependence is probably more common, judging by the high incidence of repeated prescriptions but it is also mild, as the drug-seeking behavior of patients taking these drugs has been found to be much less insistent than with other drugs. While overdosage is common, suicide rates are very low with benzodiazepine unless they are also taken in combination with other psychotropic agents or alcohol. Obviously it is recommended to avoid these drugs in people who are likely to abuse them.

Other Drugs to Treat Anxiety

During the first half of the century barbiturates were used as hypnotics and anxiolytics. Today, most clinicians have stopped using them for these purposes, confining their use to serve as anticonvulsants. Clinical trials have shown they generally compare poorly with the benzodiazepines, being less effective and with more side-effects. Chronic toxicity is common and there are many medical contraindications.

Beta-blockers, antidepressants and antipsychotics at low dosages, also have a place in the treatment of anxiety. While the former have been reported to be effective for the somatic symptoms of anxiety, it remains to be confirmed whether they really serve as general anxiolytics.

Frequently, anxiety and depression coexist. Both monoamine reuptake inhibitors and/or monamine oxidase inhibitors usually suffice. Occasionally, a benzodiazepine can be added during the first few days of treatment.

As for the antipsychotics, particularly the phenothiazines, if given at low doses for brief periods in selected patients, they may prove salutory when emotional turmoil is accompanied by agitation and anxiety.

With a reasoned approach to treatment, anxiety can be managed with medications, particularly with benzodiazepines, which despite publicity to the contrary, are neither pancrea nor poison (40).

REFERENCES

1. Lipton, M., DiMascio, A., and Killam K.F. (eds): Psychopharmacology. A Generation of Progress. New York, Raven Press, 1978.

2. Hollister, L.E.: Clinical pharmacology of psychotherapeutic drugs. New York, Churchill Livingstone, 1978.

3. Van Praag, H.M.: Psychotropic drugs. A guide for the practitioner. London, MacMillan, 1978.

4. Deniker, P.: Introduction of neuroleptic chemotherapy into psychiatry. Ayd, F.J., and Blackwell, B. (eds.): In Discoveries of Biological Psychiatry. Philadelphia, J.B. Lippincott Co., pp 155-164, 1970.

5. Carlsson, A., Lindqvist, M.: Effects of chloropromazine or haloperidol on formation of 3-methoxy-thyramine and normetanephrine in mouse brain. Acta Pharmacol Toxicol, *20:*140-144, 1963.

6. Creese, I., Burt, D.R., and Snyder, S.H.: Dopamine receptor binding predicts clinical and pharmacological potencies of antischizophrenic drugs. Science, *192:*481-483, 1976.

7. Richelson, E.: Neuroleptic and neurotransmitter receptors. Psychiatric Ann, *19:*21-40, 1980.

8. Rivera-Calimlin, L., Nasrallah, H., *et al.*: Clinical response and plasma levels: Effects of dose, dosage schedules and drug interactions on plamsa chlorpromazine levels. Am J Psychiat, *133:*646-652, 1976.

9. Davis, J.M., Janowski, D.S., Scherke, H.J., *et al.*: The pharmacokinetics of butaperazine in serum. In: Advances in Biochemical Psychopharmacology of Phenothiazines and Related Drugs, Forrest, I.S., *et al.* (eds). Raven Press, New York, 433-443, 1979.

10. Cressman, W.A., Bianchine, J.R., Slotnick, V.B., *et al.*: Plasma levels profile of haloperidol in man following intramuscular administration. Eur J Clin Pharmacol, *7:*99-103, 1974.

11. Lader, M.: Introduction to psychopharmacology. The Upjohn Co., Kalamazoo, Mich., 51-67, 1980.

12. National Institute of Mental Health: Psychopharmacology Service Center Collaborative Study Group: Phenothiazine treatment of acute schizophrenia. Arch Gen Psychiat, *10:*246-261, 1964.

13. Baldessarini, R.J.: Neurological toxicology of antipsychotic drugs. McLean Hosp J, *4:*2-19, 1979.

14. Lehman, H.E.: Psychopharmacological treatment of schizophrenia. Schizophrenia Bulletin, *13:*27-45, 1975.

15. Peroutka, S.J., and Snyder, S.: Relationship of neuroleptic drug effects at brain dopamine, serotonin, α-adrenergic and histamine receptors to clinical potency. Am J Psychiat, *137:*1518-1522, 1980.

16. Schildkraut, J.J.: The catecholamine hypothesis of affective disorders: A review of supporting evidence. Am J Psychiat, *122:*509-522, 1965.

17. Richelson, E.: Tricyclic antidepressants: Interactions with Histamine and Muscarinic acetylcholine receptors. In Antidepressants: Neurochemical, Behavioral and Clinical Perspectives, Enna, S.J., *et al.* (eds.). New York, Raven Press, 53-73, 1981.

18. Peroutka, S.J., and Snyder, S.H.: Interactions of antidepressants with neurotransmitter receptor sites. In Antidepressants: Neurochemical, Behavioral and Clinical Perspectives, Enna, S.J., *et al.* (eds.). New York, Raven Press, 75-90, 1981.

19. Iversen, L.L., and MacKay, A.V. P.: Pharmacodynamics of antidepressant and antimanic drugs. In Psychopharmacology of affective disorders. A British association for psychopharmacology monograph, Paykel, E.S., and Coppen, A., (eds.). Oxford, Oxford University Press, 60-90, 1979.

20. Fuller, R.W.: Enhancement of monoaminergic neurotransmission by antidepressant drugs. In Antidepressants: Neurochemical, Behaviorall and Clinical Perspectives, Enna, S.J., *et al.* (eds.). New York, Raven Press, 1-12, 1981.

21. Charney, D.S., Menkes, D.B., and Heninger, G.R.: Receptor sensitivity and the mechanism of action of antidepressant treatment. Arch Gen Psychiat, *38:*1160-1180, 1981.

22. Peet, M., and Coppen, A.: The Pharmacokinetics of antidepressant drugs: Relevance to their therapeutic effect. In Psychopharmacology of affective disorders. A British association for psychopharmacology monograph, Paykel, E.S., and Coppen A. (eds.). Oxford, Oxford University Press, 91-107, 1979.

23. Rish, S.C., Janowsky, D.S., and Huey, L.: Plasma Clinical Efficacy. In Antidepressants: Neurochemical, Behavioral and Clinical Perspectives, Enna, S.J., *et al.* (eds.). New York, Raven Press, 193-217, 1981.

24. Van Praag, H.M.: The Significance of Biological Factors in the Diagnosis of Depressions: I Biochemical Variables. Comprehensive Psychiatry, *23:*124-135, 1982.

25. Van Praag, H.M.: The significance of Biological Factors in the Diagnosis of Depressions: II Hormonal Variables. Comprehensive Psychiatry, *23:*216-226, 1982.

26. Raft, B., Davidson, J., Wasik, J., *et al.*: Relationship between response to phenelzine and MAO inhibition in a clinical trial of phenelzine, amitriptyline and placebo. Neuropsychobiol, *7:*122-126, 1981.

27. Paykel, E.S.: Management of acute depression. In Psychopharmacology of affective disorders. A British association for psychopharmacology Monograph, Paykel, E.S., and Coppen A., (eds.). Oxford, Oxford University Press, 235-247, 1979.

28. Monoamine oxidase inhibitors for depression. Med Lett Drugs Ther, *22:*58-60, 1980.

29. Goldberg, R.B., and Thornton, W.E.: Combined tricyclic-MAOI therapy for refractory depression: a review with guidelines for appropriate usage. J Clin Pharmacol, *18:*143-147, 1978.

30. Lewis, D.A.: Lithium in internal medicine and psychiatry: An outline. J Clin Psychiat, *8:*314-320, 1982.

31. Cooper, T.B., and Simpson, G.M.: the 24-hour serum lithium level as a prognosticator of dosage requirements: a 2-year follow-up study. Am J Psychiat, *133:*440-443, 1976.

32. Transbol, I., Christiansen, C., and Baastrup, P.C.: Endocrine effects of lithium: I. Hyperthyroidism, its prevalence in long-term treated patients. Acta Endocrinol, *87:*759-767, 1978.

33. Glen, A.J.M., Dodd, M., Holme, E.B., *et al.*: Mortality on lithium. Neuropsychobiol, *5:*167-173, 1979.

34. Hollister, L.E., Greenblat, D.J., Rickels, K., and Ayd, F.J.: Benzodiazepines 1980: Current update. Psychosomatics, *21:*1-32, 1980 (Supplement).

35. Snyder, S.H., Enna, S.J., and Young, A.B.: Brain mechanisms associated with therapeutic actions of benzodiazepines: Focus on neurotransmitters. Am J Psychiat, *134:*662-665, 1977.

36. Breimer, D.D., Jochemsen, R., and Von Albert, H.H.: Pharmacokinetics of benzidiazepines. Drug Res, *30:*875-881, 1980.

37. Greenblat, D.J., and Shader, R.I.: Dependence, tolerance and addiction to benzodiazepines: Clinical and pharmacokinetic considerations. Drug Metab Rev, *8:*13-28, 1978.

38. Rosenbaum, J.F.: The drug treatment of anxiety, New Eng J Med, *306:*401-404, 1982.

39. de la Fuente, J.R., Rosenbaum, A.H., Martin, H.R., *et al.*: Lorazepam related withdrawal seizures. Mayo Clin Proc, *55:*190-192, 1980.

40. Lader, M.: Benzodiazepines Panacea or Poison? Aust NZ J Psychiat, *15:*1-9, 1981.

18 Electroconvulsive Therapy

Pamela Wallace

ABSTRACT

Electroconvulsive therapy (ECT) is a widely used treatment modality in psychiatry and is the source of much controversy. Its exact mode of action remains unknown. Used for a wide variety of disorders in the past, ECT is today primarily indicated for the treatment of depression, in which its efficacy has been proven, and secondarily for schizophrenia and acute mania. Medical modifications have eliminated many of the risks and side-effects once associated with ECT; current risks are associated primarily with the anesthesia that accompanies the treatment. Concerns about memory loss and possible brain damage persist, and these give rise to many legal and ethical questions and suggest the need for more explicit guidelines for the use and administration of ECT.

Electroconvulsive therapy is a treatment modality that is widely used in psychiatry, about which there is an enormous amount of conflicting professional opinion and public misgiving. A random survey of 20% of the members of the American Psychiatric Association, conducted by the APA Task Force on Electroconvulsive Therapy, in 1978, revealed that 32% of the 2,973 respondents had some degree of opposition to ECT, 67% some degree of approval and 1% ambivalence. The majority of those responding agreed that ECT could be the most effective treatment for some types of patients but a majority also agreed that there is a need for more explicit guidelines for the use of ECT.

HISTORY

As early as the late 18th century, convulsions induced by lage doses of camphor were used in the treatment of mental disorders. Meduna popularized convulsive treatment in Hungary in

1935, based on the observation and belief that schizophrenia and epilepsy did not occur together in a patient and therefore might be antagonists. It was noted that some psychotic symptoms disappeared after spontaneous convulsions. In 1938, Cerletti and Bini in Italy first advanced the technique of producing convulsions by passing electrical current through the head. Their initial treatment used alternating current from a light circuit at 50 to 60 cycles per second, 70 to 150 volts, and 0.1 to 1.0 second. The initiators of convulsive therapy viewed the convulsion as the essential therapeutic element.

Over the years, many modifications have developed, including changes in the electrical current itself and medical modifications of the convulsive response. The original sine wave current has been replaced with rectangular or other steep wave unidirectional current and brief pulses that decrease the amount of current necessary to produce a convulsion. Muscle relaxation has been employed to decrease the peripheral manifestations of the seizure and reduce the risk of injury to the patient. Curare was first used for this purpose by Bennett in 1940 but has been replaced by succinylcholine to prevent the complications of prolonged dyspnea in cardiovascular collapse, which resulted in several deaths among curare treated patients.

Over the years, public opinion of ECT has been affected by sensational journalism and the biases of various subgroups within the psychiatric community. During the 1940's, many analysts believed that ECT aided repression and rendered psychotherapy useless. It was often written that the benefit of ECT stemmed from the fears and anxiety that it produced in patients before delivery of the shock. The work "shock" itself carried a connotation of punishment. Psychologists rarely made use of animal models to explain the effect of ECT with primary theories involving fear, guilt, and punishment. Some authors today believe that many of the early theories of ECT supposed the view that amnesia, pain, and punishment were central to the whole procedure and its therapeutic effectiveness.

INDICATIONS

In 1947 and 1950, the Group for the Advancement of Psychiatry reported that "ECT . . . shortened the duration of psychotic depression, involutional depression, and depression associated with organic brain disease and was beneficial for some patients with neurotic depression. ECT was recognized as effective in the manic phase of manic depressive illness, in schizophrenia with affective disorder, and in organic psychosis with excitement (e.g., catatonia), but was contraindicated for patients with psychosomatic disease, psychopathic personality, behavior disorders of childhood, and neuroses other than neurotic depression."

ECT has been used for many purposes since its introduction 40 years ago. Aside from purely psychiatric illnesses, ECT has been used in epileptics, in an attempt to increase seizure threshold, shorten epileptic twilight states, and terminate incomplete epileptic seizures. It has been used for the psychotic symptoms associated with general paresis, pernicious anemia, lupus erythematosus, multiple sclerosis, bromide intoxication, post-traumatic brain syndromes, porphyria, ACTH and cortisone treatment, and Parkinson's disease. It has also been reportedly used to treat chronic eczema and neurodermititis (the patient gets fuzzy and doesn't scratch), asthma, ulcerative colitis, intractable pain of trigeminal neuralgia and phantom limb pain, narcotic withdrawal, delirium tremens, and alcoholism with delirium tremor. There are also scattered reports in the literature of success with the use of ECT in treating anorexia nervosa, sexual dysfunctions, personality disorders, and making neurotic persons more amenable to psychotherapy. Recent reports in the literature also suggest that ECT may ameliorate phenothiazine-induced Parkinsonism, and have a beneficial effect on tardive dyskinesia.

Today, however, the primary indication for ECT is depression, and the secondary indication is schizophrenia. It is also used in some cases of acute mania. ECT has its greatest usefulness in treating endogenous depression when there is a family history of depression, a history of episodic recurring depression and the patient being treated, a history of diurnal variation with exacerbation of symptoms in the morning and associated symptoms of weight loss, terminal insomnia, and feelings of guilt, sinfulness, and worthlessness. ECT is particularly indicated in the endogeneously depressed, acutely suicidal patient. Involutional depression and unipolar or bipolar depressions, all respond well to ECT.

The results of ECT in schizophrenia are not as impressive. ECT works best in acute schizophrenia, when the illness is of short duration, when there are major affective components, and when there is an identified precipitating event in the history of a relatively well adjusted premorbid personality.

Indications for ECT have changed in recent years with the advent of lithium carbonate therapy for manic depressive illness and neuroleptic treatment for schizophrenia. ECT is still thought by many to be indicated in acute schizophrenia in hopes of obviating long term neuroleptic treatment. Most experts believe that current indications for ECT in schizophrenia include: (1) patients with episodic illness who respond well to a small number of treatments; (2) patients who have episodes of acute exacerbation while receiving neuroleptic drugs; (3) chronic schizophrenic patients who respond poorly to drugs or who may have catatonic episodes that respond well to ECT, and (4) non-compliant patients who will not use neuroleptic agents as directed. Neuroleptic agents usually represent the initial treatment of choice in schizophrenia, however. Regressive ECT — that which is given until the patient is out of contact with reality and incontinent of urine and feces, usually with daily treatments for 7 to 10 days, is recommended in catatonic schizophrenia or in patients being considered for psychosurgery as a last alternative treatment before surgery.

Electroconvulsive therapy is not recommended for use in psychoneurotic patients, although it can be useful in hysterical stupor and continues to be used for severe obsessive compulsive neuroses, even though there is not good evidence of benefit in these patients and there are some reports of exacerbation in obsessive compulsive patients. The APA Task Force stressed its clinical dictum, the observation that ECT increases neurotic anxiety. ECT has also been known to provoke overt psychosis in patients with latent schizophrenia. Post partum psychosis has a variable response to ECT.

MECHANICS OF ADMINISTRATION

Before ECT is administered to a patient, a thorough general medical examination should be done to assess the patient's ability to tolerate the premedication, the anesthesia, and the convulsion itself. The only absolute contraindication to ECT is a brain tumor or the presence of increased intracranial pressure. A recent myocardial infarction is considered an absolute contraindication by some, and Grave's disease is a relative contraindication. Age, pregnancy, cardiovascular disease, abdominal aortic aneurysm, respiratory, rheumatic, and skeletal disease, organic brain syndrome, fever, peptic ulcer, diverticula, and hernias — all of these were once thought to be relative indications, but they need not prevent the use of ECT with current modifications.

An electrocardiogram should be done to rule out recent myocardial infarction and to help with the choice of anesthetic agent, for emthyl hexatol (Brevitol) is superior to thiopenothal (Penothal) in patients with cardiovascular disease.

The patient should receive nothing by mouth, to avoid aspiration, have an empty bladder, and have dentures removed before treatment. Opinions vary greatly as to whether the use of psychotopic medication should be discontinued during the course of ECT. The APA Task Force Survey revealed 54% acceptance to some degree of concomitant drug use, 30% opposition, and 16% ambivalence. There is mounting evidence that the combination of Lithium carbonate in ECT may produce severe acute organic brain syndrome and possibly seizure activity. Physicians must make the decision for each individual patient as to whether or not there will be concomitant use of drugs and ECT. Standard atropine prophylaxis given 20 to 90 minutes before treatment was not thought by the Task Force to allow for individual variable response to the drug, and therefore intravenous atropine in 0.5 mg increments is recommended until the heart rate has increased by 10%. The use of anticholinergic agents decreases salivation and prevents reflex bradycardias resulting from vagolytic action. A short acting barbiturate has been given followed immediately by a muscle relaxant usually succinylcholine. The barbiturate prevents the patient's awareness of respiratory paralysis. Oxygen is administered until the observation of muscle tone which indicates muscle paralysis. A mouth guard is inserted and the electrical stimulus is then given via electrodes placed bilaterally over the temporal regions, or unilaterally over the temporal region and ipsilateral central parietal region. The patient is then reoxygenated until spontaneous respirations return, usually in 2 to 3 minutes. Close nursing supervision should be maintained until the patient has fully regained consciousness. Prochlorperazine (compazine) and Dramamine may be given after treatment to prevent nausea.

The short acting barbiturate is responsible for the majority of complications in present day ECT because of its effect on the cardiovascular system. In addition, barbiturates can precipitate a crisis in patients with porphyria, and one must be aware of this hazard. Complications of sodium thiopentothal include apnea, cough, chest wall spasms, laryngospasm and bronchospasm.

Succinylcholine leads to rapid paralysis and its length of action is determined by the action of a degradatory enzyme, butylcholinesterase, which is decreased in concentration in cases of liver damage, severe anemia, carcinoma, malnutrition or exposure to anticholinesterase agents present in nerve gases and weed killers. The chief complication of the use of succinylcholine is apnea; it occurs in cholinesterase deficiency or in patients with pseudocholinesterase which is inactive against succinylcholine. The problem of pseudocholinesterase which is due to a homozygous recessive trait present in 1 of every 3,000 people must be kept in mind when one administers ECT.

The APA Task Force recommended routine testing of plasma pseudocholinesterase levels in elderly or high risk patients, patients with a personal or family history of abnormal response to succinylcholine or patients with possible exposure to anticholinesterase agents.

The minimal voltage required to stimulate a convulsion is more than 80 volts and variable from patient to patient. For maximum effectiveness, the stimulus must exceed the patient's seizure threshold because subconvulsive stimuli may lead to subsequent confusion without therapeutic results. Threshold levels are greater in female and in older patients and are increased by dehydration, acute excitement, Dilantin therapy, previous seizures, and cold dry weather. The threshold is diminished by water retention, vasopressin, and hypoglycemia in the absence of coma. If within 15 seconds after the electrical stimulus has been given there is no seizure activity, a repeat stimulus should be administered.

Electro-jelly is applied to reduce the resistance of the skin and thereby decrease the threshold. The electrical resistance of the scalp, skull and meninges greatly attenuate the brain potential so that the intensity of the current is not great in any one area of the brain.

Treatment is usually given 3 times weekly or once a day in "regressive" ECT. Depressive illness usually requires 6 to 10 ECT treatments and schizophrenia, 18 to 20 treatments, although up to 40 treatments have been given in schizophrenia. In depressive illness, a positive response to treatment is usually noted after 3 treatments.

EFFICACY

Many studies indicate that ECT is superior to drug treatment of depressed patients. Two major studies of ECT and tricyclic antidepressants produced essentially the same results, showing that ECT was clearly superior to tricyclic antidepressant, monoamine oxidase inhibitors, and placebo in the treatment of depressed patients. ECT produced the quickest amelioration of symptoms, followed by tricyclic Imipramine. ECT was essentially twice as effective as placebo, which itself had a significant effect. Improvement rates with ECT averaged 70 to 80%, compared with 40 to 50% improvement with antidepressant drugs. Studies have concluded that ECT is indicated for acutely suicidal patients, with improvement expected after 3 to 6 treatments. Drug treatment is recommended for nonsuicidal patients, followed by ECT if no response is noted after 3 weeks of drug treatment.

Data suggest that there might also exist an ECT responsive, nondrug responsive population of depressed patients. Reports of the efficacy of antidepressant drugs combined with ECT are variable, although many consider this practice dangerous.

Results show that ECT has its greatest efficacy in psychotic depression with some reports of nearly 100% success with the use of ECT although there is no assurance against recurrence. Remission rates of 80 to 100% have been reported in manic depressive illness treated with ECT, again without any protection against recurrence.

Results in schizophrenia are less encouraging. There is a paucity of evidence supporting the use of ECT in schizophrenia, and many studies claiming success are subject to question because of poor controls and methods which are not technically acceptable by current research criteria. The majority of studies have found no superiority of ECT over drugs. The combination of ECT and phenothazine may be more effective than phenothazines alone, judging by the number of days of required hospital treatment. Good results with 15 to 40 ECT treatments have been reported in acute schizophrenia. It would appear that there is an inverse relationship between the duration of the schizophrenic illness and the efficacy of ECT. In patients who have been symptomatic less that 6 months, a 60% remission rate has been noted; in those symptomatic for 6 to 18 months, the remission rate was 52%; and in those suffering symptoms for longer than 18 months, the remission rate was only 10%. An early relapse following ECT is considered a poor prognostic sign. There are reports of success with ECT in some cases of drug failure. Schizophrenic patients who have a prominent affective component to their illness seemed to respond better to ECT.

Attempts to predict the outcome of treatment of depression with ECT have shown that variables correlated with favorable outcome include sudden onset of the depression, good insight, previous obsessional personality, self-reproach, duration of illness less than one year, and symptoms of early morning awakening, delusions, and psychomotor retardation. Unfavorable variables include hypochondriasis, hysterical attitude toward symptoms, depersonalization, neurotic traits in childhood, neurotic traits in adulthood, inadequate premorbid personality and emotional lability. These findings reinforce the concept that ECT is of little or no benefit in neurotic illness but is effective in endogenous and psychotic depressions.

Attempts have been made to devise a laboratory test to assess the potential benefit of ECT. The dexamethasone suppression test has been shown useful in some cases as a means to monitor the biological response to ECT, although it is not yet in widespread use. The dexamethasone suppression tests which are abnormal in many depressed patients have normalized during the course of ECT associated with clinical improvement.

OTHER EFFECTS OF ECT

One of the most consistent, often discussed and disputed effects of ECT is the memory loss sustained by patients undergoing this procedure. The complaint of memory loss is common, but it varies considerably among patients. The patients who are relieved of emotional distress are less prone to complain of memory loss. There is no good evidence for permanent loss of memory from ECT, although patients may complain of such. Patients are aware of memory impairment, or anterograde memory impairment, but not of memory loss, that is, retrograde memory impairment. Patients can judge their ability to reproduce a thought immediately, whereas forgetting cannot be judged, at least not adequately. ECT appears to have an adverse effect on retention but learning shows improvement parallel to recovery from the depressive state.

From 18 to 67% of patients complain of some persistent memory deficit after ECT, but this has not been confirmed by objective tests. Memory loss was once thought to be necessary for improvement, but it is now known that there is no correlation between memory loss and clinical efficacy. Post treatment memory loss has been objectively evaluated and it has been concluded that both retrograde and anterograde amnesia results from ECT. The retrograde amnesia may extend to events that occurred years before treatment. There is a temporal gradient, however, and most memory loss covers the period three years before treatment. This loss is largely recovered one to two weeks after cessation of treatment.

Many studies have been done comparing the effects and efficacy of bilateral and unilateral ECT. Bilateral ECT has been found to cause greater memory impairment than unilateral ECT on both verbal and nonverbal tasks and in both retrograde and anterograde memory. Complaints of persistent memory loss have also been more frequent among bilaterally treated patients (67%). Objective testing, however, has failed to disclose any difference between bilaterally and unilaterally treated patients in six to nine months of follow-up.

Unilateral ECT with electrode placement over the non-dominant hemisphere was first used by Phenon in Argentina and Lancaster in Great Britain and in 1942 by Freedman and Wilcox in the United States. There seems to be a consensus that unilateral ECT produced less memory impairment, but there is considerable disagreement as to its clinical efficacy. There is some concern that unilateral ECT may be as effective if more treatments are given, however, but it has been suggested that this is due to higher incidents of undetected "no takes" when unilateral ECT is administered.

The only explanation advanced for the memory impairment is that it is somehow related to the path of the electrical current, since there was a bilateral seizure discharge with both unilateral and bilateral ECT. Stimulation of the left hemisphere results in greater impairment on verbal tasks; with the right hemispheric stimulation, the greater impairment is for nonverbal tasks. With bilateral ECT, there is greater electroencephalographic slowing over the dominant hemisphere. After carefully weighing the existing studies, the APA test on ECT preferentially endorsed unilateral ECT.

Multiple ECT has been given at two minute intervals, with anywhere from four to ten treatments per session. Results with this method have been favorable although there are some patients who fail to respond to multiple ECT but subsequently have responded to conventional bilateral ECT.

In addition to memory loss, some patients may experience organic psychotic-like reactions to ECT, with delusional fears, hallucinations, and psychomotor excitement that may last for several days. Other patients may become combative and aggressive immediately after treatment and for up to one half hour. This reaction can sometimes be diminished in a particular patient by switching to unilateral ECT. There is a reported 0.5% incidence of spontaneous seizures in patients treated previously with ECT and this has caused some to advance the theory that ECT may "kindle" seizure foci.

PHYSIOLOGIC CHANGES

The seizure with its accompanying cerebral events is the essential process in ECT. The length of the seizure is related to clinical efficacy, as demonstrated by the fact that efficacy is diminished if the duration of the seizure is decreased by the use of Lidocaine. Brain changes are induced by the seizure, and these changes are reflected in neurologic signs and electroencephalographic (EEG) recordings.

There is an initial jerk following stimulation caused by direct cortical stimulation, followed by a latent period, followed by the tonic-clonic convulsion. The tonic phase lasts approximately 10 to 12 seconds and is followed by a clonic phase of 30 to 50 seconds. The cerebral seizure activity persists longer than the observable musculoskeletal activity. There is a period of relative electrical silence after the seizure, during which the patient is refractory to further induction of seizures.

The degree and duration of the EEG changes in ECT are directly proportional to the frequency and type of seizures, the type of current, and the technique employed. There is evidence that EEG changes persist for up to five weeks if less than six treatments are given, or up to three months after seven to twelve ECT treatments. Memory returns to normal in the majority of the patients, long before the EEG resumes a normal appearance. The nature of the EEG changes and clinical improvement remains obscure.

A prompt increase in cerebral blood flow has been noted which is maximal at three minutes and returns to normal within 30 minutes of the electrical stimulus. During and after treatment, brief capillary leakage occurs secondary to damage of the blood brain barrier. There is also an increase in intracellular free acetyl choline which may play a role in basal dilatation and increased capillary permeability. The increase in permeability of the blood brain barrier lasts longer after a series of ECT, and there is increased permeability to macromolecules. There is increased permeability to serotonin, epinephrine, and norepinephrine. There are increased acetylcholine and decreased acetylcholinesterase levels in the cerebral spinal fluid after ECT and also an increase in cerebral spinal fluid concentration of serotonin.

The exact mode of action of ECT is unknown although many investigators believe that the increased level of acetylcholine, serotonin, and norepinephrine present evidence that depression is secondary to decreased functional levels of norepinephrine and serotonin in various parts of the brain. Animal studies indicate that electrical convulsive stimuli inhibit protein synthesis by decreasing intracellular and total RNA in the central nervous system. In addition, there is an increase of sodium retention for 24 hours after ECT. Sodium transfer from the blood to the cerebral spinal fluid appears abnormally slow in depressed patients and this is reversed by ECT.

In addition to the central nervous system events accompanying ECT, there are many systemic changes, particularly involving the cardiovascular and endocrine systems. Respiration is suspended during the convulsion because of spasm of the respiratory muscles in the glottus. This results in increased carbon dioxide tension of the blood and decreased oxygen tension. The heart rate is often rapid and irregular but bradycardia may also occur. There are marked fluctuations in blood pressure which are diminished in part by the use of atropine and muscle relaxants but numerous cardiac arrhythmias are seen both with and without atropine. Observation under fluoroscopy shows that the heart may stop during the tonic phase of the seizure and the clonic phase may then be accompanied by tachycardia, fibrillations and arrhythmias. The increased salivary and bronchial secretions associated with a convulsion can be counteracted by atropine or other anticholinergic drugs.

There is a brisk outpouring of adrenal corticosteroids during the first few days of ECT followed by a return to normal despite continued treatments. The least of adrenal medullary catecholamines may contribute to hypertension and tachycardia at the time of treatment. Hypoglycemia, with glucose levels 20 to 40% above normal is seen 15 to 30 minutes after the convulsion. Although this effect is decreased by premedication with barbiturates, it may be prudent to monitor blood glucose levels of all diabetics receiving ECT as their need for insulin might increase. Serum changes include an increase in the levels of potassium, calcium, phosphorus, and protein. Menstrual changes are common in women receiving ECT, and an increase in weight and sleep time arousal are also common which may suggest stimulation of the diencephalic pituitary system. Further evidence for this is the 10 to 50 fold increase in serum prolactin concentration noted 15 minutes after electrically induced seizures and an 8 fold increase in ACTH levels after ECT.

MORBIDITY

As previously mentioned, a great deal of opposition to ECT exists both in and out of the medical community. It is estimated that 10,000 ECT treatments are given daily in the United States. Before the use of premedication, the greatest complication was vertebral compression fracture resulting from the muscular skeletal activity of the seizure. With the advent of medical modification, cardiovascular complications have predominated. They are primarily related to the use of barbiturate anesthesia and its effects on the cardiovascular system.

In some patients in whom there is a high risk of cardiovascular side-effects, a subconvulsive stimulus may be given to cause unconsciousness, before administration of succinylcholine, which will thereby obviate barbiturate anesthesia.

The fatality rate for ECT varies from 0.003% to 0.8%. The most frequent cause of death is myocardial infarction or cardiac arrest. The most extensive study of ECT related deaths showed that half of these occurred with the initial treatment and that the risk of death was 10 fold for patients more than 60 years old.

As mentioned, the only absolute contraindication for ECT is an intracranial neoplasm. Relative contraindications, however, include the following: duodenal ulcer, subdiaphragmatic hernia, abdominal aortic aneurysm, glaucoma, threatening retinal detachment, recent myocardial infarction, angina, congestive heart failure, thrombophlebitis, severe osteoporosis, major fractures, acute and chronic respiratory disease, recent cerebral vascular accident, pernicious anemia, thyrotoxocosis, pregnancy, tuberculosis, endocarditis, myocarditis, and mitral stenosis.

Frequent patient complaints after treatment include headache (29%), nausea, dizziness, drowsiness, confusion, anorexia, weakness, and palpitations. Regressive ECT leads to eventual incontinence and dysarthria.

Many persons outside the psychiatric community, and some professionals, are spreading the belief that ECT causes permanent brain damage. There are reports of ECT precipitating Parkinsonism symptoms and cognitive dysfunctions. On a pathologic level, there are reports of reticular hemorrhage, in the path of electrical current in experimental animals subjected to shock. There have also been descriptions of various cell changes in the brain as a result of ECT. There has been, however, no extensive neuropathologic study of the effects of "modern" ECT, and thus far there is not convincing evidence that ECT in a healthy ventilated subject causes more than transient alterations of cerebral function.

LEGAL AND ETHICAL CONSIDERATIONS

It is obvious that much remains unknown about ECT, but also that ECT has undisputed clinical efficacy, particularly in endogenous depressive syndromes. An overview of ECT would not be complete without a brief discussion of some of the ethical and legal aspects of the treatment.

Questions arise as a result of the physically invasive nature of the procedure, the bad reputation ECT had when it was given without medical modifications, and the potential for severe neurologic or other side-effects.

Ethical concerns arise over: (1) the right to receive ECT; (2) the right to refuse ECT or to stop it after initial consent and treatment, and (3) the nature of informed consent about ECT and its potential hazards. First of all, if one accepts the data on the efficacy of ECT, it would seem an ethical obligation to offer ECT to consenting voluntary patients, especially those who have not responded to other types of treatment or who, for medical reasons, cannot tolerate antidepressant drugs.

Secondly, the patient must have the right to decide his own destiny and refuse treatment. The dilemma comes when the nature of the patient's illness renders him incompetent to make a rational decision about his or her own well being. This brings in the concept of psychiatric paternalism and raises the question of whether the psychiatrist has the right to do more than offer treatment.

In regard to informed consent, one can query how much information is necessary for the patient, or how much the patient can understand. May one ethically treat patients on the basis of their consent when they may be incapable of fully comprehending what they are told and making a decision on the basis of it?

Efforts are currently in progress to establish ECT guidelines and to institute an annual review of the use of ECT.

One suggested set of guidelines for the use of ECT is as follows:

1. ECT should be fully voluntary whenever possible.
2. When the patient is unable or incompetent to give informed consent, a court hearing should be convened and a guardian appointed to act on behalf of the patient.
3. Informed consent should include information on (a) the increased risk of concurrent medical problems or dementia, (b) the potential for memory loss with reassurance that this is usually transient and (c) the risks of not having ECT or some other treatment or somatic therapy.

The APA Task Force advises the keeping of meticulous records by all those who prescribe and administer this admittedly effective but highly controversial form of treatment.

REFERENCES

1. Abrams, R.: Recent Clinical Studies of ECT, *Seminars in Psychiatry*, Vol. VI, No. 1, 1-10, Feb. 1972.

2. Albala, A.A. and Greden, J.F.: Case report, Amer J Psychiat, *137:* 393, March, 1980.

3. Anarth, J., *et al.*: Ameliorating Drug Induced Parkinsonism. Amer J Psychiat, *136:*8, Aug., 1970.

4. Cronholm, B. and Ottosson, J.: The experience of memory function after ECT. Brit J Psychiat, *109:* 251-258, 1963.

5. Colver, C.M., *et al.*: ECT and Special Problems of Informed Consent, Amer J Psychiat, *137:*5, May, 1980.

6. Davidson, J., *et al.*: A comparison of ECT and combined phenelzine-amitriptyline in refractory depression. Arch Gen Psychiat, *35:* 639-642, May, 1978.

7. Dornbush, R.L.: Memory and induced ECT convulsions. *Seminars in Psychiatry*, Vol. VI, No. 1, 47-54, Feb., 1972.

8. Dysken, M.W.: Serial post dexamethasone cortisol levels in patients undergoing ECT. Amer J Psychiat, *136:* 10, Oct., 1979.

9. Essman, W.B.: Neurochemical changes in ECS and ECT. *Seminars in Psychiatry*, Vol. VI, No. 1, 67-79, Feb., 1972.

10. Fink, M.: The mode of action of convulsive therapy: the neurophysiologic adaptive view. J Neuropsych, *3:* 231-233, 1962.

11. Fink, M.: Myths of shock therapy. Am J Psychiat, *134:* 991-995, Sept., 1977.

12. Fink, M.: The therapeutic process in ECT. *Seminars in Psychiatry*, Vol. VI, No. 1, 39-46, Feb., 1972.

13. Fink, M. and Abrams, R.: Answers to questions frequently asked about ECT. *Seminars in Psychiatry*, Vol. VI, No. 1, 33-38, Feb. 1972.

14. Furlong, F.W.: The mythology of electroconvulsive therapy. Comprehen Psych, *13:* 235-239, May, 1972.

15. Greenblatt, M., *et al.*: Differential response of hospitalized depressed patients and somatic therapy. Am J Psychiat, *16:* 935-943, 1964.

16. Greenblatt, M.: Efficacy of ECT in affective and schizophrenic illness. Am J Psychiat, *134:* 1001-1005, 1977.

17. Holmberg, G.: Biological aspects of ECT. Int Rev Neurobiol, *5:* 389-412, 1963.

18. Hurwitz, T.D.: Electroconvulsive therapy: a review. *Comprehen Psych*, Vol. 15, No. 4, July/Aug., 1974.

19. Kalinowsky, L.B.: ECT and other convulsive treatments. *Am Handbook of Psych*, 2nd Ed., Vol. V, 531-548, 1975.

20. Kalinowsky, L.B. and Hippus, H.: *Pharmacological, Convulsive, and Other Somatic Treatment in Psychiatry.* Grave and Stratton, New York, 1969.

21. Mandel, M.R., *et al.*: Intoxication associated with Lithium and ECT. Amer J Psych, *137:* 9, Sept. 1980.

22. O'Dea, J.P.K. *et al.*: Prolactin changes during ECT. Amer J Psych, *135:* 5, May, 1978.

23. Pitts, F.N. Jr.: Medical aspects of ECT, *Seminars in Psychiatry*, Vol. VI, No. 1, 27-32, Feb. 1972.

24. Price, T.P. and Levin, R.: Effects of electroconvulsive therapy on tardive dyskinesia. Am J Psych, *135:* 8, Aug. 1978.

25. Ruff, R.C.: A case report of cognitive impairment and movement disorder associated with ECT. Amer J Psych, *137:* 12, Dec. 1980.

26. Salzman, C.: ECT and ethical psychiatry. Am J Psych, *134:* 1006-1009, 1977.

27. Salzman, C.: The use of ECT in the treatment of schizophrenia. Amer J Psych, *137:* 9, Sept. 1980.

28. Smith, D., Surphlis, W.R.P., Gynther, M.D., *et al.*: Cited by Davis, J.M., Cole, J.O.: Antipsychotic Drugs, In: *American Handbook of Psychiatry*, Vol. 5, 2nd Ed. Edited by Arieti, S., Freedman, D.K., Dyrud, J.E. New York, Basic Books, 441-475, 1975.

29. Squire, L.R.: ECT and memory loss. Am J Psych, *134:*997-1001, 1977.

30. Squire, L.R. and Slater, P.: Bilateral and unilateral ECT: Effects on verbal and non-verbal memory. Amer J Psych, *135:*11, Nov. 1978.

31. Strain, J.J., *et al.*: Comparison of therapeutic effects and memory changes with bilateral and unilateral ECT. Am J Psych, *125:*50-60, 1968.

32. Task Force: Report 14: Electroconvulsive Therapy. Washington, DC, American Psychiatric Association, 1978.

33. Volvaka, J.: Neurophysiology of electroconvulsive therapy. *Seminars in Psychiatry*, Vol. VI, No. 1, 55-65, 1972.

34. Weiner, R.D.: The psychiatric use of electrically induced seizures. Amer J Psych, *136:*12, 1507-1517, Dec. 1979.

35. Weiner, R.D., *et al.*: Prolonged confusional state and EEG seizure activity following concurrent ECT and Lithium use. Amer J Psych, *137:*11, Nov. 1980.

36. Yudofsky, S.C. and Rosenthal, N.E.: ECT in a depressed patient with adult onset diabetes mellitus. Amer J Psych, *137:*1, Jan. 1980.

19 Psychosurgery

Gerald C. Peterson

BACKGROUND

Psychosurgery is the most ethically and morally controversial treatment in psychiatry. It is the cutting, removal, or coagulation of brain tissue to produce a change in emotion or behavior. The procedure was first reported by Egas Moniz, a Portuguese psychiatrist, in 1936. Thousands of procedures were performed between that time until the early 1950's. The purpose of the procedure was to reduce intractible, aggressive, and severely disturbed behavior in chronically ill psychiatric patients. The popularity of the procedure and the zeal of the psychiatrists and neurosurgeons performing the procedure during those years is understandable when one realizes effective antipsychotic and antidepressant medications were not available until the 1950's. The popularity of psychosurgery has declined dramatically since the 1950's and currently only between 200 and 300 procedures are done each year in the United States.

THEORETICAL BASIS

The majority of procedures done today are aimed at disruption of nerve tracks between the frontal portions of the brain and the deep, midline limbic system or within the limbic system itself. The limbic system, consisting of amygdala, cingulum, fornix, cingulate gyrus, and portions of the thalamus and hypothalamus, is the area of the brain involved in production of emotional response. The cingulum is the primary nerve fiber bundle carrying messages within the limbic system, and it is postulated that interruption of the cingulum bundle will reduce the intensity of emotionality.

The frontal area of the brain is involved in such high level psychological functions as anticipation of how a person's behavior will affect his environment, insight, foresight, and modification of responses to fit the person's social situation. It has long been observed clinically that damage to this area of the brain results in reduction of worry, pessimism, anxiety, the person is less concerned about past or future consequences of his behavior and at times may become crude, impulsive, and childish. Patients who are excessively worrisome, depressed, anxious, and over-react to environmental events would be most likely to benefit from surgical interruption of inputs from the prefrontal area of the brain into the limbic system.

PROCEDURES PERFORMED

In the early years of psychosurgery, a lesion was made to interrupt fibers passing from the prefrontal area to the limbic system by inserting a leukotome through burr holes in the frontal area of the skull. Freeman, an American psychiatrist, popularized a procedure involving puncture of the superior, orbital plate with an ice pick and producing a lesion in the inferior, medial portion of the frontal lobe. These early procedures resulted in a significant morbidity with mortality rates ranging as high as 5% and production of postoperative epilepsy in up to 15% of patients. With these procedures, larger areas of brain were affected and sometimes resulted in production of a frontal lobe syndrome with crude impulsive behavior, childishness, overeating, obesity, and lack of motivation. In recent years, much more limited procedures on the frontal lobe have been undertaken.

Lesions of the cingulum bundle may also be produced with a wire leukotome or by electrocoagulation using stereotactic placement. The lesions are small, generally about 1 cm in diameter bilaterally. Modified frontal leukotomy is done stereotactically using a wire loop leukotome with the extent of the lesion variable depending on the severity of symptoms presented by the patient. The morbidity to the patient is much less with these procedures with the mortality rate generally below .1% and an epilepsy rate of about .7%. The production of a "frontal lobe syndrome" is almost unheard of following a cingulotomy and is relatively infrequent with limited frontal leukotomy. Areas of the brain involved in motor control, vision, sensation, memory, and language are avoided and general intelligence is not impaired in complicated cases. It is not unusual to see an improvement in IQ scores following the procedure as the patient is less troubled by anxiety and difficulty concentrating while performing intellectual tasks.

WHO IS LIKELY TO BENEFIT

Because of other effective treatment available today, psychosurgery is generally reserved for those patients who have been refractory or only temporarily improved with the use of psychotropic medications, psychotherapy, or electroconvulsive therapy. Generally, the procedure is done on these highly selected patients only after months or even years of intensive psychiatric therapy. People who show excessive concientiousness, excessive drive, severe obsessiveness, and excessive anxiety as part of their basic personality are more likely to have a beneficial outcome. People who are schizoid, paranoid, have a schizophrenic illness, or are tempermentally very changeable are more likely to have an unfavorable outcome. Generally, schizophrenic patients do not benefit greatly from psychosurgery, particularly those who have blunting of their emotions. Thought disorders, delusions, and hallucinations are not improved by psychosurgery, although some schizophrenics with marked excitability or depression may benefit by reduction of these symptoms. Severe incapacitating anxiety, unrelenting depression, severe phobias, and severe persistent obsessive compulsive disorders all have been benefited by psychosurgery. The presence of severe chronic pain also responds well to cingulotomy or modified, prefrontal leukotomy. Psychosurgery has been proposed for other psychiatric disorders including drug addiction, alcoholism, severe personality disorder, or sexual deviance, but the outcome with these patients is variable. An ideal candidate for psychosurgery would be a patient who has always been overly conscientious, worrisome, and compulsive who has developed a severe, anxiety state, depressive state, or obsessive compulsive disorder that has been unresponsive or only briefly responsive to other therapy and has been treated by competent psychiatrists for an extended period of time.

SPECIFIC NURSING CONCERNS

Because of the irreversible nature of the procedure, the behavior of the patients must be well documented prior to surgery and reassessed postoperatively. Observation of the patient over an extended period of time is essential and basic psychological testing of intelligence, personality characteristics, and a complete neurological evaluation are essential. The relatives and the patient must be advised preoperatively of the nature of the procedure and the risks involved. Options for other therapy should be discussed and the patient and relatives should enter into the procedure fully informed and with mutual consent. The patient should be allowed to express his own thoughts and feelings about the procedure and especially his expectations of outcome.

The patient may ask to talk to someone who has had the procedure and this can be reassuring and helpful. However, because of issues of confidentiality, this is often not possible. The patient should be told he will have a moderate headache for a few days postoperatively and will receive medication to control it. The scalp will be shaved above the forehead for the burr holes and he or she should be informed that there will be two small depressions in the skull with small scars where the burr holes are made. The patient can be reassured that he or she will function as well after the surgery as before and hopefully better because of a reduction in his symptoms, but that it may take up to six months for complete improvement to be noted.

Usually, the patient is in the hospital for only a short period of time (usually less than a week) for the procedure, and he will be prepared for surgery and followed on a neurosurgical unit where the nurses are familiar with neurosurgical patients and procedures. He or she can be informed that four out of five patients with severe anxiety and depression are improved by the procedure, but ocasionally it is not helpful and some patients may eventually relapse. Occasionally, after a cingulomotomy procedure, patients have urgency of urination for approximately three days postoperatively and should be informed and reassured about this. In general, preoperative and postoperative care is the routine for any neurosurgical patient, although obviously a psychosurgery patient may require more intensive psychiatric support and will need psychiatric follow-up.

ETHICAL AND LEGAL CONSIDERATIONS

Because normal tissue is operated on and the procedure is irreversible, ethical issues arise concerning alteration of the patient's personality. Usually, basic personality characteristics are affected to a minor degree and the overall long-term effect of better adaptation and freedom of psychiatric symptoms must be considered. As in all surgical procedures, harm may result but the overall harmful effects of the procedure are very low as previously noted. Generally, the patient is most concerned when the procedure has been ineffective in reducing his symptoms or he has recurrence in the future following relief of his discomfort postoperatively. It is imperative that the patient is well informed of the procedure and potential for improvement and he should enter into the procedure being completely informed and having given freely his consent. Under no circumstances should the patient's civil rights be abridged.

Legally, the patient should sign a prepared consent form for his procedure acknowledging his concurrence and that he has been informed of the risks. If the patient is incompetent to give consent, occasionally this can be obtained through court appointed guardians. Most states have now set up psychosurgery guidelines considering the procedure experimental, stating that it should only be performed in patients who are refractory to all other forms of psychiatric therapy. A psychosurgery committee to review the indications for the procedure and to interview the patient is set up by the hospital and includes an uninvolved psychiatrist, a neurologist, and a neurosurgeon. This review panel should discuss the case at length and concur with the decision to proceed with psychosurgery. Adequate documentation of the patient's psychological functioning and psychiatric disturbance must be demonstrated and documented prior to surgery and adequate provisions must be provided for follow-up observation and testing. Both the commission established by the United States Congress in 1974 on the use of psychosurgery and the APA Task Force have rejected the proposal that psychosurgery for therapeutic reasons be prohibited by law.

THE FUTURE

The place and usefulness of psychosurgery has still not been clearly established in psychiatric treatment. The procedures undertaken currently are limited and safe and as more well-documented follow-up studies are done, the usefulness of the various procedures should become clearer. As more becomes known about the function of various areas of the brain, more specific procedures may become available. Even though currently limited to a highly select group of patients, psychosurgery could conceivably be performed more frequently in the future as more specific information becomes available. On the contrary, if psychotropic medications become more effective, the number of procedures may diminish. Because it has been demonstrated to be effective in certain patients, psychosurgery should continue to be considered as highly effective therapy in a selected group of patients.

20 Family Therapy

Larry Goodlund and Diane Goodlund

Family therapy is a process of intervention designed to decrease stress of symptom formation within a family. Family therapy differs from other treatment modalities fundamentally in that it views the family, not the individual, as the basic unit of pathology. It is a relatively new form of therapy arising in the '40's and '50's, but not becoming a required part of psychiatric training until the late 1970's (AMA Directory of Residency Training Programs 1979–1980). While a comprehensive historical review of the subject is beyond the scope of this chapter, interest in the family as a pathological unit began in 1937, when Nathan Ackerman published, *The Family as a Social and Emotional Unit.* Gradually, in the 1940's and '50's, the momentum increased, with a number of research centers being formed throughout the United States. Often, the researchers worked in complete isolation of each other, and as a result, today there continue to be multiple schools of family therapy relying on differing theoretical bases. Guerin (1976) provides an excellent historical review of the development of family therapy and the interactions between early pioneers, who by the strength of their personalities have tended to dominate the field for over 25 years.

Traditional psychiatric therapy has tended to rely heavily on the medical model, or the treatment of a disease process in an individual. In varying degrees, family therapy has diverged from this model, borrowing from a wide variety of theoretical backgrounds, communications theory, learning theory, general systems theory, and traditional theories such as psychoanalysis. In general, the person's behavior is viewed in the context of the family, and the meaning of behavior comes from its usefulness to the family. Families are seen as desiring stability or homeostasis. Stress arises when the family is unable to deal with such problems as financial crisis, the changing developmental needs of the children, death, or medical illness.

Family therapy may be divided into several major theoretical orientations. These include the following: behavioral, analytical, or insight; communications, structural, and strategic theory. Behavioral family therapy relies heavily on social learning theory. Patterson (1971) in essence, teaches families the techniques of behavior modification. The role of reinforcement, contracts, and negotiation are all taught to family members. Change occurs with increased consistency in the parents, increased structure within the family, and more straightforward communication. It is perhaps the simplest form of family therapy to learn, and is useful with families in which the pathology is not profound. Highly disorganized families in which the pathology revolves around noncompliant children and parents with inconsistent discipline approaches are often helped by this method.

Insight oriented family therapy has its origin in psychoanalytic theory. Nathan Ackerman was, until his death, the leading spokesman of this theoretical position. The individual members of the family are seen as carrying a series of incorrect or irrational beliefs about themselves and other family members. It is theorized that if these beliefs are uncovered, the family members will be able to interact on a higher plane.

Family therapy's advantage over individual therapy is that it allows the therapist the opportunity to see the interactions directly, rather than through the distortions of the family members. In addition, it tends to bring the conflicts from the past into the present. Individual conflicts are analyzed as to the impact they have on the overall family functioning, and communication is interpreted. Feelings are elicited in an attempt to bring them into conscious awareness, and transference is analyzed.

An example of therapy with an insight orientation is that of a middle class family of four: the father is a highly trained professional who is moderately depressed and who prides himself on being able to take criticism from the other family members without being affected personally. His two sons and wife were increasingly concerned about his withdrawal. During a session in approximately the middle of therapy, his wife initially confronted the therapist with his lack of sensitivity towards her in a previous session. She then attempted to withdraw from further discussion of the subject but it became apparent to the therapy team that this pattern was a reaction of a recurrent lack of conflict resolution between the husband and wife. During the course of therapy session, this transference to the therapist was interpreted. The family members were allowed to convey their concerns toward their father/husband and he was helped to talk about his depression.

The proponents of communications include such diverse theorists as Bateson and colleagues who in 1956 published the controversial work, *Toward a Theory of Schizophrenia*, in which they described the "double bind." The "double bind" is a situation in which one person, defined as the victim, through repeated experiences, is given by other family members a primary injunction followed by a secondary conflicting injunction at a more abstract level. For example, a primary statement "come hug me," followed by the secondary communication in which the parent receives the child in a stiff, unloving manner. This communication is followed by a yet third negative injunction prohibiting the victim from escaping. Over a period of time, this pattern was believed to lead to the development of schizophrenia. Later, John Weakland, a member of the Bateson team (1974), wrote concerning the relationship between behavior and communication. He saw the main function of this controversial article as a step in the formation of communications theory.

Virginia Satir, as much as anyone, has popularized the communications theory of family therapy through numerous demonstrations across the country. She uses sculpting, a technique in which family members are arranged in physical positions as a way to visually demonstrate the family's communication problem. In a family with a rigid, noncompromising father and a passive son, the dyad might be cast with the father standing scowling with his arms across his chest looking down on a kneeling, begging son. Also, Satir uses clarification, simplification and role play as tools to improve communication and to point out disguised emotional content.

Watzlawick formulated a structured family interview consisting of 8 tests including defining the families' main problem, planning something together, and describing each person's positive and negative points. He used a basic communications theory technique which has great diagnostic value and can be a powerful tool especially when combined with video tape replay. Later work by Watzlawick seems to fit in the strategic group.

It is probable that communications theory is a special case of insight oriented psychotherapy. It was included here as a separate technique because of it's differences from classic analytical approaches.

Structural family therapy has been popularized by Minuchin, its primary theoretician. In Minuchin's approach, he sees the individual in his social context and uses a technique for changing the basic organizational system of the family. He believes that if the family structure is changed, the positions of each of the members of the group are also changed. This process leads to a change in a person's experiences and perceptions. Minuchin sees the individual's psychic life as being constantly influenced by interactions between people. He feels changes in the family structure lead to changes in behavior and in the internal psychic processes. He also sees the therapist as becoming, in part, enmeshed in the family. More recently, he has begun to point out to the therapist the need for theoretical change in view point. Traditionally, therapists have looked at the pathological family interactions. He emphasizes the positive aspects in family relationships to improve self-esteem. Proponents of the structural school tend to form a "therapeutic alliance" with the family using the technique of "joining" in which the therapist reaches out to family members and empathizes with the individual. Also, the technique of "accommodation" is used, in which the therapist adjusts his own personality in order to achieve "joining." Clearly "joining" and "accommodation" require high levels of self-awareness on the part of the therapist. This awareness is usually gained by holding supervised sessions with an experienced therapist watching from behind a one-way mirror. The structuralist believes these techniques must precede restructuring.

Minuchin is an extremely active therapist who will move from chair to chair, redefining pathologic behavior, and at times takes on the characteristics of one of the family members. Tasks or homework are assigned to test the flexibility of the family. The tasks are straightforward and have a high degree of face validity when compared to the tasks used in strategic therapy. Perhaps his most famous task is asking the family with an anorexic member to eat together during the therapeutic session.

In structural family therapy, it is not essential for each family member to be present for each session. At times, subgroupings are used to achieve specific goals; for example, the marital partners may be separated from the rest of the family in an attempt to improve their interactions.

The strategic group is a rather diverse collection of therapists including such people as Haley (1963), Palazzoli (1974), and Watzlawick (1974). Therapists of this school tend to see problem resolutions through the paradoxical manipulation of power. They see the system as being composed of active participants with no true victims. They tend to seek out the rules of "the family game" in an attempt to change the rules to stop the maladaptive patterns. Insight is not seen as important for change; movement is. As opposed to the structurist who tends to use straightforward homework assignments, the strategic therapist will use what seem to be illogical or paradoxical assignments. For example, a child with separation anxiety is told not to attend school, so that she may stay home and give comfort to her lonely mother. The direction to stay home is called a "symptom prescription." In addition, the symptom is redefined in the form of it's usefulness to the family. This has the advantage of allowing the therapist to ally himself with the family's attempt to solve a problem, and not having to challenge one or another member of the family directly. Strategic therapy has a special usefulness with a rebellious and negativistic teenager because of rebelling against the symptom prescription, movement is in an adaptive direction.

At this point in time, all of the theories of family therapy are only partial answers to complex questions. There is, as yet, no comprehensive theory of family therapy. Some theories have been generated from relatively limited samples of patients, or types of family pathology. There continues to be a wide interest in theory formation, and it appears that some of the theories are at least able to have limited predictive success.

Family therapy is primarily a therapeutic modality, but it has other uses. It is widely used in evaluation. While most practitioners see a need for individual interviews, it is becoming increasingly apparent that such diagnostic work is incomplete without observations of the family acting together. In the simplest form, this may be asking the family to define the problems while they are together, or in a more complex form, such techniques as a structured family interview may be used. No matter what the therapist's orientation, being able to see the family interact as a unit provides valuable information. Even brief encounters could give necessary evidence in planning the proper therapeutic modality. For example, the author in working with a young girl with anorexia nervosa saw, during a diagnostic session, that it would be premature to involve her in family therapy. Rather, she was placed in a homogenous group of adolescents, all suffering from eating disorders. The girls talked about common family problems, and at the end of a session the patient requested family therapy which was then initiated. Resistance was thereby avoided.

Family therapy can be combined successfully with individual sessions, group sesseions, or with the use of medication. Too often, the beginning family therapist feels that he or she must conform exactly to a particular model or technique. Oberfield (1980) presented a case of a teenage girl in which he used insight, structural, and strategic techniques at various times in the therapy to deal with resistance. In addition, there are times when it may be desirable to separate family members in an attempt to work on specific problems which may be a contraindication to working with the entire family.

The indications and contraindications for family therapy continue to be a highly controversial area. McDermott (1981) points out that this controversy is intricately related to the controversy over diagnosis and whether or not diagnosis is a meaningful concept. Workers opposed to diagnosis see it as antiethical to a systems approach.

Haley (1971) felt the question of diagnosis is irrelevant, as did Auerswalk (1979). Both authors see family therapy as a way of thinking, rather than a therapeutic option. Wynne (1965) taking a more moderate approach, felt that the contraindications for family therapy decreased as a therapist became more experienced.

Interpersonal conflicts, marital disturbances, delinquency, and sexual acting out are seen as indications by Ackerman (1966), Kramer (1970), Maline (1979), and Schechter (1980). Separation problems of the young child are seen as an indication for family thrapy by both Brown (1972) and Malone (1979). In separation problems of the older adolescent, attempting to disengage from the family, the situation becomes more complex. Adolescent separation is seen as an indication by Wynne (1965) and Ackerman (1966) but it is seen as a contraindication by Maline (1979) and Schechter (1979). Primary concern appears to be whether or not the family therapy will aid the adolescent's separating from his family, or whether the closeness generated by therapy will further enmesh the adolescent in the family. A solution to the problem, forwarded by McDermott (1981), is that if the conflict appears to be an intrapsychic conflict then individual therapy may be a more effective approach, but if the family is not permitting the adolescent to separate, family therapy seems to be the treatment of choice.

The treatment of psychosomatic illness is a highly controversial area. Ackerman (1966) and Schechter (1980) both see it as a contraindication, for fear that it will precipitate a medical crisis. Conversely, in a series of articles written in 1974, Liebman, Minuchin, and Baker took the position that family therapy is the treatment of choice and perhaps the only treatment for a series of psychosomatic illnesses. They focused on asthma, diabetes, and anorexia nervosa, in fact implying that family therapy is essential in the treatment of anorexia nervosa. In their work, they described a psychosomatogenic family. Such families are characterized as being overly close, overly protective, rigid, and lacking in conflict resolution. Minuchin's technique with such families has been to substitute one symptom for another, for example, not talking for not eating. He then redefines the problem as an issue of control within the family. The family becomes the focus of treatment, not the child. Regardless of theoretical position on the subject of psychosomatic illness, a close working relationship with the patient's physician is a necessity, as it is not uncommon for the family's physician to become enmeshed in the family's conflicts.

A divorced or divorcing family also appears to be an area of controversy. Ackerman in 1966 felt that an irreversible trend toward a family breakup was a contraindication and his views were echoed by Kramer (1970) and Maline (1979). As a result of research into divorcing families by Wallerstein and Kelly, Robertson has taken the position that family therapy has an important role to play in the prevention of long-term disability in the children of the divorce. It has been found that in those families unable to give up the conflicts after the original divorce decree, who continue to remain deeply enmeshed and angry, family therapy appears to provide the only hope of resolution, leaving the child with access to both parents.

To a large degree, family therapy grew out of research into schizophrenia in the early 1950's, and yet, the role that family therapy plays in the treatment of that disorder remains controversial. Ackerman (1966) saw a family member with a progressive paranoid condition or extremely rigid defenses against psychosis as a contraindication for family therapy. Guttman thought that it was not helpful and could be harmful with the prepsychotic or postpsychotic young adult. Wynne (1965) lists acute schizophrenia as a contraindication and Kramer lists chronic schizophrenia as a contraindication. At the present time, it would appear that schizophrenia is best treated with antipsychotic medication, family therapy being used in helping the family cope with the problems that arise from having a schizophrenic member.

Ackerman (1966) found the inability of a family member to be honest, a contraindication to therapy. Severe psychotic depression is seen as a contraindication by Wynne (1965), Kramer (1970), and Offer (1975). The lack of sufficient family structure is a contraindication to treatment according to Wynne (1965) and Offer (1975) as is the refusal of a significant family member to participate. The fear that a dominant family member will physically rataliate because of material discussed within the family setting is a valid reason not to enter into family therapy until safeguards have been created.

In the clinical setting, families tend to present with a problem which they may have previously defined. They expect, through the course of therapy, some resolution to that problem. The general problem is not perceived as having it's origin in the overall functioning of the family but rather it is perceived as arising from one or more of the family members. In a sense, the therapist is asked to "fix" the deviant family member. As a consequence, the therapist's first task is to redefine the problem, at the same time, being sensitive to the families' overall expectations. Insensitivity to expectations will often result in the family leaving therapy prematurely. It is not uncommon for the therapist to have a different perception of the problem, and to abruptly confront the family members, thus increasing their resistance. A major pitfall occurs when the therapist sides too directly with one or more of the family members, against a dominant member. As in other forms of therapy, the therapist needs clear-cut goals and therapeutic maneuvers need to be clearly understood.

After the goal has been redefined, the next phase is often a struggle for power in the family. During this stage, hostility is brought out. This hostility needs to be explored and worked through with the hope that after the initial anger has cleared, the family can begin to work on underlying problems. At times the family may show resistance or tire of the struggle, and it is often a necessity for the therapist to help bring them back to the task at hand. It is through problem solving that the family is able to develop a new sense of self-esteem and to prepare for the final task, that of separation from the therapists. This should be done in an active way, rather than simply allowing the family to slip away. Ideally termination is agreed upon by all family members and the therapist.

REFERENCES

Ackerman, N.: *The Family as a Social and Emotional Unit.* Bulletin of the Kansas Mental Hygiene Society, 1937.

Ackerman, N.: *Treating the Troubled Family,* New York: Basic Books, 1966.

Auerwald, E.: Personal Communication quoted by J. McDermott in Indications for Family Therapy, J Am Acad Child Psychiat, *20:*409-419, 1981.

Bateson, G., Jackson, D., Haley, J., and Weakland, J.: Toward a Theory of Schizophrenia. Behav, Sci, *1:*251-264, 1956.

Brown, S.: Family Group Therapy In: *Manual of Child Psychopathology,* ed. B. Wolman. New York: McGraw-Hill, 969-1009, 1972.

Guerin, P.: Family Therapy: The First Twenty-Five Years. In: *Family Therapy, Theory, and Practice,* ed. P. Guerin, New York: Gardner Press, 2-22, 1976.

Guttman, H.: A Contraindication for Family Therapy. Arch Gen Psychiat, *29:*352-355, 1973.

Haley, J.: *Strategies of Psychotherapy.* New York: Grune & Stratton, 1963.

Haley, J.: Family Therapy. Int J Psychiat, *9:*233-242, 1971.

Kramer, C.: Psychoanalytically Oriented Family Therapy. Family Institute of Chicago, Publ No. 1, 1-42, 1970.

Liebman, R., Munuchin, S., and Baker, L.: Integrated Treatment Program for Anorexia Nervosa. Am J Psychiat, *131:*432-436, 1974.

Malone, C.: Child Psychiatry and Family Therapy. J Am Acad Child Psychiat, *18:*4-21, 1979.

McDermott, J.: Indications for Family Therapy: Question or Non-Question? J Am Acad Child Psychiat, *20:*409-419, 1981.

Minuchin, S.: *Families and Family Therapy.* Cambridge, Mass.: Harvard University Press, 1974.

Oberfield, R.: Family Therapy with Adolescents: Treatment of a Teenage Girl with Globus Hystericus and Weight Loss. Read before Am Acad of Child Psychiat, 1980.

Offer, D., and Vanderstoep, E.: Indications and Contraindications for Family Therapy. In: *The Adolescent in Group and Family Therapy,* ed. M. Sugar. New York: Brunner/Mazel, 145-160, 1975.

Palazzoli, M.: Self-Starvation: *From the Intrapsychic to the Transpersonal Approach to Anorexia Nervosa.* London: Caucer, 1974.

Patterson, G.: *Families: Applications of Social Learning to Family Life.* Champaign, IL: Research Press, 1971.

Robertson, A.: Personal Communitacion, 1981.

Satir, V.: *Conjoint Family Therapy.* Palo Alto: Science and Behavior Books, 1967.

Schechter, M.: Indications and Contraindications for Marital and Family Therapy, In: *The Family,* ed. C. Holfing and J. Lewis. New York: Brunner/Mazel, 240-270, 1980.

Wallerstein, J., and Kelly, J.: *Surviving the Breakup.* New York: Basic Books, 1980.

Waltzlawick, P., Weakland, J., and Fisch, R.: Change: *Principles of Problem Formation and Problem Resolution.* New York: Norton, 1974.

Weakland, J.: "The Double-Bind Theory" by Self-Reflexive Hindsight. Fam Proc, *13:* 3, 1974.

Wynne, L.: Some Indicationa and Contraindications for Exploratory Family Therapy. In: *Intensive Family Therapy*, ed. I. Boszormenyi-Nagy. New York: Harper and Row, 289-322, 1965.

21 Behavior Therapy

Joyce Keen

INTRODUCTION

The *Zietgeist* which allowed the growth of behavior therapy is very different from the era and aura surrounding Freud. Mysterious hidden meanings and associations with past traumas are replaced by changes in frequency counts. That history affects current behavior change is not questioned, but rather, that emphasis placed on current behavior change is more efficient than delving at length into the past. Efficiency from the patient's standpoint is defined as cost in acquisition of coping skills, and from the therapist's standpoint as ability to observe rather than interpret. As might be expected, these skills can be more easily transferred to the patient as behavioral self-management than can lengthy hypothetical interpretations of meanings. Insight is nice but whether it is necessary to adaptive behavior is questionable.

Behavior therapy applied to inpatient psychiatric settings is much more prevalent in mental hospitals than in psychiatric units of general hospitals (1). Nurses employed in the latter setting, therefore, face a greater potential challenge. Knowledgeable psychiatric nurses may have the opportunity to teach, not only patients and their concerned persons, but also physicians. One textbook written in the late fifties included as principles of psychiatric nursing a chapter dealing with nursing care through understanding (2). Emphasis was placed on " . . . what the nurse believes to be the reason for the patient's behavior (p. 59) . . . seeking the 'why' behind the patient behavior . . . (p. 60) because . . . the behavior itself is seen as symptomatic of the patient's difficulties, not as the determinant of what the patient needs" (3). What an unfair responsibility to place on a nurse, or any human being! The underlying assumption of "whys" and "needs" may not even exist, at worst, and at best, may be attributable to one of a thousand or more "causes." Obviously, an operational definition of need was not stated. Therefore, if a patient reports that the behavior was necessary to fulfill a need, who can argue? On the other hand, if emotional or psychological needs were operationally defined, like biological needs, i.e., something without which the organism will cease to exist, then therapists would have a better foothold from which to challenge or confront the patient. Unfortunately, few researchers have addressed such a difficult task. Therefore, options are limited to accepting as fact any verbalization which begins with, "I need . . .," or choosing to redirect the focus of therapy. Herein lies the skill of the knowledgeable psychiatric nurse who does not wish to be caught helpless and reflective, but effective in contributing to productive change conducive to the patient's well-being. Behavior therapy provides the vehicle for achievement of this goal.

HISTORICAL PERSPECTIVE

Behavior coincides with existence, which is the meat of philosophy. Your guess is as good as Carl Sagan's if you exert as much energy as he in gathering data to explain how "it" all began and progressed to now. Something did something, behaved in a certain way, which appeared to be related to consequences of that doing. Jumping eons, one finds human beings recording observations attempting to connect the happenings. Most writers begin somewhere around 300 B.C. with the Greeks, emphasizing Aristotle, Plato, or Socrates. Aristotle recorded his search for causes of body movements, discriminations, and categories of behavior and was cited two thousand years later by Millenson in a text about the scientific approach to behavior (4). Unobservables such as "mind" became worthy of mere black-box discussions and researchers were reinforced who recorded and reported data.

Followers of Aristotelian logic can be traced through Descartes (1596–1650), Whytt (1750), Darwin (1859), and many others. The major complications arose by way of Wertheimer (1938) with gestalt theory and Freud (1895) with psychoanalysis, and their respective followers. Most basic textbooks, therefore, include theoretical techniques derived from gestalt, psychoanalysis, and behavioral orientations with many combinations and permutations. This chapter selectively presents techniques which behavioral research has validated through diligent adherence to the scientific method. Prolific research can be found describing reflex (elicited) behavior, conditioning of those reflexes through classical Pavlovian methods, and operant (emitted) behavior which can be strengthened or weakened by various paradigms. The basic scenario encountered by the psychiatric nurse involves operant behavior of inpatients. The consequences of those operants have resulted in their becoming inpatients. Therefore, learning to behave differently increases the probability of the inpatient being discharged. But do they feel better and think differently? Behavior therapy has provided the means by which such a question can be answered more truthfully. Feelings and thoughts can only be guessed or assumed until the patient behaves. Behavior is lawful, i.e., follows certain rules. The psychiatric nurse who knows the rules, truly can provide nursing care through understanding — not passive sympathy for some "underlying" difficulty, but active intervention.

Two basic simple rules have been derived from many complex experiments. The first is called stimulus response (SR) behavior and the second is response stimulus (RS). The S represents environment and the R represents behavior in both rules. SR behavior describes reflexes. Examples include the knee jerk, muscle contraction to shock, or quick removal of the finger from fire. The individual does not pause to decide whether to respond to the stimulus. Responses are predictably automatic. But even these behaviors can be conditioned, i.e., changed or modified. However, the second rule is the focus of this chapter. A behavior (R) occurs and is followed by a stimulus (S) which determines whether R will continue, increase, decrease, or cease. In other words, operant behavior is controlled by its consequences. An operant can be strengthened (occur more frequently) or weakened (occur less frequently) by reinforcers. Identification of desirable or undesirable operants (pinpointing) and finding reinforcers is the heart of behavior therapy. Failure on either task will complicate treatment and lengthen a hospital stay.

Operant, a term coined by Skinner to replace older terms such as *purposive* or *instrumental*, derives from operate. Thus, behavior which "operates" on the environment and appears to have the "purpose" of being "instrumental" in obtaining consequences is called operant behavior. Apparent elicitors of operants can rarely be found, so the term "emitted" more accurately describes the behavior; whereas, reflexes are obviously "elicited."

The procedure of waiting for an operant to be emitted and following it immediately with a reinforcer is called the operant paradigm. Thus, a reinforcer is a stimulus which, when it follows an operant, strengthens that operant. Walking, talking, smiling, looking, and playing are examples of operants.

Reinforcers may be tangible or social and are highly individualized. What reinforces one person may be aversive to another. Effective behavior therapy, therefore, requires knowledge of the patient reinforcement history independent of the therapist's value system. Reinforcers fall into two categories: primary reinforcers such as food, water, and sex; and secondary reinforcers, such as money, music, or clothes. The former are common to all people, and the latter have acquired the capacity to reinforce by having been associated with primary reinforcers in the past. Presenting a reinforcer is called positive reinforcement; taking away a reinforcer is the procedure of extinction. Removing an aversive stimulus is called negative reinforcement; presenting an aversive stimulus is punishment. Schedules of reinforcement describe timing of presentation of the reinforcer. In ratio schedules, the reinforcer is presented after each response (continuous), after a specified number of responses (fixed ratio), or randomly after an unspecified number of responses (variable ratio). Interval schedules involve reinforcing behavior by the clock. Intervals of time may be fixed or variable. Variable schedules are extremely powerful in that behavior thus conditioned maintains at a high frequency and is very resistant to extinction. Superstitious behavior occurs when responses are accidentally reinforced by an untimely presentation of a reinforcer. Most compulsive behaviors were inadvertently conditioned in this manner.

One other concept, shaping, is essential for successful application of behavioral principles in psychiatric nursing. Shaping, also called successive approximation, is the procedure by which an ultimate goal is obtained via reinforcement of well defined increments. For example, if the desired goal is walking, then reinforcing standing, then stepping, would be appropriate shaping. These behaviors are necessary prerequisites, successive approximations, to the final behavior. Common sense would presumably dictate such a simple principle, but mother's methods have been polished. "Be good and I'll take you to the movies" sounds very different from "make your bed, carry out the trash, hang up your clothes, and we'll go to the movies at four o'clock."

TECHNIQUES

Techniques presented in the following section are derived from the above principles. Both group and individualized programs will be discussed although the economic reality of psychiatric hospitalization usually means that the techniques applicable to groups are more frequently used.

Token Economy

Quite simply, a token economy program is exactly what the name implies: an economic system whereby patients earn payment (tokens) for desired performance. Tokens are exchangeable for goods or privileges. Tokens may be points on a chart, poker chips, or any tangible countable item. Desired performance may include individualized behaviors highly specific to one patient's treatment or applicable to the entire unit. Accumulated tokens are then used by patients to purchase items from a "store" such as snacks or toiletries, or to buy privileges such as telephone, television time, or weekend passes. The system theoretically resembles real life situations in which a person has a job for which he is paid and then can buy whatever is wanted with the money earned. Ward-wide token economy was first reported by Ayllon and Azrin in 1965 (5) and further elaborated in 1968 (6). The goal is to increase the occurrence of everyday adaptive behaviors by shaping small specific increments of those behaviors. Success depends upon reliable specification of behaviors, observation, recording, effective reinforcers, and a reasonable balance between payment and prices. Human rights issues of an ethical-legal nature emerged forcefully in the '60's directing public attention to potential social inequities toward minority groups, including patients. Wexler carried the banner in protest against token economy as a threat to patient rights (7). Therefore, it is not advisable to deprive a patient of such basic items as clothing, food, and bed as part of any behavior modification program. The general rule of thumb is not to include as purchasable reinforcers items which patients are accustomed to having for free.

Token economies have not been used extensively for modification of psychotic "symptoms" because the elimination of bizarre behavior does not automatically restore appropriate behavior. Furthermore, eccentric behaviors are more likely to be tolerated by society if the individual is otherwise self-sufficient, functional, and seemingly harmless. Modification of hallucinatory behavior or incoherent speech, for example, is usually accomplished by individualized programs.

Individual Programs

All staff members involved in caring for a patient should be aware of particular programs designed to change that individual's behavior. The patient chart would seem to be a logical place to record data so that all shifts have access to it. Specialized forms kept in the front of the chart are often helpful but may eventually make the chart too bulky. A notebook or Kardex file is frequently used to solve this problem with brief summary notations of progress made in the chart. Even housekeeping staff can innocently sabotage a program if not adequately informed. For example, if cigarettes are being used as a reinforcer and the patient is crafty enough to "bum" from uninformed employees, the program obviously will not work. The team approach to designing and running a program ideally facilitates staff communication and understanding. However, the overall responsibility for coordination, data acquisition, and analysis of progress should be assigned to one person for best results.

Systematic desensitization is probably the most famous individual technique in behavior therapy (8). Reciprocal inhibition, the underlying principle, means simply that a person cannot be both relaxed and anxious simultaneously. Therefore, achievement of deep muscle relaxation (9), the opposite response to anxiety, will inhibit the fear associated with a particular event, situation, or person if properly applied. Usually, the therapist and patient together build a hierarchy of scenarios related to the anxiety provoking stimulus beginning with low anxiety items and progressing to the specific high anxiety item. First, the patient is trained in progressive relaxation techniques using taped or personal instructions to tense, then relax, major muscle groups until the patient reliably reports low tension levels.

Biofeedback equipment provides objective physiological confirmation data but if such instruments are not available the patient can report a number between one and one hundred to quantify degree of relaxation from extremely tense (100) to extremely relaxed (1) with 50 describing the patient's perception of an average in-between state. After the patient consistently reports low levels, the lowest anxiety provoking scene is imagined. At this stage, the patient is instructed to lift a finger to indicate anxious feelings. If relaxation is maintained, then the next item in the hierarchy is presented in imagery. Whenever relaxation is inhibited, visualization of a lower item is again presented. Once the entire list has been imagined with maintenance of relaxation, the procedure can progress to include *in vivo* experience, whereby the patient gradually approaches the feared stimulus in real life while practicing the relaxation techniques previously learned. Disadvantages of using systematic desensitization in psychiatric inpatient settings are obvious. Lengthy one-to-one sessions are necessary, the patient must be intact cognitively, and the identified problem fairly well circumscribed. Phobias are particularly amenable to this individualized procedure.

Other individual techniques include implosion, flooding, reinforced practice, and modeling. Implosion (10) involves repeatedly imaging the worst possible exaggeration of the feared event, object, or situation with discussion of feelings which arise during the session until the scenes are ineffective in producing anxiety. Flooding (11) is similar to implosion except that exposure to the disturbing situations is performed in reality, prohibiting the usual avoidance behavior. Both implosion and flooding should be used with caution and ample time for reassurance.

Reinforced practice and modeling are gradual techniques designed to keep anxiety at a minimum, in contrast to implosion and flooding which deliberately provoke and maintain high anxiety. Reinforced practice (12) is essentially the same as shaping. The desired behavior is broken into small steps, each of which is practiced and reinforced. Modeling procedures (13) add to any technique the advantage of vicarious learning through observing another person's behavior and the consequences of that behavior.

Group Techniques

Group therapy has obvious cost-benefit ratio advantages over individual therapy. One or two therapists can treat eight or ten patients at a time. Components of the individual techniques mentioned above, such as relaxation training, can be applied in a group setting. A few general guidelines for group work will be mentioned. If both sexes are included as group members, then a male/female pair of co-therapists gives all group members the opportunity to observe and model appropriate behavior. The number of patients in a group may vary, but seven to ten usually is best. Group sessions should last about an hour and a half and meet as frequently as needed to accommodate the group members. Some groups may meet daily and others only once a week. Therapists should be trained in group techniques; less experienced therapists should be paired with therapists who have had more experience until they feel comfortable leading a group. The room should be enclosed such that auditory and visual distractions from other patients and unit activities do not interfere with therapy. Chairs should be comfortable and arranged in a circle or semicircle. A large writing pad with magic markers and/or a blackboard is often helpful for displaying information to the group. If any type of recording equipment is used, all patients must give informed consent. Lastly, the group members may wish to establish guidelines governing such activities as smoking, eating, and drinking during group; whether to have a break, how to "claim time" to speak, with special emphasis on confidentiality.

When a group is new, making such rules is often the first therapeutic activity because a group decision with consensus must be reached which requires communicating one's agreement or disagreement with ideas presented. Trust and cohesiveness are also enhanced by this first group activity resulting in a group decision. For an ongoing group, older group members may take turns sharing the rules of the group with a new member and obtain an agreement to abide by the rules. A group contract stating rights and responsibilities of members, including leaders, can be a helpful tool for obtaining consent and informing the patient. It should be signed by both patient and group leaders and may be referred to at a later time as a method of assuring compliance. The atmosphere should be warm, friendly, informal, and conducive to personal sharing yet structured by preplanning and post-discussion by the group leaders. Assignments to group are a staff decision based on behavioral observation which suggests a need to obtain the skills offered by a particular group.

Comprehensive planning for several groups adds the benefit of being able to accommodate various levels of patient functioning. Whatever the type of group, the vehicle for application of behavior therapy is goal setting and progress checks. An exemplary progression into group might include the following sequence: at session one the patient is introduced briefly, group rules are explained, a contract is signed and the remainder of the session is spent observing. During session two, goal setting would be done.

Subsequent sessions would include progress checks of those goals with periodic goal review during which additions or deletions are considered. Group input is extremely valuable for each of these stages. With knowledge from staff meetings, the group leaders can guide the input until the goal is stated in observable, specific, behavioral terms. For example, group members might report that "Mr. Jones smells bad." The goal would then be stated as "take a shower" and a minus recorded if he has not. Social approval for the pluses magnifies the reinforcing effect. All pluses could then later be calculated and exchanged for various privileges or items. Making a goal sheet using a large piece of paper and magic markers with the patient's name at the top and dated progress checks enhances group participation as they are able to see progress, or lack thereof, with consequences. Satisfactory achievements of all goals on the chart might be rewarded with a graduation ceremony and celebration, with subsequent assignment to a higher level group.

Lower level groups are designed to facilitate the learning or relearning of basic skills or aids to daily living including grooming, dressing, eating, cooking, or cleaning. Tasks should be simple and concrete with some being easier in order to ensure success and some slightly more challenging. Other groups would then include social skills, communication, advancing on to vocational or occupational training and personal growth. Relaxation, assertiveness, leisure time and recreation as well as more creative activities such as art, drama, or music round out a well designed program preparing the patient for real life after discharge. The final group may be entirely devoted to after treatment planning with progress checks made by telephone or outpatient visits. It is highly beneficial to involve family members or concerned persons in the patient's treatment during this group. They can provide data regarding the environment to which the patient will be going thereby increasing the probability of setting realistic goals.

One other point regarding group composition should be addressed. Most general psychiatric units include patients whose ages range from adolescents to geriatrics. It is not always possible or desirable to separate groups by age. One solution might be to include all ages in regular groups with an occasional special group formed to discuss problems related specifically to that group. Occasionally, it is therapeutic to form a short-term homogeneous group to deal with adolescent problems, women's issues, men's issues, parenting problems, or senior citizens' issues, for example.

Usually, however, it is unrealistic to separate out specific groups in a general population setting. Whether a person is sixteen or sixty, certain behavioral skills are required in finding a job. However, retirement or unwanted pregnancy may be highly specific issues for certain groups. Collateral educational groups are also highly beneficial, especially for maintenance of progress after discharge. Many units set aside an evening called "family education night" during which families and concerned persons are encouraged to attend. They learn what is happening to the patient as well as what to expect from the patient's behavior. Family involvement also facilitates post-treatment recommendations for ongoing outpatient family or individual therapy.

CURRENT TRENDS

Behaviorism has changed. To tough-minded Skinnerians, the evolution may appear broader, softer, less measurable and more similar to other psychological orientations, and even discouraging. Research purists who dreamed of defining behavior as only that which can be publically observed may have lamented the explosive entry into the literature of studies in covert sensitization and cognitive behavior therapy during the seventies. "Covert" implies private, hidden, and unseen actions, and "cognitive" is a throwback to black box phenomena. The trend began around 1965 when Homme suggested that thinking is a behavior, a covert operant of the mind which he coined "coverant" (14). Caupela (1966) demonstrated an applicable technique based on this idea to treat obesity by using aversive imagery (15). For example, imagine that spaghetti is a mass of wiggly, bloody worms crawling around on the plate. It worked. At seven months follow-up subjects were maintaining weight losses.

Common sense dictates the necessity to recognize as real, if difficult to measure, the content of thought. *Cognitive* is the term used to describe mental processes. Apparently, cognitive behavior can be conditioned (16). The generally acceptable manner of describing this procedure is the modification of self-statements. What a person says to himself or herself is observably relevant to a multitude of other complex behaviors. "I can't" versus "maybe I can" may determine whether a person initiates a new activity. Many strategies for encouraging positive self-statements are currently being developed. Asking the patient to simply tell you something positive and personal can be a beginning. Another giant step from behavior modification as a procedure applied by an outside person is the increasing emphasis on self-control. Patients are taught the principles of behavior therapy and then arrange self-presented consequences in the form of self-reinforcement or self-punishment. Harris reported such a strategy for weight control (17). A program monitor who participates in planning and carrying out the design is helpful.

Predictably, as private events become scientifically popular, a technology for measurement of these events arises. Biofeedback is considered an operant paradigm which facilitates the learning of voluntary control of physiological variables such as heart rate. blood pressure, galvanic skin response, or brain waves. Kamiya, considered by many the father of biofeedback, reported operant control of alpha waves measured by electroencephalogram and fed back to the person (18). Visual and/or auditory displays of electronically amplified and filtered signals picked up by surface electrodes provides information to the individual. Such information is equivalent to reinforcement. Kamiya included the effects of increased alpha output reported by subjects as altered states of consciousness, a hot topic for symposia in the eighties. This is a far cry from early behaviorists who said that consciousness, even if it exists, is irrelevant to the study of human behavior! Schwitzebel summed up current trends very nicely when he said "a primary goal of behavior technology is to expand our individual and collective capacity for self-programmable psychological adventures" (19). One could stretch the imagination to envision a psychiatric unit as a super scientific playground where not only do sick people get well, but well people get better!

The role of the psychiatric nurse as medication dispenser and patient as passive receiver is changing. The approach to mental health is veering from the medical/disease model of "treat-the-symptom" toward prevention. Requirements for training care givers must change to accommodate vastly greater knowledge in lay persons.

Television routinely includes health spots which often deal with psychological topics, and Dear Abby is one of many newspaper advice givers. Many patients read home magazines which discuss sophisticated treatment, and then question their therapists and physicians.

Principles set forth early in this chapter have not changed. But where, by whom, and to whom may change considerably.

The natural setting has been a favorite longing for the site of therapy, administered by a variety of professionals, to an entire group. Psychologists in the classroom are a familiar example. Psychiatric nurses in the home working with families are less familiar, but very possible. If the entire environment, both persons and objects, is taken into consideration, changes are more likely to occur and continue. A new discipline called behavioral medicine encourages interaction among many professions and is likely to result in more mental health workers in hospital settings. Discovering how thoughts, actions, and emotions interact with physical illness crosses many professions and requires a holistic, multidisciplinary approach to treatment.

Broader issues of a political and philosophical nature will be faced in the very near future. National health insurance, if legislated into existence, could increase the number of patients who seek or are referred for treatment, since prohibitive cost would be reduced. If, simultaneously, educational assistance for professionals is reduced, the quality of care is likely to suffer. Technology, again, may fill the gap. Already, computer assisted diagnosis, as well as more direct computer controlled treatment, are available. Remote mobile health care units now deliver service to isolated or emergency populations while maintaining audio-visual contact with a physician located miles away. With the increasingly common use of home computers, it is conceivable that many services previously obtained in the office or hospital could be delivered in the home with paraprofessional assistance. Strangely enough, early accusations that behaviorism was mechanistic may turn out to be literally true.

Recent success in the launch and return of the space shuttle expands the study of human behavior to new conditions. As a wider variety of people become outerspace travelers and workers, the effect of weightlessness, crowded confinement, and perpetual life threatening hazard will require more research. Since federal funding for research is diminishing, the private sector will be encouraged to enter the market. With profit as the reinforcer in free enterprise, it is difficult to predict the course of future behavioral research. A good guess would be the rise of private shuttle companies which produce the hardware and then, by necessity, conduct the research to allow comfortable, safe human use. Treatment of space related disorders, both physical and mental, is no longer the province of science fiction.

Ethical issues have been, are now, and must be addressed continually in behavior therapy. Controversy centers around the use of direct observation. If a patient knows he is being observed, behavior may be affected by the very awareness of observation. Yet, whether it is ethical to observe and record another person's behavior without his knowledge is questionable. Confidential storage and communication of information also presents ongoing ethical discussions. Dramatic entertainment such as the movie "A Clockwork Orange" has sparked fear and criticism directed at the idea of control of behavior. Skinner's unfortunate choice of titles is often interpreted as control of human behavior *without* "freedom and dignity" of the individual. All practitioners of behavior therapy must remain acutely aware of the social impact of their interventions.

In summary, the goal of behavior therapy is to improve human adaptation to environment by changing the environment or by changing response to the environment. Successful adaptation includes cognitive, emotional, and motor activity conducive to an individual's well being; environment includes everything outside the person, both animate and inanimate. Such a comprehensive task cannot be accomplished without knowledge derived from scientific research and training in application of that knowledge.

REFERENCES

1. Agras, W.S.: "Behavior Modification in the General-Hospital Psychiatric Unit," In: *Handbook of Behavior Modification and Behavior Therapy*, H. Leitenberg (ed.). Englewood Cliffs, New Jersey: Prentice-Hall, Inc., 547-565, 1976.

2. Matheny, R.V. and Topalis, M.: *Psychiatric Nursing*, St. Louis: The C.V. Mosby Company, 1957.

3. Matheny, R.V. and Topalis, M.: *op cit.*, 59-60, 85.

4. Millenson, J.R.: *Principles of Behavioral Analysis*, New York: The MacMillan Co., 1967.

5. Ayllon, T. and Azrin, N.H.: "The measurement and reinforcement of behavior of psychotics," *Journal of the Experimental Analysis of Behavior*, 8, 357-383, 1965.

6. Ayllon, T. and Azrin, N.H.: *The Token Economy: A Motivational System for Therapy and Rehabilitation*, New York: Appleton-Century-Crofts, 1968.

7. Wexler, D.G.: "Token and Taboo: Behavior modification, token economies, and the law," *California Law Review*, 61, 81-109, 1973.

8. Wolpe, J.: *Psychotherapy by Reciprocal Inhibition*, Stanford, California: Stanford University Press, 1958.

9. Jacobson, E.: *Progressive Relaxation* (2nd edition), Chicago: University of Chicago Press, 1938.

10. Hogan, R.A. and Kirchner, J.A.: "Preliminary report of the extinction of learned fears via implosive therapy," *Journal of Abnormal Psychology*, 72, 106-109, 1967.

11. Baum, M.: "Extinction of avoidance responding through response prevention (flooding)," *Psychological Bulletin*, 74, 276-284, 1970.

12. Herzberg, A.: "Short treatment of neuroses by graduated tasks," *British Journal of Medical Psychology*, 19, 19-36, 1941.

13. Bandura, A. and Walters, R.H.: *Social Learning and Personality Development*, New York: Holt, Rinehart and Winston, 1963.

14. Homme, L.E.: "Perspectives in psychology, XXIV. Control of coverants, the operants of the mind," *Psychological Record*, 15, 501-511, 1965.

15. Cautela, J.R.: "Treatment of compulsive behavior by covert sensitization," *Psychological Record*, 16, 33-41, 1966.

16. Meichenbaum, D. and Cameron, R.: "The clinical potential of modifying what clients say to themselves," In: *Self-Control: Power to the Person*, M.G. Mahoney and C.E. Thoresen (eds.). Monterey California: Brooks/Cole, 1974.

17. Harris, M.B.: "Self-directed program for weight control: a pilot study," *Journal of Abnormal Psychology*, 74, 263-270, 1969.

18. Kamiya, J.: "Operant control of EEG alpha rhythm and some of its reported effects on consciousness," In: *Altered States of Consciousness*, C. Tart (ed.). New York: John Wiley, 1969.

19. Schwitzebel, R.L.: "Behavior technology," In: *Handbook of Behavior Modification and Behavior Therapy*, H. Leitenberg (ed.). Englewood Cliffs, New Jersey: Prentice-Hall, Inc., 1976.

22 Nurses and Psychoses

Lloyd A. Wells

The nosologic issues, diagnostic considerations, descriptions of syndromes and overall treatment measures for psychotic patients of different types have been discussed elsewhere in this book. Actual clinical intervention on the daily ward level with such patients requires a great deal of creativity and flexibility, and this brief chapter will attempt to address some of these issues.

By definition, all psychotic patients are out of contact with reality as it is interpreted by those around them. While several different conditions can lead to psychosis, many of the symptoms of psychosis are shared by those several conditions. The most common causes of psychosis are drug-induced, physical illness, depressive, manic, schizophreniform and post-partum. We shall attempt to differentiate some of the different approaches required by these different conditions.

Although it is always reassuring to have a set of general rules available for dealing with people who are so very different from most of what we consider to constitute humanity, the major rule is to be willing to be flexible.

Every patient is different. A patient who is psychotic because of LSD intoxication will react very differently and will need very different nursing care than a patient who is confused and disoreinted because of open heart surgery. General rules rigidly applied make the nursing staff feel more comfortable but usually are of little use to the patient. Thus, the first rule needs to be flexibility.

It is important with each psychotic patient to have some comprehension of the type of psychosis and the type of specific problems the patient is experiencing. Nursing care for the patient who is terrified by persecutory delusions will be very different from nursing care of a patient who is mildly euphoric because he thinks he has died and gone to heaven. It is, therefore, necessary to make an assessment of the components of the patient's psychotic process and then to develop management priorities within a nursing framework for each such patient.

The third general rule, after deciding to be flexible and making some general patient management priorities, is to develop acceptance of the patient within the context of his or her psychotic system. Psychosis is alien to most of us and makes us uncomfortable. It is extremely easy to reject a psychotic patient, and many psychotic patients, particularly schizophrenics, are exquisitely attuned to subtle rejection. Acceptance of the patient does not mean endorsing his psychotic world view but merely acceptance of him as a human being and a certain tolerance toward the psychotic world view. One of the primary functions of the nurse in dealing with such a patient is to be the patient's representative of a non-psychotic world. To enter the patient's psychotic world with this representation of a non-psychotic world requires acceptance of the patient, and little can be done in terms of establishing a relationship without such an acceptance. Of course, this does not mean that the nurse has to like the patient. Counter-transference to psychotic patients can be extremely strong in either a positive or negative way. There is nothing wrong with such counter-transference feelings, but it is important to be aware of them in order to achieve a professional type of acceptance.

Fourth, the nurse has a major role in developing a reality orientation for the patient. In the context of the inpatient unit, the nurse can be accepting of the patient and his delusions but also point out to the patient the reality of his existence on the ward. It is all very well that the Nazis are sending the patient telepathic messages, but at 12 noon it is time to have lunch. The nurse is the stand-in for reality in the patient's world. It is far more helpful to the patient that the nurse establish a sense of reality by her actions and expectations — i.e., eating lunch, going to activities, etc. — than that the nurse consistently tell the patient he is wrong. Arguing with a psychotic patient about the specific content of his psychosis is usually self-defeating. Representing reality to the patient and making as many reality-oriented demands on the patient as he can tolerate, give him a much more internalized sense of reality.

Fifth, it is a major function of the nurse to assess on an ongoing basis the degree of the patient's capacity for control. If it is a function of the nurse to make expectations of reality to the patient the nurse must also be aware of how much the patient can possibly comprehend and participate in this reality. Thus, it makes no sense at all to ask an actively hallucinating patient to be in enough control to go to a lecture on parapsychology. As the patient's representative of reality, the nurse must also be willing and able to assume whatever amount of control is necessary. It is important, too, for the nurse to be aware that psychotic patients' degree of control can change very rapidly, and the nurse must be ever vigilant regarding this process.

Sixth, it is the task of the nurse to develop a trusting relationship with the patient as far as this is possible. Trust is not a one-way type of relationship. For the patient to actively develop a trusting relationship with the nurse, the nurse must reciprocate the trust. This does not mean that the nurse assumes the patient is in control; the two issues are completely different. For the nurse to trust the patient means essentially that the nurse is willing to view the patient as a human being having problems with perception and control but as a human being, nevertheless, who at some level wishes to have a positive relationship with the nurse. To develop a trusting relationship the nurse must be consistent in her demands of the patient and her motive relating to the patient. A trust relationship between the nurse and psychotic patient does not mean that the nurse is the repository of the patient's secrets or that she conceals what he tells her in confidence from other members of the treatment team. This must be specified to the patient. It is, of course, gratifying to any mental health professional to be viewed by the patient as the most important member of the treatment team and the only one the patient can "trust." In the rare event that this trust appeals excessively to our narcissistic needs, however, patient care can be greatly harmed. The nurse, for example, who sets up a contract with the patient that he will call her before attempting suicide and who then goes off the shift and cannot be reached can cause grievous harm to the patient's physical well-being and to his future capacity to trust.

Seventh, it is the task of the nurse to attempt to bolster the patient's self-esteem. Again, this is not done by unrealistically praising the patient and telling him or her that he or she is a wonderful person. It is done far more by showing the patient that the nurse does have expectations of him which he or she feels the patient can carry out. As the patient improves, the expectations increase and this gives the patient evidence that he is improving, which often is helpful to his self-esteem. Relating to the patient as a human being in spite of his psychotic process, is usually perceived by the patient and also helps to bolster self-esteem. In spite of his craziness, he is also a human being, and the nurse's acceptance of that fact and emphasis of it in her relationship with the patient is often immensely helpful to the patient's self-esteem.

Eighth, the nurse should be cognizant of the patient's interpersonal relationships, both in his family and on the ward. The nurse is in an excellent position to observe interactions between patient and family and patient and other patients. The nurse can notice major problems in interpersonal relationships and bring them to the treatment team. In addition she can help the patient to strengthen his interpersonal relationships wherever possible.

Ninth, the nurse should be aware of the defense mechanisms being used by the psychotic patient. While defense mechanisms can be assessed on the basis of reports, subtle defense mechanisms often become apparent only in the context of an ongoing relationship. It is not necessarily the task of the nurse to interpret the defense mechanism to the patient. On the other hand, it is very helpful to the treatment team and to the nurse to be aware of the particular type of defense mechanisms being used because they will modify the approach of the nurse, particularly in her discussions with the patient.

Tenth, the psychotherapeutic approach of the nurse to the patient with a psychosis is primarily through the means listed above. Many people would also include psychotherapy as a major component of the treatment plan for the nurse. In my view, formal psychotherapy with a psychotic patient in a supportive manner can be extremely helpful, but it remains less important than the other nine tasks listed above. If these are carried through, they are psychotherapeutic. If they are not carried through, the patient will not be accessible to any kind of supportive therapy and it will be a waste of the patient's and the nurse's time. If the other nine components of nursing treatment are carried through, the patient may also derive some benefit from talking about his view of the world with the nurse. Should this become part of the treatment plan, it is extremely important that the nurse be aware of the patient's defense mechanisms. It can be extremely harmful to a patient to have a nurse miss his defenses of projection and introjection and to become caught up in the patient's psychotic world. This can cause great fright to the patient and can be harmful not only to the patient but to the nurse, the treatment team, and indeed the entire ward milieu.

Specific techniques of dealing with individual behaviors of psychotic patients could be listed, but for the most part it is wise not to have a cookbook approach to such patients. That approach makes the staff comfortable without adding significantly to the care of the patient and also tends to cause the staff to pigeonhole the patient rather than to see him as an individual. Far more useful is to set up treatment goals, list the ten priorities of nursing care for the psychotic patient as provided in this chapter, and attempt to develop a reasonable plan for implementing each of them for the individual patient. This requires a good deal more work than using a standard and stereotyped approach but its rewards in terms of patient improvement and increased ward morale are great.

23 Nursing Care for the Hospitalized Patient with Psychotic Symptoms

Marcia Justic

This chapter addresses the role of the nurse in caring for hospitalized, psychotic patients. It provides some specific approaches to various features of psychosis, but it also provides a general model of approach to any hospitalized psychiatric patient.

ASSESSMENT

Introduction

In accordance with the Nursing Process, conducting a thorough psychiatric evaluation is essential in order to develop a comprehensive nursing approach for the patient and family (1). The psychiatric evaluation includes a mental status examination as well as a psychosocial history. The data gathered should serve as a baseline for ongoing assessment and history taking. Patients who exhibit psychotic symptoms often experience very frequent changes in mental state including varying levels of orientation and communicativeness. Noting such changes will provide insight into numerous areas including: the nature of the patient's illness, stimuli which precipitate symptoms, and effective interventions which lead to symptom reduction. The initial psychosocial data available may be vague or incomplete. Further contact with the patient and family as well as tapping other information sources may be valuable. Additional resources include charts and histories from previous treatment, including non-psychiatric treatment, friends, clergy, work supervisors or co-workers.

The psychiatric evaluation provides a framework for organizing a multitude of data. It serves to define the scope of the patient's problem thereby providing a basis for the initial states of interdisciplinary planning. In addition, the psychiatric evaluation is the first step in establishing a therapeutic relationship with the patient.

Techniques

Since the psychiatric evaluation provides the opportunity for contact with the patient, it is important for the nurse to utilize an effective approach. Such an approach involves developing a sense of timing and a supportive demeanor, establishing a comfortable environment, and interviewing skillfully. In order to develop a sense of timing, the nurse needs to recognize that in order to conduct an in-depth interview, the patient must have a manageable level of anxiety. This will enable him to cooperate by recalling past material and responding coherently to questions. If the patient is agitated, extremely anxious or frightened, the nurse should postpone the interview and attempt to make the patient more comfortable. Initial physical and psychological assessments can be made as the nurse spends time with the patient attempting to reduce his anxiety level. In addition, other information sources including the family may be available to provide data. Conveying concern for the patient's comfort and security may help to assure the patient that he is in a safe environment where people are concerned about his well-being.

Once the nurse determines that the timing is appropriate, a setting should be chosen which allows for privacy, comfort, and few distractions or interruptions. The patient should be told the purpose of the interview, stressing the need to understand his perceptions of his illness and goals for treatment. It is important that the nurse explain to the patient that many questions will be asked in an attempt to understand many areas of his life both past and present. The nurse should offer encouragement and understanding about the difficulty which may be encountered as the patient describes painful events and problems. Many patients may not understand the relevance of certain questions or may be frightened or suspect of others. Therefore, it is helpful to stress that the patient, too, may ask questions or decline to answer certain questions if he wishes. It is important to let the patient set the limits on time and the depth of information even though this may require that the interview be conducted at various intervals. The patient may not verbalize these limits directly, but the nurse can be aware of certain cues, i.e., asking how many other questions will be asked, commenting on fatigue, increase in body movements or decrease in attention span.

As the nurse conducts the interview, it is important to be goal directed as to the type of data to be collected and to provide some structure to the questioning. However, it is best to ask broad questions and allow the patient to tell his story rather than asking numerous specific questions which require only a "yes" or "no" reply. For example, phrases such as, "What brings you to the hospital?" or "Tell me about the problem you've been experiencing" are usually more effective than direct questions such as, "Are you experiencing anxiety?" This type of interviewing will enable the nurse to gather data as well as assess the patient's mental status. The patient's responses will yield important clues to the nature of his thought processes, thought content, level of insight and judgment, orientation, memory, and feeling tone.

As the nurse listens attentively to the patient's responses and offers support, the patient may become more comfortable and open. With this in mind, it is helpful to structure the interview to proceed from the least threatening to increasingly personal topics. For example, areas related to sensitive family topics or sexuality should generally not be addressed in the beginning of the interview unless the patient initiates them. The nurse should try to attend to themes which may become apparent as the patient talks (2). For example, in reviewing significant history, the patient may discuss difficulties in grade school, adjustment problems in adolescence, the absence of a peer group and numerous job changes in addition to a lack of close friends. All of this information lends itself to a theme of failure, isolation and lack of self-esteem, although the patient may not recognize this. Identifying such themes will help in formulating a clinical picture of the patient and the problems he encounters. Documentation is important to determine whether such themes are recurrent and significant throughout the patient's hospitalization.

Psychosocial History

In gathering psychosocial data, there are a few areas which can be of special significance in interviewing patients who are experiencing psychotic symptoms. Perhaps the first is the patient's perception of the presenting problem(s) followed by his expectations of hospitalization. The patient's responses offer a wealth of information including: his insight into his illness, willingness to be hospitalized, sense of responsibility for change, motivation and hope regarding treatment, and sense of power and control over life events. A patient who states that no one has cured his problems before, but he's willing to try once more, will require an entirely different approach than a patient who asks for assistance so that he can control his symptoms. This discussion of the patient's presenting problem(s) should include a history of the present illness as well as a description of the symptoms and their onset and duration. The history of the illness should also include any changes in weight, appetite or sleep patterns. Prior hospitalizations and treatment should be noted with attention to psychotropic medications used to treat the patient. The nurse should attempt to have the patient describe current medication usage in detail as to how and when it is taken and if the patient ever experienced any side-effects. With regard to previous hospitalizations, it is important to try to elicit the patient's attitudes and feelings about the treatment. Additionally, it is helpful to determine whether the patient can identify his coping measures. For example, a hallucinating patient may discuss the problem he is having with hearing voices and how they developed from friendly to angry and frightening voices. He may be able to identify that the voices are worst at night when he is alone, but during the day he can avoid them by watching television or talking to a friend.

This data would be important when planning strategies for the patient to gain control over the hallucinations. Another area to explore is that of the patient's daily activities, including his ability to perform self-cares, usual household chores or routines, and job related activities. Any changes which have occurred will give the staff an idea of the extent of disruption in daily living which the patient and his family have experienced. An illustration of this might be a situation in which a wife and mother states she isn't able to do her daily chores and that friends and family are coming in to help. Upon further questioning, the nurse discovers that other people are doing laundry, child care and meal preparation. This data would help to elucidate the level of the patient's immobilization and disorganization as well as family stress. In a more positive direction, the nurse should attempt to have the patient discuss personal strengths, areas in his life which may be satisfying, and future goals. The patient's ability or inability to respond will give staff an idea about the patient's self-esteem and motivation to return to his previous life sytle. The area of interpersonal relationships is also very important in order to determine the nature and extent of the patient's illness. It is essential to assess any recent changes in socialization such as increased isolation, distrust of friends, family or fear of going out of the home alone. Other areas related to interpersonal relationships include past and current friendships and the amount of closeness which may or may not have existed in these relationships. Family or friends may describe a patient as being "to himself" with no one ever knowing how the patient feels or what he may be thinking. This data will help staff form a sketch of the patient's developmental history and current functioning related to interpersonal relationships. Whether or not these have been satisfying and ego building or a source of failure will provide clues about the patient's illness and the symptomatic behavior exhibited.

The family history and assessment provides a great deal of information about the patient's interpersonal development. The staff can develop some insight into the family's dynamics by observing the following: the attitude of the family toward the patient and his hospitalization; the family's communication style including channels and rules; mutual expectations among members; and family roles. These are just a few areas which will unfold if the nursing staff spends time with the patient and his family. The nurse may observe many different dynamics, such as a mother always making demands of her husband by speaking through their son who is the identified patient. Observing these dynamics can have important implications for the patient's therapy. The formal family interview should be directed toward identifying the family's perceptions about the patient's illness, their goals for treatment, the family's coping style and reactions to stress, and any changes which may have occurred as a result of the illness of the identified patient. A family genogram can be a useful tool in developing a picture of the family structure and dynamics both historically and currently (3). A few areas which can be explored and illustrated via the genogram are: significant relationships within the family, both conflictual and collusive; personality descriptions; the patient's placement in the sibling group; relationships with extended family members; geographical and ethnic origins; family tragedies and triumphs; and significant illnesses including psychiatric illness. Working with the family for several sessions to develop a genogram often helps to decrease the family's anxiety and stimulate more open discussion about the patient and family.

Beyond the family assessment and history, the patient's academic and occupational record can be significant. Academic success or failure and any changes in such patterns provide data about the patient's level of adjustment during adolescence and early adulthood. The occupational history offers similar information about the patient's ability to function in a work setting and relate to co-workers and supervisors. A gradual decline and poor adjustment in these areas over a long period of time indicate a more serious level of pathology than perhaps a sudden, recent change in performance (4).

The area of psychosexual development can be a sensitive one especially during an initial interview. However, exploring the patient's sexual development, present sexual functioning and any sexual concerns can be helpful in a number of ways. If the patient does experience troublesome sexual thoughts, guilt feelings, delusions, etc., the nurse's direct and open approach may encourage the patient to discuss sexual content. If the patient does not respond or does so in a guarded fashion, the nurse is still indicating that discussion of sexual material can be important and appropriate. The patient may remember this when he feels more comfortable with staff or when he is particularly troubled by sexual issues.

Gathering a drug history can have special importance when a patient is psychotic. Determining whether the patient previously or currently abused alcohol and/or chemicals can be very difficult, yet it is essential in order to discover if there is an organic basis for the patient's symptoms. If the staff does not feel the patient is reliable, friends or relatives should be questioned or a drug screen may be ordered by the physician.

A final area which can be very significant is seeking information about the patient's general health. In many instances, psychosis is related to a physiologic cause such as an electrolyte imbalance, head trauma, tumors, various medications and numerous other organic factors. As a nurse providing a holistic approach, all avenues should be explored in order to gather a complete and accurate history.

Mental Status Examination

All areas of the mental status exam are important when assessing a patient displaying psychotic symptoms. The areas to be assessed include: appearance and general behavior, stream of thought, speech, affective responses, thought content, sensorium, intellectual functioning, judgment, and insight (5, 6). While the patient is responding to questions during the psychiatric interview, the nurse can assess the extent of disturbance in the patient's stream of thought as evidenced by such phenomena as loose associations, flight of ideas, blocking, perseveration, or other such symptoms. The content of the patient's thoughts can also be noted at the time to determine if the patient experiences delusions, ideas of reference, preoccupations, obsessions, ruminations, or perceptual disturbances including any type of hallucinations. Although the patient may not readily admit to such experiences, his behavior (i.e., looking around the room or whispering in responses to voices) and his perceptions of many life events will provide cues which indicate that the patient may be experiencing such symptoms. It is usually not difficult to determine if the patient's affective responses and mood are appropriate for the circumstances and subject matter. Patients may exhibit a wide range of responses from inappropriate laughter and elation to a flattened bland affect. Other areas such as intellectual functioning and insight may be more difficult to assess if the patient is unable to respond to questions in an organized, appropriate manner.

Whether the psychiatric evaluation presents a clear or confusing picture, psychological testing can be invaluable in validating or challenging the staff's assessment of the patient. Tests such as the Minnesota Multiphasic Personality Inventory (MMPI), Weschler Adult Intelligence Scale (WAIS), Bender Gestalt and Rorschach can offer data related to the patient's personality, affectual tone, thought processes, intellectual functioning and signs of organic brain involvement. If the patient is extremely disturbed or resistant the tests may be invalid and should be repeated at a later time by a psychologist or psychometrist. In other instances, some forms of testing can be repeated to determine whether the patient is progressing. Psychological tests should not be used in isolation to assess a patient; used in conjunction with other forms of evaluation, however, they are invaluable in completing a clinical picture of the patient.

PLANNING

Introduction

The assessment phase of the nursing process is followed by planning which involves the development of patient goals and the nursing approach. This planning is not done in isolation from the rest of the mental health team. This team usually includes representatives from psychiatry, psychology, social work, recreational/

occupational therapy and nursing. The nurse is often in the unique position of coordinating the patient care planning with the mental health team, nursing staff and the patient. The kind of planning which is done is dependent upon the types of services and programs provided by the agency. Brief therapy centers, crisis intervention units, long term residential treatment facilities, and day or night hospitals vary in their approach to treatment. While some aim to quickly return the patient to the community with outpatient follow-up, others provide treatment which makes it possible for the patient to be more completely rehabilitated before discharge. Another factor which will affect the team's planning is related to the patient's entry into the health care agency (7). Whether the patient is receiving treatment voluntarily or under duress will have an impact on his goals for treatment as well as his response.

Team Approach

Initially, members of the mental health team will usually share observations and information from their assessments of the patient. The team must then identify its goals for the patient with the approach and evaluative criteria based upon its concurrent clinical impressions. All of this is subject to periodic reevaluation and modification. The team should have a well established plan for meetings and channels of communication to insure consistency of care and patient evaluation.

Nurse-Patient Planning

The nursing staff is responsible for establishing nursing diagnosis, patient oriented goals (sometimes referred to as expected outcomes) and a nursing approach which will be consistent with the planning of the mental health team. Nursing diagnoses are initiated which identify and prioritize patient problems appropriate for nursing intervention. These diagnoses usually focus on patient behaviors and needs rather than medical diagnoses and provide a framework for subsequent planning. The patient oriented goals should be both short and long term. Goals should be dated, concrete, and stated in a manner which is measurable. For example, contrast the goal, "the patient will feel more comfortable on the unit by 8/27," to the following goals which are measurable:

1. "The patient will talk with nursing staff by 8/22,"
2. "The patient will eat meals in the dining room by 8/23,"
3. "The patient will begin to converse with one or two other patients by 8/25."

The latter set of goals is observable, while "comfort" can only be subjectively assessed without specific criteria. The nursing staff should include the patient in setting goals for his treatment. This collaboration between the nurse and patient will often involve negotiating as well as prioritizing goals. If the patient is able to engage in goal setting, even in a very superficial manner, a great deal is being taught and conveyed including a sense of patient responsibility, hope, realistic self-expectations, staff interest and appropriate treatment expectations. It is obvious that severely disorganized patients may not be able to discuss treatment goals initially. However, the nursing staff should try to include all patients in planning as soon as possible. The patient's goals will usually focus on symptom alleviation. The nurse should be prepared to assist the patient to identify short term goals necessary to attain in order that the patient's "curative" goal will be reached. For example, a patient may verbalize that she "wants the voices to leave me alone and this is my only goal." The nurse can help the patient to recognize that an initial goal may be, "seeking out the nursing staff when voices begin" which will help her establish a sense of control. A long-term goal may involve the patient identifying stressors which create anxiety and result in the hallucinations.

Specific Areas of Planning

After goal establishment, there are three areas which require special planning as the mental health team develops an approach. These include the involvement of the patient in milieu therapy, family intervention, and patient/family teaching. Most patients will be involved in milieu therapy to some extent since most agencies consider the hospital environment to be therapeutic in itself. Intrinsic to the concept of a therapeutic milieu, however, is the philosophy that all aspects of daily living on the unit can be therapeutic and that patients have strengths to be tapped and utilized in their own treatment as well as treatment of fellow patients (8). All levels of staff have talents which contribute to a therapeutic milieu. In addition to the patient's exposure to the therapeutic environment, planning should focus upon the patient's involvement in specific programs or activities which will meet specific needs. Hospitals offer programs which help patients develop interpersonal, occupational and leisure skills. A research study was conducted by Beard, Enclow and Owen which reported positive changes related to the involvement of chronic psychiatric patients in structured activities including reality orientation groups, remotivation and resocialization activities (9). They found an increase in social competence as well as prevention of detrimental repression. The mental health team should mutually plan what activities and groups would benefit the patient; the team should then consistently encourage participation. The patient's progress should be frequently evaluated to determine if the groups are appropriate for the patient's level of functioning and current status. Group leaders should be included in planning and evaluation meetings which involve patients participating in their groups.

Another area requiring special planning is that of family involvement. Usually, all staff nurses are involved in family assessment and have frequent contact with the family, although special preparation and training is essential for the nurse who will be conducting family therapy. The nurse will often be a cotherapist in family sessions with another member of the mental health team. The team needs to recognize that its interactions with the family may lay the groundwork for the success or failure of subsequent family therapy sessions. The goal is always to involve and engage the family by offering support and teaching. All too often, the entire family or a specific family member may sense that the staff blames or holds them responsible for the patient's illness. This only serves to solidify family defensiveness and pathology. If limits need to be set for the family related to interactions or visiting, it should be done in a way to enlist the family's help rather than demanding compliance. Instead of alienating the family, strategies should be developed to engage the family. Minuchin refers to "joining operations" which are applicable not only to family therapists but also to the nursing staff who may have the most frequent contact with the family (10). "Joining" requires that the nurse adapt to the family's interaction style and tempo, experience the family, and follow them with interest and empathy (11). Eventually, therapy may be directed toward changing many family operations; such change, however, cannot be attempted initially. Many agencies may begin family therapy during the patient's hospitalization while others focus mainly on supporting the family until discharge when a referral may be made for family treatment. In either case, the nurse should begin teaching and preparing the family by exploring family stressors and emphasizing possible positive outcomes of family sessions.

Another area of family involvement is related to the teaching which will be done with the patient and family. The development of a teaching plan is an important aspect in the overall planning. The nursing staff is responsible for assessing the patient and family's knowledge base with regard to mental health, the nature of the patient's illness, treatment, medications, communication skills, as well as many other areas. Once learning needs are assessed, the nurse should develop a plan which specifies content to be taught, appropriate teaching strategies, and timing. Developing guidelines for timing is essential; otherwise, the teaching will not be helpful. For example, attempting to teach the patient and family about group therapy is not appropriate when they are still in a crisis state due to the patient's admission. Therefore, the nurse should provide teaching when the patient and family show signs of readiness such as asking questions related to content which has been identified as part of the teaching plan. Teaching techniques are most effective when the material is delivered in a manner which is not too simplistic yet not beyond the learner's level of comprehension. Various strategies should be utilized including pamphlets, learning packets, videotapes, individual teaching sessions, and groups. Many agencies have specific groups which give patients and their families an opportunity to learn about mental health, family dynamics, medications, interpersonal skills and numerous other areas. These groups encourage the participants to share knowledge and offer support to each other. Teaching is not a one time activity; instead, the nurse should repetitively assess the patient's and family's level of knowledge.

Discharge Planning

It may seem premature to begin discharge planning during the early stages of the patient's hospitalization. Yet, whenever discharge needs are identified, they should be documented and interventions to meet these needs initiated. Follow-up treatment is a discharge need which requires anticipatory planning and patients who experience psychotic symptoms usually require such follow-up. Agencies or specific therapists who have previously provided treatment or will offer future services should be contacted and periodically updated about the patient's status. Many patients have additional needs such as housing, vocational rehabilitation, and financial counseling, which should be identified early in the hospitalization. Otherwise, the necessary arrangements may be prolonged beyond the patient's actual discharge, which can cause the transition back into the home and community to be very difficult.

IMPLEMENTATION OF NURSING CARE

Introduction

In providing nursing care for patients with psychiatric disorders, a first concern should be that of maintaining the patient's rights. Nurses' attitudes toward patients determine if they can provide truly humane care. It can be easy to fall into the trap of thinking of patients in terms of their symptomatic behaviors or diagnoses, for example, "Mary, the schizophrenic." Although patients may display characteristic symptoms at times, these patients are unique individuals who are not unintelligent, criminal, or evil. Their lives and experiences are often more similar than different from ours. The behavior of psychotic patients may at times be difficult to manage, confusing, and quite disturbing, but mental health professionals should not judge or treat patients in a harsh manner because of their symptoms (12). In order to cope with this stress peer support should be available through care conferences or groups so that staff can ventilate their concerns and frustrations. This is not to say that all nurses can be therapeutic for all patients. However, the nurse that finds herself constantly angry or anxious with patients should seek peer support to review her feelings and level of job satisfaction.

The rights of psychiatric patients are protected by law. States vary in the legislative acts which they implement to protect patients, yet there are certain rights which seem to be protected fairly consistently such as: communicating privately with people outside the hospital, carrying out legal activities, reviewing one's status or examination by a psychiatrist of choice, the provision of treatment in the least restrictive environment, and the right to informed consent for specifically designated treatments or therapies (13). This list is not all-inclusive, but these are rights retained by all voluntary patients as well as committed patients in some states (14).

General Principles of Therapeutic Intervention

Aside from developing a sensitivity to patients' rights, there are a few principles which characterize therapeutic nursing intervention. These principles include staff acceptance of the patient, consistency in the treatment approach, and the provision of a safe environment. In addition, other principles involve meeting needs such as physical and reality orientation which are prevalent among patients experiencing psychotic symptoms. These patients also require assistance in working on "here and now" problems of living.

Conveying acceptance and empathy toward patients is very important. This acceptance should be expressed in a nonpatronizing and nonparental manner. Although the nurse may not agree with a patient or may find his behavior disturbing, care can still be given with respect and concern. Psychiatric patients cannot be easily categorized into "good" or "bad" patients since expression of anger — even when inappropriately displayed — and a lack of cooperation are often signs of health, while passive acceptance may indicate regression and despondency.

Providing consistency in the treatment approach and expectations of the patient is essential. This can be particularly difficult with the psychotic patient whose behavior, at times, may be quite changeable and confusing. Documentation of behavior in the patient's progress notes and plan of nursing care is invaluable. The patients' goals and treatment, including effective management and routines, should be clearly described. Disagreements among the nursing staff may be quite common when deciding upon an approach. However, these conflicts should be confronted and negotiated so that a plan of care is developed which will be consistently followed by everyone caring for the patient. Consistency in staff assignments is also important since patients cannot be expected to adapt frequently to unfamiliar caretakers. In order for a patient to develop a sense of trust and security, there should be a few staff members who are consistently involved.

Safety is also a general principle in providing therapeutic nursing care. The nursing staff is responsible to provide an environment which is safe for all patients including those in danger of harming themselves or others. This can be quite challenging particularly with newly admitted patients who are often frightened and seem quite unpredictable to the staff. Since the patient has the right to treatment in the least restrictive setting, staff should attempt to help the patient maintain self control and develop a sense of security. If a patient does begin to strike out or injure himself, the staff must quickly intervene. A patient requiring seclusion and/or restraint should be monitored closely. Often, closed circuit television systems are useful for constant observation. It is not therapeutic for a patient to be continuously controlled by the use of these measures. The patient's uncontrollable behavior usually lessens as his anxiety, fear, and confusion decrease. This often occurs as the patient begins to trust the staff and as the use of neuroleptic medicines reduces the patient's discomfort. At this time, alternative measures such as verbal control, limit setting, and positive reinforcement should be utilized to help the patient regain self-control.

Patients with psychotic thought disorders are often quite confused and need reality orientation. This can be described as a concentrated effort on the part of the nursing staff to work with the patient to increase his awareness of person, place, time, and situation (15). Every contact with a patient presents an opportunity to assess the patient's level of confusion and to intervene when there is a need for reality orientation. The staff must also work with the patient's family to help in the orientation effort. Reality orientation does not involve arguing with patients who are hallucinating or delusional about the reality of their experiences. Instead, with many psychotic patients, a brief interchange can divert them from hallucinations, delusional ruminations, and preoccupations. With patients suffering from organic brain disorders, consistent, 24-hour orientation can be appropriate since the patient may have difficulty remembering from one moment to the next. The nursing staff can also manipulate the environment so that orienting cues such as clocks, calendars, and door tags are visible to confused patients (16).

In developing a therapeutic approach with a patient suffering from a psychotic disorder, psychodynamic therapies which lead to the uncovering of unconscious processes are usually not beneficial (17). The *Statement on Psychiatric and Mental Health Nursing Practice* identifies, "working with clients concerning the here-and-now living problems they confront," as a major nursing activity

(18). This activity is particularly effective with many psychotic patients since the focus of therapy is often to provide a supportive relationship which encourages the patient to verbalize and learn to cope with stressors. The patient should be assisted to identify and explore his feelings in order to learn to deal with them appropriately. Likewise, self-esteem and identity are important, and the nurse needs to consistently work with the patient to develop a positive sense of self. Family relationships should be explored so that interventions can be implemented. Although all of these issues should be explored, this type of approach differs from a purely psychodynamic one in that the focus is on present issues only, rather than their relationship to past relationships and experiences which may have contributed to the patient's illness.

One of the most consistent physical needs of patients suffering from psychosis is that of monitoring the effects of drug therapy. Psychotropic drugs are usually valuable in interrupting psychotic thought processes and altering the patient's level of anxiety and discomfort to a more tolerable level. The nurse should be acutely aware of the patient's response to such medications including any untoward effects. Many patients can be particularly sensitive to certain chemical agents, and the nurse is often involved in monitoring the patient during numerous drug trials. Side effects such as extrapyramidal symptoms, oversedation, anticholinergic effects, and allergic reactions should be addressed immediately (19). These symptoms can be extremely uncomfortable and distressing to the patient. The patient can become quite frightened and resistant in the future to drug therapy. Therefore, the nurse should observe for initial cues that the patient is developing side effects, i.e., slurred speech, lethargy, fine tremors and an inner jitteriness.

Communication

Effective communication techniques are essential when working with patients experiencing psychoses. It is important that the nurse recognizes that patients want to communicate even though their fears may inhibit them from doing so (20). Their inability to verbalize thoughts and feelings is not usually a result of conscious resistance. There are usually times when the patient can more easily talk with staff since patients are rarely out of touch with reality at all times. Therefore, while the nurse should consistently try to establish contact with the patient, particular efforts should be made during the patient's more lucid, rational moments.

The nurse-patient relationship usually progresses through predictable phases delineated as the introductory, working and termination phases (21). In the introductory phase, the nurse should be aware of the patient's need to maintain emotional distance and a sense of control over the relationship. Common facilitative techniques such as active listening, the use of broad, open-ended questions, clarifying, and silence may be effective. Even these techniques may not be effective unless combined with empathetic caring, honesty, and consistency over a period of time. The psychotic patient may be slow to develop trust, particularly since he has usually experienced many interpersonal difficulties. In order to progress to a working stage, the patient and nurse must identify problems in the patient's life and begin to establish goals. The working phase usually focuses on assisting the patient to re-establish a secure sense of identity and explore his thoughts, feelings, and behavior (22). The nurse will also help the patient to evaluate his thoughts, feelings, and behaviors by providing feedback and supportive confrontation (23). This approach can lead to mutual problem-solving, with the nurse offering encouragement as the patient strives to meet his goals and develop effective coping behaviors.

The last phase, that of termination may be difficult for the patient and the nurse. Frequently, patients display anger and regression. The nurse should attempt to work through these feelings with the patient and convey a sense of confidence in the patient's abilty to cope with termination. In addition, there should be ongoing arrangements to transfer the patient's intimacy, dependency, and other needs to appropriate individuals and/or a therapist who will be available for the patient upon discharge.

Throughout the phases of the nurse-patient relationship, a climate of acceptance should be maintained. An effective nurse will recognize that sharing can be quite threatening for a patient. It can be difficult for the patient to tolerate physical or emotional closeness. Oftentimes, the patient will act out his fears and expect to be rejected. The nurse may unexpectedly find the patient to be silent, using obscene language, gesturing bizarrely, or verbalizing hostile feelings. The patient's expectations of rejection should not be met; instead, the nurse should remain undemanding and should tolerate such behavior within limits, thereby conveying acceptance. In addition, the patient should always be allowed an adequate sense of personal space. Touch and physical closeness can invade the patient's fragile ego boundaries (24).

In working with psychotic patients, the symbolic nature of the patient's communication can be puzzling. Although the nurse attempts to decipher this communication, it is not always appropriate to confront the patient with possibly correct interpretations. Instead, such unstated interpretations may help the nurse understand the nature of the patient's conflicts. In addition, the nurse can assist the patient to communicate more clearly and directly. In doing so, the patient may uncover thoughts and feelings which have been blanketed in psychotic verbalizations. In her article, "Nursing Intervention with Patients with Thought Disorders," Patricia Schroder identifies many common language forms typical of patients with psychotic thought processes (25). She discusses the use of global pronouns and generalizations to project internal feelings about self such as "They hate me, they think I'm a bad person." A psychotic patient often believes that his thoughts are automatically known by others so he may frequently state, "you know" or leave sentences unfinished. A patient's ambivalence may be noted as he uses many "qualifiers" which enable him to avoid making a definitive statement (26). For example, "It may be good if I go to activity therapy, but sometimes when I'm there I get bothered. To get bothered is really upsetting so I really should wait to decide. On the other hand, I'm not sure." Symbolism is often manifested by "condensing" thoughts or reactions into a single symbol (27). An example which illustrates this concept is a woman who repetitively wears a wig when feeling agitated and depressed. When hospitalized, she continues wearing the wig until she begins to feel less depressed and more in control of her life. The patient condenses all of her negative thoughts and feelings into the wig, which she removes as her pain and discomfort decreases. Autistic language is usually symbolic of a patient's inner world and the people within it (28). Neologisms and word salads are sometimes verbalized and indicate the presence of autistic thinking.

The purpose in attempting to understand psychotic communication is that the nurse can then assist the patient to recognize and clearly express his verbal and nonverbal messages. This is much more therapeutic than ignoring the messages, assuming that they have no meaning, or feigning understanding. The nurse should convey a wish to understand the patient and should model clear, directive communication.

INTERVENTION

Withdrawn and Depressive Behavior

Patients who are withdrawn and experiencing depression are often immobilized and unable to meet their own physical or psychological needs. The observable "vegetative signs" include: a change in appetite, difficulty sleeping, weight changes, slowed thought processes and speech, and a lack of interest and energy. The patient often isolates himself, and personal cares which affect his appearance and hygiene may be neglected (29). These symptoms and behaviors usually further erode the patient's self-esteem so that he feels worthless and hopeless.

Often, nursing interventions initially focus upon the patient's physical needs (30). The staff should identify the problematic areas such as nutrition, sleep, elimination, or hygiene. The patient often requires encouragement to resume meeting these needs with as little assistance as possible. Some patients become so regressed that it is necessary to feed and bathe them. These physical cares should be provided in a nurturing manner, and measures which may be perceived as punitive and/or infantilizing such as tube-feedings, should only be implemented in life threatening situations. At times, a patient's refusal to eat or his difficulty in sleeping may occur because of delusional fears. For example, a patient may believe that he is being punished for his unpardonable sins and that people are planning to harm him.

It is often difficult to determine the source of the patient's fears since he may not be verbally interacting with the staff, yet it is essential to try to determine if fears and delusional ideas do exist.

It is important to assess the patient's sleep patterns and intervene if insomnia is a major problem. This symptom is very troublesome for a patient since it results in exhaustion and since the sleepless hours are often filled with depressive thoughts and self recrimination. Medication is often increased or added to end the sleeplessness cycle. However, when additional medication is not appropriate other methods to induce sleep may be attempted. Often, just staying with a patient until he is able to sleep seems to have a calming effect. In addition, a warm bath, soft music, reading to the patient or television watching may be useful.

The patient's psychological needs during this period of withdrawn behavior can be quite complex, particularly if the patient is not interacting with the staff. The patient does need the security of an accepting, non-demanding relationship. Although the staff should encourage the patient to verbalize thoughts and feelings, a nurse should be available to sit quietly with the patient even if he is unable or unwilling to talk. Sitting in silence can be anxiety-provoking for the nurse, yet it is often very comforting for the patient, particularly if the nurse conveys that this is acceptable and that he/she wishes to spend this time with the patient. When time is spent with the patient consistently, this often confirms that the staff does care and communicates to the patient that he is a worthwhile individual. The patient may then begin to respond to the staff. Initially, his repsonse may be very subtle and the nurse should be acutely aware of facial expressions, body movements, posture, and eye contact. Any type of response should be acknowledged in a positive way.

Reality Orientation may be a significant psychological need. The nurse can orient the patient by referring to the time of day, month, season, current events, etc. during the course of conversation. Items from home such as a radio, clock, family pictures, favorite clothes or other familiar articles may help the patient remain oriented and also lift his spirits.

Maintaining a level of activity can also help with the patient's reality orientation. It is important to insist upon activity even if the staff accompanies the patient or provides a wheelchair. Although the fearful patient should not be forced to be with other patients, the staff can take several walks with the patient so that he is out of his room periodically. As the patient becomes mobilized, activities can be planned which are non-threatening and rewarding, such as short term projects, non-competitive games or listening to music. If the patient has any interests or hobbies, related activities can be provided. These activities may help the patient with tension reduction as well as lead to an increase in socialization. While engaging in activities, the patient may face a need for decision-making which may be difficult and threatening. Deciding which dress to wear or whether to bathe in the morning or afternoon can be overwhelming. The nurse can assist the patient initially by offering limited choices. For example, the patient may be encouraged to select one of two dresses which may be less anxiety provoking than facing a closet with numerous outfits.

As the patient is being assisted with activity and decision-making, the timing may be appropriate to encourage the patient to identify feelings and sources of stress. The staff may need to help the patient channel his feelings appropriately and also determine if ventilation is therapeutic. With some patients, verbalizing negative thoughts and feelings is non-productive, anxiety provoking, and depressing without offering any relief. In contrast, other patients are able to identify feelings and problem areas in a constructive fashion. In either situation, the staff should respond to the patient in an adult and genuine manner. While false assurance and patronizing behavior are to be avoided, the staff should acknowledge the patient's smallest efforts.

When caring for patients with withdrawn and depressive behavior, it is especially important to establish short term reachable goals with the patient. As the patient works to meet these goals, the staff can identify the changes in his behavior and attitudes. This type of realistic feedback can begin to help the patient rebuild ego strength and a sense of self-esteem. It may also provide an opportunity for reality testing for the patient whose self-deprecatory thoughts are of a delusional nature. It is a sign of progress when a patient can identify his own strengths and successes.

When working with patients who have become regressed and withdrawn, dependence can become an issue. Initially, the staff must allow a great deal of dependent behavior and meet many of the patient's basic needs. However, the staff should be astute in their assessments of the patient, observing for signs that he is able to handle independent activities. This may vary throughout the patient's hospitalization, but periods of increased withdrawal should not be viewed as failures or signs of relapse. Instead, the patient and staff should expect difficult days. The staff may still insist that the patient maintain a certain level of independent functioning while offering additional support and encouragement.

As the withdrawn, depressed patient becomes increasingly mobilized, the staff should be aware of a heightened suicide potential. Assessments should include direct questioning as well as observation. It is not safe or acceptable to allow a patient to leave the hospital unit unaccompanied until the staff is confident that the patient is not suicidally depressed. Classic signs indicative of suicidal intent are a marked change in mood and behavior which may include a sudden lifting of depressive symptoms, a sense of purpose, or an interest in resolving family matters. These are only a few cues; the staff's knowledge of the patient and his individual situation will offer more sound criteria for assessment.

Bizarre Behavior

Patients with a variety of psychiatric illnesses may exhibit bizarre behavior. Wild laughing, loud inappropriate speech, posturing, hurling oneself around the room are a few of the behaviors which the nursing staff may need to manage. It is difficult to determine the nature of such behavior since at times it may seem very purposeful and attention seeking while at other times appear to be the result of the patient's loss of control. It is essential that the staff respond in a non-punitive manner and assist the patient to control his behavior. Many times, bizarre behavior is the product of disintegrative thought processes; in other instances it is a desperate attempt on the patient's part to get certain needs met. In either situation, this type of behavior requires firm yet supportive intervention. The behavior has meaning, but often the nurse must respond before the meaning is clear.

Comfort and safety may become important issues with extremely regressed patients. For example, a patient who is posturing in awkward positions may need body supports for his extremities. Allowing the patient to assume these positions may be more therapeutic than restraining the patient in a supine position.

Reality orientation may also be a need of regressed patients. Consistently offering information about their person, the place and time may be helpful. In addition, if they are confused about past events or present circumstances, the staff should correct their misperceptions.

It is always important to respond quickly when the patient begins to behave bizarrely, not only on the patient's behalf, but also for the other patients who may be disturbed or frightened by the behavior (31). Offering a calm but firm approach may assist the patient to regain control. Since such behavior is often a response to anxiety and the environment, it is often helpful to reduce the stimuli by directing the patient to a quiet setting. When the staff determines that the patient is able to cooperate and the potential for destructive behavior is not a problem, spending time alone with the patient can be helpful. Once the patient has become reintegrated and is calm, it is useful to discuss thoughts or feelings which may have precipitated or been associated with the behavior. If anxiety-provoking thoughts can be identified, it is often possible to establish mutual goals so that the patient can begin to control behavioral responses. For example, a patient may be willing to seek out staff members when he begins to feel frightened by other patients. When a patient is not able to follow through with a goal which requires so much self control and initiative, the staff can offer to check with the patient at specific times if the patient will agree to honestly share his feelings and level of anxiety. Whatever efforts may be necessary on the part of the nursing staff, if it provides an initial basis for the patient recognizing his feelings and gaining control over his response, it is worthwhile.

As the patient begins to gain control over his behavior, it is important that he become aware of other people's reactions to his behavior. This information may be an important part of the patient's reality testing and may also help the patient with interpersonal relationships since he will begin to recognize how others are affected by his actions. For example, a patient may have no awareness that his pacing, grimacing, and hair pulling are frightening to other patients.

Often, it is necessary to repeat the process of identifying troublesome feelings, reality testing, and goal setting before the patient begins to feel a sense of control. Periods of regression may follow periods of integration. Specific events may lead to the resumption of regressive, bizarre behavior. The meaning of the events and resulting behavior should be explored with the patient. For example, a patient may resume posturing and screaming after difficult visits from her family as a way to communicate her anger and pain.

When bizarre behavior is the result of an intentional striving to get needs met, the staff should openly discuss their desire to understand the meaning of the patient's behavior. The patient should be acknowledged when he appropriately verbalizes his feelings and needs. It is not therapeutic to reinforce the inappropriate behavior by giving the patient the attention and nurturance he is seeking if he will not cooperate and try to identify his needs with the staff. However, this requires trust on the patient's part and can be quite painful since there is a risk of rejection. The patient's needs, once identified, may be unrealistic and/or overwhelming for the staff. However, the staff can discuss what they can realistically provide and attempt to negotiate this with the patient. For example, a patient may eventually recognize that she grabs the nurses and sits on the floor in the middle of the unit in order to get their attention. She verbalizes that she wants a nurse to be with her all the time. The staff can discuss the times when a nurse can be with the patient, offer her activities which will keep her near the nursing desk and begin to explore her fears of being alone and assure her support when she is frightened. This type of attention may temporarily meet her needs until she becomes more stalibized.

Bizarre behavior often serves as a protective mechanism for coping with fears associated with delusions, hallucinations, or confusion. It is important that the staff should help the patient to establish alternative coping mechanisms before trying to extinguish the behavior. Negative reinforcement or other purely behavioral techniques may lead to the cessation of a specific behavior; without adaptive alternatives, however, the patient can become overwhelmed and regress even further.

Manic Behavior

Manic patients frequently display bizarre behavior; therefore, in providing nursing care, the interventions described in the previous section are relevant. When mania has escalated to a level where the patient is psychotic, the patient's thought processes are usually greatly accelerated and may involve grandiose delusions and hallucinations (32). It is difficult to reach a therapeutic balance when the patient is channeling his energy effectively yet not being overstimulated to the point of mental and physical exhaustion.

One aspect of nursing care of manic patients is similar to the care provided for other patients experiencing psychosis. The patient's physiologic needs for nutrition, sleep and hygiene must be considered. Often, a manic patient cannot follow through with self care or respond to internal cues such as hunger or sleep deprivation. In order to assist the patient, the nurse may need to be creative in her strategies. For instance, with a patient who is having difficulty sitting down to eat a meal because of constant movement and speech, finger foods can be offered which can be eaten while the patient is active. The patient can be assisted to care for personal hygiene and wash clothes by being structured to do these tasks for short periods of time. For example, in performing morning cares, a patient may brush his teeth before taking a short walk and then return to wash the upper part of his body. He may need to leave his room several times before completing his cares. Although this demands a great deal of nursing time and coordination, it may be more effective than attempting to get the patient to follow through with activities in a concentrated routine manner.

Sleep is usually a major problem for these patients. Even with appropriate pharmacotherapy, a patient may only sleep for short periods. Expecting the patient to lie quietly while awake is usually unrealistic. During the night the staff can plan a quiet activity to help the patient channel his energy while not disturbing others. The patient may engage in repetitive activities such as folding clothes or hoarding articles. During the night as well as daytime, allowing the patient to carry out these activities may have a calming effect (33).

Activities which do not require constant concentration and can be completed in a short period of time, usually provide diversion for the patient. It is best to avoid engaging the patient in competitive team activities which can lead to overstimulation, frustration and irritability. Physical exercise and movement activities can be therapeutic. Staff must constantly observe the patient for signs of overstimulation and agitation. Finding a place for the patient where stimuli are reduced and he can calm himself is important. Secluding such a patient frequently leads to further agitation and even panic. Rarely does seclusion successfully reduce stimulation unless a patient willingly goes to the room to be alone. It is often beneficial for the patient to have a single room in a quiet area on the unit (34). The staff can then work with the patient to identify when he is becoming agitated and to demonstrate that this uncomfortable feeling can be reduced by going to a quiet area such as his room. He can then engage in activities which calm him.

Frustration, anger, and irritability are often displayed by the manic patient. The patient is often very egocentric during acute phases of his illness: he feels very powerful and important. He usually ignores social cues and the feelings of others. While the staff can respond neutrally to the patient who is angry. there may be a need to protect other pateints from verbal abuse, hostility, or even physical abuse. If such incidents occur and the patient cannot be controlled verbally, physical intervention may become necessary. During the course of the hospitalization as the patient begins to gain control over his thoughts and behavior, the nursing staff can work to help the patient express anger and frustration in an appropriate manner, since this is often a chronic problem for this patient who is struggling against inner self-directed anger and aggression.

The patient's manic behavior, which may be loud, boisterous, sexually oriented and demanding, can be very disturbing to other patients. The patient may become a scapegoat on the unit and the source of ridicule and hostility. The staff may need to try to shield the patient from this process by limiting the patient's activities in large groups or by working with the other patients to express their feelings directly and appropriately.

Limit setting often becomes a constant source of frustration for the nursing staff as well as the patient. The nursing staff should make every attempt to meet the requests and demands of the patient which are reasonable. Limits should be reserved for behaviors which are impulsive and self-defeating, for instance spending large sums of money or arranging business transactions. The nursing staff will also need to limit behaviors which are intolerable for other patients. It is best to approach the patient firmly, using brief, simple explanations in contrast to allowing the patient to start a lengthy discussion or argument. It is often easy to divert a manic patient from troublesome behavior since his attention span is quite limited. Power struggles should be avoided as much as possible since the patient will become extremely angry if he feels his desires are being thwarted. However, consistent limits and expectations may promote feelings of safety as well as decrease manipulative behavior.

The staff should work with the patient to establish mutual goals which will lead to esteem building and feelings of security. These are important patient needs even though his behavior gives no indication that these are problem areas. Conveying that the patient is responsible for his behavior is essential since patients often see the staff's limit setting as very controlling and parental. Responses to the patient's behavior such as shock or anger should be avoided since they only serve to enforce inappropriate behaviors. Neutral responses are more often therapeutic, as is the approach of offering positive reinforcement when the patient attempts to control his impulses and follow through with goals.

Patients who exhibit mania may be treated with lithium carbonate, which is indicated for the control and prevention of manic episodes in manic depressive illness (35). The nursing staff should be concerned with the side effects and toxic effects of this drug. Lithium blood levels are usually ordered by the physician every other day when trying to stabilize the patient. It is often difficult to determine therapeutic dosages for patients since individuals vary in their sensitivity to lithium. The patient's weight as well as fluid intake and output should be monitored since normal excretion depends upon a well balanced diet. The diet should provide adequate sodium and fluid intake but not an excess of either, which could lead to decreased lithium levels (36). If the patient manifests symptoms such as anorexia, diarrhea, muscle hyper-irritability, nausea, blurred vision, or confusion, the patient may be toxic and blood levels should be drawn (37). Such symptoms can escalate to the point of seizures and coma, so toxicity must be prevented. Patients may also complain of side effects such as mild thirst, hand tremor, mild nausea, and headache. The nurse is also responsible for providing thorough medication teaching and discharge information for patients receiving lithium. The patient should be informed about diet, lithium blood levels, side effects, contraindications, and signs of toxicity.

Delusional Thinking

The following section will discuss nursing interventions with patients experiencing delusional thinking. Delusions may be characterized as being paranoid, grandiose, or somatic (38). Depressed patients often experience delusional thinking about having "committed the unpardonable sin" or being povery striken. The patient's delusions serve as a maladaptive coping mechanism in the face of overwhelming anxiety. His behavior may be condescending and hostile in an attempt to protect himself. In response, the nurse should use a calm, self-assured, yet supportive manner. Angry responses and the use of confrontation, logic, or argument to dispel delusions are never successful (39).

Although patients' delusional ideas and fears may seem quite bizarre, such fears should not be treated in a callous or demeaning manner. For example, patients may believe that they are religious figures such as Jesus Christ or Ghandi, and that they are being persecuted and plotted against. The nursing staff should never agree with the patient's ideas but they can convey that although they don't share the patient's beliefs, they understand that the patient is sincere as he shares his perceptions. In addition, the staff can acknowledge the fear, pain, and hurt which must accompany certain ideas and beliefs. When the patient's anxiety and fears are creating a sense of panic, the patient may respond to reassurance and reality orientation. In the case of a patient who thinks that his wife and child have been killed in a car accident, the staff can attempt to assure the patient that his family was not in an accident. A phone call or visit by the family would then support the staff's assurances. As quickly as possible, the nursing staff should identify the behaviors which are precipitated by the patient's delusional thinking. For instance, a patient's refusal to eat or take medications is often associated with the idea that someone is trying to harm or kill him. This should not be interpreted as a lack of cooperation; instead, the staff can acknowledge the patient's fears and offer to taste the food or prepare the medication in the patient's presence.

Unlike patients who require guidance and structure for many aspects of their daily living, many delusional patients respond well when they are given the opportunity to exert control over their environment, schedule, activity, or meals. This may result in the patient developing a sense of personal esteem and security since the staff is conveying an attitude of respect, concern and the recognition of the patient's rights. For example, flexible meal times may allow a patient the comfort of eating alone instead of being forced to eat with other patients which may create anxiety and agitation. Encouraging the patient's sense of control can also help the staff avoid power struggles with the patient which may erode trust levels which have been established.

Patients who have delusions that are not of a paranoid nature may be comfortable in sharing and socializing with staff and patients. These patients may continually focus on delusional materials. Once the patient's ideas have been thoroughly reviewed, it may be helpful to divert the patient so that he will focus on other ideas and activities in order to socialize in a more appropriate manner. At other times, the staff can attempt to have the patient identify feelings which accompany his beliefs instead of dwelling on their content. Examining these feelings and developing goals to handle them appropriately are optimal, long-term goals. Lack of a secure ego identity and self-esteem is usually a major issue and the staff may need to help the patient develop goals in this area.

Patients who experience delusions of a paranoid nature may have many additional needs. Respecting the patient's need for territorial space by not touching or cornering the patient is necessary to prevent fear and agitation. The staff should approach the patient by using clear, simple language in a straight-forward manner while avoiding overfriendly or patronizing behavior.

Psychiatric patients benefit from consistent staff assignments and this is particularly true with patients experiencing paranoid delusions. With a limited number of staff providing care, there is potential to build a trust relationship. The patient must be allowed to set the pace of the therapeutic relationship since his symptoms often provide a mechanism to avoid intimate contact. Honesty within the relationship is essential; any attempts to force the patient's cooperation through half truths or trickery can be extremely damaging. The patient should not be forced to interact with other patients. Activities can be planned which involve only the patient or trusted staff. Solitary activities requiring concentration often provide a source of diversion. Demanding that the patient socialize with other patients can lead to panic and extremely aggressive or self-abusive behavior. As the patient becomes more comfortable and trusts at least one staff member, other staff and patients can be introduced gradually.

When the patient's delusional ideas involve a fear of persecution and rejection, the potential for violence is great (40). The staff should monitor the patient closely to prevent suicidal, self-abusive, or aggressive behavior. A restricted environment may be necessary to protect the patient as well as other patients.

Perpetual Disturbance-Hallucinations

Hallucinations are a complex phenomenon which nurses and other mental health professionals seek to understand in order to provide effective intervention. Hallucinations describe the experience where the patient hears, sees, tastes or feels something which does not exist. This experience is described as having three basic characteristics: the created perception, projecting this perception onto reality, and the patient's belief that this perception is real and not self-created (41). The most common form of hallucination which patients experience is auditory. The other types are usually associated with some type of organic involvement which may result from drug usage, drug withdrawal, injury to the brain or some form of organic brain disease (42). Since auditory hallucinations are the most common, they will be the focus of this section; however, many nursing interventions can be easily generalized to patients who experience any type of hallucinations.

It is important that the nurse recognize how hallucinations develop. Premorbidly, the patient is usually an individual who has been isolated, withdrawn and extremely anxious. Initially, the patient invents a friend or helper through auditory hallucinations (43). This experience offers comfort in the face of anxiety and conflict. The patient begins interacting with the voices repeatedly. According to Arieti, the hallucinations are composed of sensory and perceptual material from the past or present (44). With repeated interactions with the voices, the individual begins to isolate himself more and his behavior usually comes to the attention of others, i.e., family or friends. Eventually, the invented voices become negative and frightening. The individual projects his concept of self as bad and unacceptable onto the voices as well as other inner conflicts such as anger and rejection (45). Instead of offering a comforting experience, hallucinating becomes anxiety-provoking, and the voices may threaten the patient or demand violent behavior. The individual's behavior will become more bizarre and he will feel as though he is being controlled by the voices. Usually at this time the patient is brought for some type of treatment (46). Recognizing how hallucinations develop may help the nurse to comprehend the fear and loneliness associated with this experience. Such recognition also serves as a basis for intervention since the development of a therapeutic relationship can help the patient control the hallucinatory experience and eventually replace hallucinating with personal contact and human relationship.

In assessing the presence of hallucinations, a direct statement such as, "are you hallucinating?" may be frightening to a patient. The patient may interpret this question in a way that indicates that the nurse is mind reading or also hears the voices. Many times, patients may fear that such a revelation will lead to punishment by the voices. Less direct statements may be more effective when the nurse suspects that the patient is hearing voices. Examples of such statements are: "Do you ever become so anxious that you have unusual experiences like hearing or seeing things that perhaps other people don't?" "Are you feeling anxious?" "What happens to you when you feel so uncomfortable?" "What's happening now, you seem to be giving attention to something other than your voice or mine?"

Once the nurse has determined that a patient does experience hallucinations, it is important to assess the impact that environmental stimuli have on the hallucinating patient. Patients may hallucinate when alone due to the anxiety produced by certain thoughts; however, other patients may experience more discomfort when they are surrounded by other patients. The patient's immediate environment should be altered as he begins to feel anxious and hallucinates. For example, a nurse may accompany a patient to his room from a noisy unit lounge and stay with him until their talking reduces the patient's anxiety and the voices.

The staff should acknowledge that the patient's experience is real and frightening to him, while insisting that the voices don't exist for them. Questioning the logic of the voices or arguing is not helpful. Many patients may be reassured if the staff supportively state that the voices do not exist and are a part of the patient's illness which he can learn to overcome. It is essential that the patient begins to identify and verbalize the relationship between his feelings, i.e., anxiety, fear, loneliness, and the hallucinations. This then leads to the recognition that the voices are from within himself and are related to internal rather than external causes.

Patients may become agitated and extremely uncomfortable when actively hallucinating. In addition to altering the environmental factors which may have precipitated anxiety, the nurse should redirect the patient to reality. Interrupting the hallucinatory experience by: talking and engaging the patient in conversation, touching, or activity may help divert the patient. Secluding a patient who is hallucinating often increases the patient's fear and agitation. Instead, staying with the patient while attempting to calm and divert him is usually more effective. While avoiding making any demands on the patient, the nurse may have the patient accompany her as other daily tasks are performed. Often, encouraging the patient to sing, creating competitive sounds, or verbally insisting that the voice go away, will help the patient refocus his attention and begin to feel some control over the voices (47).

Staff members who are frightened by the hallucinating patient should seek assistance since these patient are very sensitive to the feelings of others, and staff anxiety may lead to increased fear and loss of control. The staff needs to be caring yet in control to prevent the patient from harming himself or others if the voices are commanding dangerous or aggressive acts. A supportive yet firm approach is essential in order for the patient to regain self control.

Patients experiencing hallucinations related to alcohol withdrawal, drug intoxication, or drug withdrawal require intensive management. A nurse should remain with the patient to insure safety and monitoring of his physiologic status. During this time she can attempt to orient the conscious patient to reality, explain in detail procedures being performed and assure the patient that the symptoms are related to chemical intoxication or withdrawal. It is helpful to have the room lighted so that shaded shadows and figures do not provide stimuli for frightening visions. However, the most difficult tasks often involve physiological stabilization. The nurse is an integral part of the team as it intervenes by administering medications and other treatments to prevent life threatening complications from occurring.

Inappropriate Sexual Behavior

Psychotic patients often exhibit inappropriate sexual behavior which may be very disturbing for the staff as well as other patients. Such behavior is often symbolic and is usually related to sexual conflicts. The patient's disordered thoughts may focus on sexual material, hallucinatory voices may demand bizarre sexual acts, or delusions may involve fears of homosexual encounters. Frequently, inappropriate sexual behavior is manifested when the patient is quite regressed, i.e., public masturbation, shouting sexual words and ideas.

On the basis of the patient's history, including current interpersonal dynamics, the meaning of the behavior should be explored. At times, acknowledging the underlying conflict which the patient is acting out may help the patient identify and verbalize his feelings. For example, the nurse might help the patient recognize that his inappropriate seductive behavior with every female patient stems from his fears of homosexuality. Encouragement to talk about these fears may help the patient control his behavior and work on the actual conflict.

Patients may not understand that discussing sexual material is acceptable and productive during appropriate times.

At times, the nurse may be approached with sexual appeals or seductive behavior since she/he may be viewed as a safe person who won't reject the patient. Patients may not be able to differentiate between professional concern and caring and sexual feelings. The response to sexual requests from either male or female patients should be firm yet gentle, trying to help the patient understand the nature of the nurse–patient relationship. Although the patient may react in an angry, rejecting manner, it is essential that the nurse continue to approach the patient and attempt to re-establish contact.

When a patient's sexual behavior is socially inappropriate, it is important to interrupt the behavior in a firm yet non-condemnatory manner. Patients who are confused may require close observation so that staff can help them control their behavior as well as protect them if they are responsive to sexual approaches from other patients.

Often, patients who do have control over their behavior become sexually involved with one another. Such a couple may respond to a discussion exploring their own vulnerability during their hospitalization. They may be able to recognize the negative impact this relationship could have on their therapy. The nurse can help them identify alternative ways to express comfort and concern. Patients who are sexually involved with one another pose a difficult problem for staff since a parental approach usually involves secretive, rebellious behavior yet the staff feels responsible for the patient's behavior. Every attempt should be made to approach the problem in a supportive fashion while insisting that the patients should assume responsibility for their involvement and the possible consequences.

If a patient is engaging in solitary masturbatory behavior, the staff can protect the patient from exposure by working with him to limit the activity to the privacy of the room and to appropriate times. When patients are extremely regressed, behavioral techniques based upon positive reinforcement can be implemented to help the patient limit his activity. For example, favorite activities or foods may be offered when a patient does not openly masturbate for a specified period of time.

The nursing staff should develop a matter-of-fact yet understanding attitude when discussing sexual behavior. It is essential that the patient is not made to feel guilty or ashamed of sexual feelings and desires. In order to insure this type of approach, nurses should explore their own level of comfort and anxiety related to sexual issues. If this is a sensitive, difficult area, the nurse's assessment of his/her feelings and subsequent responses to patients is necessary in order to avoid rejecting, punitive attitudes to the patient's inappropriate sexual behavior.

The Confused and Disoriented Patient

Patients of all ages may suffer from confusion and disorientation. Often the confusion is acute in nature and will disappear as the patient's thought processes begin to clear. Confusion and disorientation which result from drug intoxication or withdrawal are also usually time limited. Other patients may manifest these symptoms chronically as a result of irreversible organic brain impairment. The impairment may be due to degenerative, vascular, traumatic, metabolic, or neoplastic causes (48).

In caring for these patients, it is important to note that patients often vary in their level of cognitive functioning according to the time of day, anxiety level, environmental stimuli, and individual factors. Astute assessment is necessary since many patients will cover this confusion by appearing calm and quiet while answering questions with vague responses (49). Pursuing the patient's responses with more specific questions may reveal that the patient is quite confused and in need of reality orientation.

Insuring that the patient's physiologic needs are met is very important. Unlike other patients who can often follow through with daily activities once reminded, severely confused patients may not be able to carry out even simple tasks. Consequently, the staff may need to provide continual assistance in order for the patient to eat, bathe, and dress. Incontinence is often a problem: frequent checks and bathroom visits may be effective. Otherwise, the patient should be cleaned promptly to prevent skin breakdown and rashes. Sleep can also become a major problem since confused patients often suffer from "sundowning" when they become more active and agitated at night while napping during the day. Providing for mild sensory stimulation often has a calming effect and maintains orientation to reality, i.e., a radio played softly or a night light. Other comfort measures to induce sleep include: back rubs, warm baths, offering milk or a warm liquid, quietly reading to a patient or staying with him for a short time. Medications such as hypnotics and sedatives frequently create further confusion and agitation.

Additional physiologic needs may be directly related to the patient's ability to perceive reality. The staff should assess the patient's need for glasses, hearing aid or mobility aids which help the patient maintain contact with his surroundings. If patients have hearing or vision deficits, the staff should approach the patient so they can be easily seen or heard.

Confusion is usually exacerbated by the unfamiliar or unexpected. Consistency of staff caring for the patient as well as predictable routines can afford the patient a degree of security which leads to optimal functioning. A calendar, clock, daily schedule and door tag may help the patient maintain orientation and a degree of independence. Familiar objects from home such as family pictures, certain clothes, and favorite possessions also serve to orient the patient. Similarly, limited numbers of close friends and family members who visit often have a positive effect. In contrast, large numbers of visitors may provide sensory overload and confuse and frighten the patient.

In addition to personal objects and daily routines, discussing topics which are familiar to the patient may help to decrease the patient's confusion and provide a sense of satisfaction for the patient since he can communicate knowledge and expertise (50). For example, the nurse can discuss crops and weather with a retired farmer or rock music with a young adult who shows interest in current music. All contacts with the patient, including physical cares, present the opportunity to orient the patient. For instance, while assisting a patient to bathe, the nurse can discuss familiar subjects or orient the patient to person, place, and time by frequently using the patient's name, mentioning the hospital and unit activities, and talking about season-related topics (51).

In working with confused patients, it is important that the staff should recognize the anxiety and fear that the patient experiences and provide a calm and supportive approach. Talking down to patients, calling elderly individuals "grandma" or "grandpa," or conveying a patronizing, parental attitude can create hostility in some patients while reinforcing regression in others. When communicating with confused patients, it is helpful to face the patient at a close but comfortable distance. Touch can indicate sincere interest and may help to maintain the patient's attention (52). Using brief, simple statements and explanations allows the patient more easily to interpret the nurse's message. Bombarding the patient with questions to stimulate his memory may serve only to confuse and agitate the patient. Family members may need to be advised not to use this approach since they often believe that if they are able to stimulate the patient's memory, he will return to "normal." The staff can help the family by encouraging them to provide the patient with reality oriented information, answer questions even if they are repetitious and correct misinformation in simplistic terms. For example, a patient asking for his deceased wife should be reminded of his wife's death and the time of her death as well as any other details which may be helpful.

When a confused patient is verbalizing fear and anxiety, it is usually therapeutic to acknowledge his feelings. However, dwelling on these may lead to an increase in anxiety and depression rather than relief. Therefore, at times, moving the conversation along to a familiar but different topic may be more beneficial than allowing the patient to ruminate.

Motivating the patient to be active can be difficult, yet it is important for physical and psychological well-being. Arguing and forcing the patient to leave his room are usually not effective: activity becomes synonymous with punishment. Instead, stimulating the patient with a favorite hobby, visitor or even a favorite snack to be eaten in the activity room may be more successful It is often necessary to leave the patient for a time if he is refusing to go out of his room and approach later in a positive manner. Group activities may serve as a source of stimulation as can interpersonal contact such as reality orientation groups, music or movement therapy sessions, or leisure groups. Despite the staff's efforts, patients may have periods when they are more confused, withdrawn and inactive. During these times, a level of stimulation should be maintained and bed exercises or passive range of motion exercises may need to be initiated to prevent any physiological complications.

Violent, Aggressive Behavior

The potential for violence directed toward self or others is high when patients are actively psychotic. Hallucinations and delusions can lead the patient to act in an impulsive, destructive fashion without external provocation. The need for continuous assessment is obvious if there is any indication that the patient might behave violently. If a patient does act on these impulses, seclusion and restraint should be used judiciously. Extended periods of seclusion may not be appropriate since the patient may respond to intervention and may quickly resume self control. Staff need to observe for early signs of agitation such as pacing, loud talking, repetitious or aggressive body movements. Such early detection can allow for preventative interventions including talking with a patient in a quiet area or diversional activity.

Psychiatric unit should have Standards of Nursing Care which identify procedures for intervening with a violent or suicidal patient. The standards should describe assessment, levels of precaution, and intervention. In addition, criteria and procedures for patient restraint and seclusion should be developed so that the staff is consistent in their approach.

With patients who are potentially violent or suicidal, concern for the patient should be expressed with the assurance that the staff will provide security and safety. This attitude contrasts with a suspecting, punitive approach which often provokes violent or suicidal acts as the patient expresses his anger. Long term mutual goal setting may be possible as a patient regains control, so that he attempts to verbalize thoughts and feelings rather than act them out.

The nursing staff may need a safety mechanism to help it deal with feelings which may arise after facing crises in which patients are aggressive, suicidal, or inflicting self-harm. Such experiences can be very frightening and depressing. Without a source of support, staff members may withdraw emotionally from patients in order to avoid these overwhelming feelings. Preventive strategies should be developed so that mutual staff support is available through staff meetings, short term support groups, or staff oriented conferences and seminars.

EVALUATION AND MODIFICATION

In the ongoing process of evaluation, the staff should continually assess the patient's response to the mental health team's approach according to the criteria established. Often, in the initial phases of the patient's hospitalization, the focus will be on symptom relief. This may be realistic since the patient's symptoms often need to be controlled before any type of meaningful therapy can be initiated. However, there is a danger if symptom relief becomes the long term focus of the patient's hospitalization. Patients who have experienced psychotic symptoms usually need assistance to manage many areas of their life including interpersonal relationships, occupation, family relationships and day-to-day activities.

The mental health team will evaluate the patient's progress and care periodically while the nursing staff is responsible for evaluation on a shift by shift basis. It is imperative that such evaluations be documented and relate to the established nursing diagnosis. The nursing staff should also give special attention to the goals which are mutually developed with the patient. The patient's subjective assessment of his status is extremely valuable and important although in many instances it is overlooked. The patient's evaluation will also offer the nursing staff insight into the appropriateness of their goals for the patient. Although usually well-meaning, it is common for the nursing staff to attempt to initiate behavior and life changes which are not even remotely desirable to the patient. In order to insure active collaboration between the nursing staff and the patient, periodic evaluation sessions may be scheduled. Some institutions have initiated nursing rounds in which the patient is interviewed by a nurse consultant or head nurse (53). The patient is questioned about his progress, productive and non-productive experiences in the hospital, and nursing care in the presence of the nurses involved in his care (54). This provides an opportunity to collaborate about goals and elicit feedback about the patient's perceptions of the nursing care provided. In addition, final evaluations with the patient should always be conducted when the patient leaves the hospital.

An important aspect of evaluation relates to the nurse-patient relationship. Members of the nursing staff should continually assess the nature of their relationships with their patients by requesting peer feedback and supervision to validate their self evaluations. Hildegard Peplau has discussed "illness-maintaining behaviors of nurses with inpatients" (55). She encourages nurses to become responsible to identify such behaviors in their daily work and to alter them in order to become true change-agents. Illness maintaining behaviors which nurses may manifest are usually unique and too numerous to mention. However, a few danger signals may include: making "pets" of a few patients, becoming so close to a patient that the nurse loses objectivity so that the patient is no longer a patient, viewing the patient in a possessive way, responding to dependent behavior by confirming the patient's "helpless" self-view, choosing sides with a patient against friends, family members or other staff, arguing with a patient, or immediately responding to a patient's anxiety or troublesome behavior with over-medication or seclusion rather than exploring the underlying problems and dynamics (56, 57). Many of these behaviors may result from countertransference. The countertransference response may be related to previous relationships, unresolved conflicts or past experiences. The patient is usually perceived in a very positive or negative manner. Other staff members can often identify danger signals with objectivity. Therefore, their perceptions are valuable even though they may not seem accurate to the nurse initially.

In discussing evaluation, it is essential to consider evaluation measures and criteria for all the nursing care delivered on a specific unit. The nursing staff usually develops Standards of Nursing Care. The Standards describe nursing activities which are required when providing care for specific patient populations. For example, there may be standards for the hallucinating patient, manic-depressive patient, paranoid patient, or schizophrenic patient. The categories may be determined by psychiatric diagnoses or patient symptoms and behaviors. Usually, more than one standard may be utilized since patients may manifest a combination of symptoms. Nursing audits should be frequently conducted by the staff to determine if the Standards are being implemented. The patient's plan of care should reflect these Standards although they will be individualized according to the needs of a specific patient. This type of broad evaluation insures feedback for the nursing staff and provides for continuous improvement in the quality of nursing care.

DISCHARGE PLANNING

Patients who have experienced psychotic episodes usually have many discharge needs. Whether the patient is discharged after receiving maximum benefit from treatment or prematurely, against medical advice, the nursing staff should attempt to help the patient in his re-entry into the community. With patients who are legally committed, discharge is often conditional. The patient is required to continue some type of therapy or contact with the treatment facility. Conditional discharge often provides a mechanism to bridge the gap between hospital and community living since the patient and staff evaluate the patient's ability to adjust to a more independent life style (58).

Discharge planning should occur throughout the patient's hospitalization. Follow-up treatment with continued pharmacotherapy and psychotherapy is usually a discharge need for patients who have been psychotic. In addition, patients may require vocational counseling, financial and housing assistance, and medical care. The nurse often coordinates the patient's access to agencies providing these services. The patient should be involved in discharge planning and should independently arrange for meetings and appointments whenever feasible. Initiating these contacts when the patient still has staff support may help to insure that the patient will follow through when he must do so independently.

The patient and his family have many teaching needs at the time of discharge. Often, the family does not know what to expect from the patient; they may be confused about behavioral changes and frightened that the patient will regress. The patient and family should be assisted to mutually explore these issues. Often, the staff will need to provide information about normal phases of reintegration, symptoms which may require medical attention and the follow-up activities which have been planned. Medication teaching is usually an important area for both the patient and family. Information about the effects of the medication, dosage, administration, side effects and any special precautions such as blood tests and diet should be reviewed until the patient and family show evidence of comprehension. Many hospitals give the patient the opportunity to self administer medications for several days before discharge so that the patient can establish a routine. Medication compliance after discharge continues to be a problem. Patients are frequently re-admitted to the hospital for symptom recurrence because of the patient's discontinuing his medication. It is important that the patient is taught that although he may not feel the effects of medication, it is helping him to remain stabilized even if he experiences anxiety or depression at times (59). Comparing the patient's need for medication to that of the diabetic or hypertensive patient often helps dispel fears of addiction. The patient should be assured that side effects can be managed once brought to the attention of medical personnel. Often, aftercare medication groups provide a chance for patients to discuss concerns and encourage one another to continue taking their medications.

Termination is an important aspect of nursing intervention during discharge. The patient and nurse face various tasks which are necessary to complete before discharge is appropriate. It is important that the patient evaluate his therapy, review his successes and verbalize negative experiences (60). With particular nurses, the patient may feel a loss of a significant person in his life and he must work through the feelings associated with this including grief, anger, and ambivalence. The staff should work to transfer the patient's dependence to another support system that will be available to the patient (61).

Adequate time should be available for the patient and staff to work through termination issues. As dismissal approaches, patients may go through periods of regression, acting-out, anger and denial. Ideally, the patient should feel comfortable by the time of discharge. If the patient is unable to get to this point, follow-up treatment becomes even more important. There should be a sense of finality to the hospitalization and the nurse-patient relationship (62). If continued contact or treatment is planned, the nature of the relationship should change and there should be an understanding that the treatment process is entering a different phase which will necessitate separation and independence on the patient's part.

Termination can be a difficult process for the nurse. It is important to refrain from establishing a friendship which will be maintained after discharge in order to avoid termination. Such relationships are rarely therapeutic and reinforce the individual's dependence. Frequently, such a relationship sabotages the efforts of the patient's new therapist and the patient does not successfully reintegrate with family and friends. The nurse is usually meeting her own needs in this situation rather than those of the patient.

In order to facilitate termination and the discharge process, many inpatient units provide discharge groups. Both the patients and family members may be involved in such groups. The group members usually share their feelings and concerns related to discharge. In addition, problem solving may occur as patients discuss their fears about such issues as: returning to work, what to tell family members and friends, symptom recurrence, and seeing a new therapist. Discharge groups provide an opportunity for patients to support one another and acknowledge that their feelings and fears are not unique or abnormal. If the patient has been participating in any type of therapy group, it is important that he work through termination with group members. Even though this may be a painful experience, the other group members may offer helpful feedback for the patient and his sense of group "belongingness" may motivate him to seek similar support in outpatient groups.

In summary, the discharge phase of hospitalization provides many opportunities for the patient to grow, to cope with difficult feelings and to prepare for everyday living. Patients need a great deal of direction and guidance as they face discharge, and the staff should not be tempted to prematurely separate from the patient even though he no longer manifests troublesome symptoms. Instead, energy must be directed toward teaching and supporting the patient and family so that they feel a degree of security and assurance as the patient leaves the hospital.

REFERENCES

1. Stuart, G. and Sundeen, S.: *Principles and Practice of Psychiatric Nursing.* St. Louis: The C.V. Mosby Co., 295, 1979.

2. *Ibid.*, pg. 296.

3. Carter, E. and McGoldrick, M.: *The Family Life Cycle: A Framework for Family Therapy.* New York: Gardner Press Inc., pg. xxiii, 1980.

4. Lieb, J., Lipsitch, I., Slaby, A.: *The Crisis Team.* Haberstown, Maryland: Harper and Row, 45, 48, 1973.

5. Freedman, A. and Caplan, H.: *Modern Synopsis of Psychiatry.* Baltimore: William and Wilkins Co., 347-353, 1976.

6. Eaton, M.T., Peterson, M.H., Davis, J.M.: *Psychiatry,* Third Edition. New York: Medical Examination Publishing Co., 43-47, 1976.

7. Wilson, H. and Kneisel, C.: *Psychiatric Nursing.* California: Addison-Wesley Publishing Co., 367, 1979.

8. Benfer, B.: "Defining the Role and Function of the Psychiatric Nurse as a Member of the Team." *Perspectives in Psychiatric Care, 18:*172, 1980.

9. Stuart, G., and Sundeen, S.: *op. cit.* pg. 569.

10. Beard, M., Enelow, C., Owen, J.: "Activity Therapy as a Reconstructive Plan on the Social Competence of Chronic Hospitalized Patients," *The Journal of Psychiatric Nursing and Mental Health Services.* Feb., 33-41, 1978.

11. Munuchin, S.: *Families and Family Therapy.* Cambridge: Harvard University Press, 123, 1974.

12. Wilson, H. and Kneisel, C.: *op. cit.* pp. 364-368.

13. McGarry, L. and Kaplan, H.: Cited by Stuard, D. and Sundeen, S. *Principles and Practice of Psychiatric Nursing.* St. Louis: The C.V. Mosby Co., 1979.

14. *Ibid.*, pp. 276-277.

15. Scarbrough, D.: "Reality Orientation: A New Approach to an Old Problem." *Nursing, 74:*12-13, 1974.

16. Hahn, K.: Using 24-Hour Reality Orientation." *Journal of Gerontological Nursing, 6:No. 3:*130-134, 1980.

17. Wilson, H. and Kneisel, C.: *op. cit.*, pg, 364.

18. *Ibid.*, pg. 364.

19. Stuart, G. and Sundeen, S.: *op. cit.*, pp. 260-262.

20. Wilson, H. and Kneisel, C.: *op. cit.*, pg 365.

21. Sundeen, S., Stuart, G., Rankin, E., Cohen, S.: *Nurse-Client Interaction.* St. Louis: C.V. Mosby Co., 134-151, 1981.

22. Stuart, G. and Sundeen, S.: *op. cit.*, pp. 123-128.

23. *Ibid.*, pg, 126.

24. *Ibid.*, pg. 157.

25. Schroder, P.: "Nursing Intervention with Patients with Thought Disorders." *Perspectives in Psychiatric Care, 17: No. 1:*32-39, 1979.

26. *Ibid.*, pg. 36.

27. Robinson, L.: *Psychiatric Nursing as a Human Experience.* Philadelphia: W.B. Saunders Co., 146, 1972.

28. *Ibid.*, pg. 149.

29. Aquilera, D.: *Review of Psychiatric Nursing.* St. Louis: C.V. Mosby Co., 65, 1977.

30. Payne, D.: *Psychiatric-Mental Health Nursing,* 2nd edition. New York: Medical Examination Publishing Co., 76, 1977.

31. Aquilera, D.: *op. cit.*, pp. 76-77.

32. Pasquali, E., Alesi, E., Arnold, H., VeBasio, N.: *Mental Health Nursing: A Bio-Psycho-Cultural Approach.* St. Louis, C.V. Mosby Co., 394, 1981.

33. Wilson, H. and Kneisel, C.: *op. cit.*, pg. 378.

34. Aquilera, D.: *op. cit.*, pg. 60.

35. Dixson, D.: "Manic Depression: An Overview." *Journal of Psychiatric Nursing and Mental Health Services, 19:No. 6:*28-31, 1981.

36. *Ibid.*, pg. 29.

37. *Ibid.*, pg. 30.

38. Stuart, G. and Sundeen, S.: *op. cit.*, pg. 147.

39. Payne, D.: *op. cit.*, pg. 96.

40. *Ibid.*, pg. 96.

41. Arieti, S.: *Interpretation of Schizophrenia.* New York: Basic Books, 250, 1955, In: Field, W. and Ruelke, W. "Hallucinations and How to Deal with Them." *American Journal of Nursing,* April, 1983.

42. Field, W. and Ruelke, W.: *op. cit.*, pg. 250.

43. *Ibid.*, pg. 638.

44. Arieti, S.: *op. cit.*, pg. 247.

45. Field, W. and Reulke, W.: *op. cit.*, pg. 639.

46. *Ibid.*, pg. 639.

47. Field, W. and Ruelke, W.: *op. cit.*, pg. 640.

48. Trockman, G.: "Caring for the Confused or Delirious Patient." *American Journal of Nursing,* 1495, September, 1978.

49. Sandok, B.: "Organic Brain Syndromes." *Comprehensive Textbook of Psychiatry,* Second Edition. Freedman, A., Kaplan, H., Sadock, B. eds. Baltimore: Williams and Wilkins Co., 1060, 1975.

50. Trockman, G.: *op. cit.*, pg. 1496.

51. Hahn, K.: "Using 24-Hour Reality Orientation." *Journal of Gerontological Nursing, 6:No. 3:*131, 1980.

52. Trockman, G.: *op. cit.*, pg. 1496.

53. Hahn, K.: *op. cit.*, pg. 133.

54. Stuart, G. and Sundeen, S.: *op. cit.*, pg. 563.

55. *Ibid.*, pg. 563.

56. Peplau, H.: "Psychiatric Nursing: Role of Nurses and Psychiatric Nurses," *International Nursing Review, 25:*44, 1978.

57. *Ibid.*, pg. 36.

58. *Ibid.*, pg. 44

59. Manfreda, M.: *Psychiatric Nursing*, Edition 9. Philadelphia; F.A. Davis Co., 23, 1973.
60. Reid, L.: "Approaches to the Aftermath of Schizophrenia." *Perspectives in Psychiatric Care, 17:No. 6:*258, 1979.
61. Wilson, H. and Kneisel, C.: *op. cit.*, pg. 143.
62. *Ibid.*, pg. 143.
63. *Ibid.*, pg. 143.

24 Hospitalized Children with Psychiatric Disorders

Lloyd A. Wells

In this chapter, I shall briefly attempt to address the nurse's range of responses to the myriad of syndromes found in children who are psychiatrically impaired. Before one can consider current appropriate responses to children, it is often of interest and value to consider a historical perspective on the way children have been treated through the ages.

The history of childhood, though romanticized by so many of us, is in fact a rather steady and tragic account of the neglect and abuse of children by societies which do not value them. Indeed, it is an ironic fact that as we document more and more cases of child abuse now in the last third of the 20th century, the rate of child abuse is probably actually lower than it has ever been, at least in the last 6,000 years. Infanticide even occurs in some nonhuman primates, and certainly we have an historical record of legiticized infanticide in Western soceity. Less than 2% of families in the Greek classical period had more than one daughter reach adulthood. The exposure of children was considered to be not very chic, but at the same time not morally reprehensible, in the classical age of Greece. Children were seen as the property of their parents and particularly their fathers. Routine sexual abuse of Greek children by their teachers was considered part of the experience of growing up.

Through the first ten decades of Christendom, the fate of children was a bit better, but many were sold by their parents, and they continued to be considered parental property. With the Renaissance, there was a dawning of intellectual realization that children deserved better treatment but in fact society became increasingly ambivalent toward children, and this somewhat ambivalent approach continued until the mid-19th century when it was gradually replaced by a mode of socializing children and attempting to make them responsible (1). This has largely continued to the present with considerably more effort being devoted to helping children. Nevertheless, representatives and representations of all of these various historical modes of child rearing are easily found in our time.

It is always important for the treating professional to realize that the child of whatever age has both legal and ethical rights. These include in most cases the right to confidentiality of privileged communications. The immediate impulse to regard the child's statements as not having the same kind of fiduciary bearing as statements of an adult patient show a certain insensitivity to the human rights of the child. Obviously, when not sharing confidential information could result, in the judgment of the professional, in serious harm to the child, then the professional has to make a reasoned judgment about sharing that information; but in other situations the child's communications should be regarded as privileged.

The child, too, has a right to legal counsel in matters related to involuntary mental hospitalization and placement both inside and outside the parental family. The concept of the guardian *ad litem* is extremely important in the advocacy of children, and children who are in a court related system should know about the availability and responsibility of such a guardian.

Children who face certain intrusive treatments, including surgery and psychopharmacologic intervention, have a right to express their discontent about such a procedure, and if their discontent is great enough, again, a judicial framework may be necessary to solve the dilemma. In the enormous majority of cases, however, a mature, well meaning professional talking to the child will help the child to make a reasonable decision in his own behalf.

Any consideration of a nursing or other psychiatric intervention with children requires some comprehension of the patterns of parenting involved in that child's family. It is found frequently that children who become psychiatric patients have had poor experiences of parenting. For many years, it was thought that a rather simplistic relationship existed in which bad parents produced bad children. It is not, however, so simple.

Nothing is more tragic than blaming innocent people for the vagaries of childhood behavior, and it is indeed a sobering thought that until fairly recently the parents of children with infantile autism and Gilles de la Tourette's syndrome were blamed as the cause of these syndromes. Today, we make elegant psychodynamic arguments that patterns of parenting cause schizophernia, delinquency and other severe syndromes of childhood and adolescence. Perhaps at some future date we will consider these allegations as preposterous as those regarding infantile autism and various mental retardation syndromes.

There are, however, several vagaries of patterns of parenting of which the psychiatric clinician should be aware. First, there is the very complicated situation in which a cycle of positive feedback is set up between parent and child. Often, the child is a premature or ill baby with whom it is very difficult to bind. The child does not do anything to improve this process: he is neither cute nor cuddly nor particularly gregarious. The child may also have some physical defects which make him somewhat less attractive than the normal child. Such a child, in spite of excellent efforts on behalf of the parents, may not develop normative attachment behavior and may develop several behavioral deficits as he ages. It is difficult to say that this disorder is caused by the child's parents. Rather, it is a lack of interaction between the child and his parents at what is probably a critical period. Syndromes like this become perpetuated in vicious cycles of positive feedback and are very hard to break.

Another type of parental pattern which is found in the families of several delinquent children is the pattern in which there is what Adelaide Johnson and Szurek called *fostering*. In this syndrome, the child is committing an act which is unconsciously desired by the parents. Often one or both parents has some latent antisocial impulse which the child acts out. Study of the family will reveal several very subtle and largely preconscious or unconscious cues to the child to act in a certain way.

The author believes that projective identification on the part of the mother and occasionally by the father is a major cause of maladaptation in childhood and adolescence. In this situation, the parent identifies very strongly with certain aspects of the child and then places on the child the onus of living up to the parents' identification with the child. In the healthy situation, the child identifies with the parent. In this maladaptive situation, it is the parent who is identifying with the child, often looking to the child to serve in a paternal or maternal role or often asking of the child that he or she be a perfect, grandiose self for the parent. Such expectations are impossible to meet and set up an incredibly harsh chain of guilt, depression, dysphoria, and self-destructive behavior.

These maladaptive patterns of parenting are not the only maladaptive patterns of parenting, but they are fairly common and the psychiatric clinician should be familiar with them.

Once a child or adolescent has been hospitalized, it is important to have certain expectations of the child and certain roles for the staff to fulfill in the hospital situation. It is important to first of all realize when a child or adolescent should be hospitalized. It seems to the author that the child should be hospitalized when an emergent situation has occurred in which the child's life or health is imminently threatened. Similarly, a child should be hospitalized if the pattern at home or in a foster home is so unproductive that the child's developmental tasks are being interfered with in a very significant way which would impair his development into a mature individual, and where there is reason to believe that separation from the home and intensive psychotherapeutic work will allow the child to develop more normally.

Once the child has been admitted, it is important that the ward environment be as secure as possible and as home-like as possible. It is important that treating professionals not try to be parents to the child or try to become the child's confidant but rather that they be friendly and supportive, with expectations of the child but without punitive affects toward him. Expectations must be spelled out to the child, and a treatment plan must be individualized in detail for the child. Children do very poorly if they are placed in a lock-step, rigid kind of environment. They will often adapt well to the environment while they are in it, but on release from the hospital the older maladaptive patterns may become even worse.

Some specific problems encountered in hospitalized children and adolescents are considered below.

In the case of a child who is hospitalized in an emergency type of situation, such as a suicidal threat or attempt, or massive misuse of a substance, it is necessary to perform a thorough evaluation. One of the major hazards of this evaluation is that it will be made too brief or that it will be made too long. In general, it is impossible to evaluate the extent of a child's psychiatric syndrome and social situation in a matter of just a couple of interviews. The adolescent will usually not allow the treating person to really get to know him during that period because adolescents are by nature very defensive and need to protect their perceived vulnerability. Usually, a period of at least 10 days is required for an adequate in-hospital assessment of such a patient. Once this assessment has been made, however, there is no need to incarcerate every adolescent who has had suicidal ideation or used too many street drugs. It is certainly possible to plan an appropriate and helpful outpatient program for many such youngsters. This must be a decision made by an entire treatment team. It is very difficult to make this assessment on the basis of spending an hour a day with the patient, but if input is gathered from psychiatrists, psychologists, psychiatric nurses, child care workers, and others who have had intimate contact with the patient over a period of several days it is usually quite possible to arrive at a knowledge of the extent of the person's psychological and social functioning and malfunctioning.

The long term treatment of an adolescent or child is a very different proposition.

In-hospital treatment of adolescents is a very difficult task. It is necessary to be aware of each such patient as a unique individual. This frequently becomes difficult because in adolescence patients frequently act as if they were caricatures of certain affects and alloplastic states. Nevertheless, under the alloplasticity frequently lurks depression and low self-esteem. One must also be aware of the individual variations in growth and development among adolescents. Two 15-year-old boys or girls may be very different in their physical and emotional degree of development.

For many years, it was thought that adolescence was a time of storm and stress for all individuals, that all young people in this age group had what was known as "adolescent turmoil" (2). In fact, the kind of strife referred to does not occur in all adolescents in their adaptation to society and their family. It is my belief, however, that most adolescents, at least intrapsychically, experience a great deal of turmoil, and that this is a necessary part of the process of growing and separating from the family. One very difficult feature in dealing with this age group, however, is to ascertain when the relatively normal turmoil becomes abnormal, when it is no longer an unpleasant but basically healthy coping mechanism and becomes a maladaptive mechanism or even part of a mental illness.

Once an adolescent is hospitalized, particularly for any kind of long-term treatment, the issues that have been discussed about adult inpatients become very important, and the adolescent is, if anything, more sensitive to many of them than most adult patients are. When a child is placed in the hospital, he is almost inevitably homesick even if this is not admitted. In addition, the child's family, though ostensibly happy that he is being hospitalized, has an unconscious issue, usually, to keep the child as part of the family so that the family members will not need to feel guilty. Thus, often, the child is given a strong unspoken message that he should not cooperate with the treatment or should not be involved in any type of criticism of the family (3). These issues of homesickness and covert family agendas must be addressed directly by the treatment staff throughout the patient's hospitalization, but particularly early on.

All the issues of resistance and transference/countertransference which apply to adult patients apply to adolescents. Very often, people who work with adolescents have several unresolved adolescent issues, themselves — as do most of us. Nevertheless, staffs of adolescent units have particular problems with countertransference and often have covert agendas with certain patients who act out. Often, the behavior of a treatment team toward such patients is rejecting without any conscious awareness of this on the part of the team. As with adult patients it is necessary for the treatment professionals to be consistently vigilant regarding their countertransference feelings, and to talk about these within the team setting.

In addition to the rejecting type of countertransference mentioned above, a parental countertransference is almost inevitable on an adolescent unit, and many nurses and other health care professionals will react to the patients in a very parental way. Often, there is an attempt to overprotect the patient, to minimize expectations of him, and, in fact, to infantilize him. Along with this, there is often an attempt to make the unit "perfect." I think that the concept of good enough mothering developed by Winnicott and others can be applied to running an adolescent unit. One should not strive for a perfect unit because this would isolate the patients from the world and make it intensely difficult to return. One should, however, strive for a good enough unit — a place that is fair and with caring professionals in a clear cut chain of command. Adolescence is not a time for experiments in democracy, and adolescent inpatients on psychiatric units are not capable of making binding decisions about important features of the ward milieu. Thus, while some issues may be negotiable and flexibility about them must be maintained, there are some issues which are non-negotiable: use of alcohol and drugs on the unit, sexual relationships among patients, etc.

Many adolescents lack the capacity to describe their affects and reactions. An effort must be made not only to help the patients identify and express affects, but also to teach patients in a more didactic way about affects and their vicissitudes. Group therapy and assertiveness training can often be helpful in this regard. Nevertheless, many adolescent patients do not develop the capacity in the hospital to talk about their conflicts and instead act them out. Acting out is a universal phenomenon on adolescent units and is to be expected. The staff should do everything in its power to prevent acting out of a serious nature, but it should not be self-recriminative when it occurs, because it is, indeed, inevitable. One should, however, examine the acting out behavior, because behavior does have meaning, and sometimes we can even discover what that meaning is. The metaphor which the patient expresses through the acting out often has reference to his transference with the unit, his primary nurse, and his psychotherapist.

It is important to involve the families of adolescents when they are in the hospital, and while formal family therapy may not be indicated or helpful, some kind of family program and some sort of involvement of parents with their children is certainly helpful and necessary.

Flexible nursing approaches are necessary for pregnant adolescents, depressed children and adolescents, children with physical illnesses who are also severely stressed, and children with phobias. A schizophrenic youngster also needs an extremely flexible, individualized approach.

With all these *caveats*, there may be a fear on the part of the reader to become involved in the psychiatric care of children. The rewards, however, are far greater than the many frustrations.

REFERENCES

1. deMause, L.: The evolution of childhood, History of Childhood Quarterly: The Journal of Psychohistory, *1:*503, 1974.

2. Freud, A.: Adolescence, Psychoanal Study Child, *13:*255, 1952.

3. Rinsley, D.B. and Hall, D.D.: Psychiatric hospital treatment of adolescents: parental resistances as expressed in casework metaphor, , Arch Gen Psychiat, *7:*286, 1962.

25 "Special" Patients

Lloyd A. Wells

Psychiatric nursing and all mental health professions are replete with dilemmas involving patients with particularly severe psychopathology or patients whose psychopathology causes particularly severe reactions in caretaking personnel. In this chapter, we shall discuss this phenomenon in general and pay particular attention to patients who have problems of dependence, borderline patients, V.I.P.'s and "special" patients, along with patients who are mute, retarded or hallucinating. Suicidal patients will also be considered.

Although many people have attempted to anticipate every possible clinical situation and devise a treatment plan, it is best to try to approach each individual problem patient in his or her own right as a separate entity and not to try to memorize a lockstep approach to such a patient. Each clinical situation is in fact unique and different. The capacity for empathic contact with a patient, which is frequently lacking, is totally ruled out and impossible if one is attempting to relate to a patient as a syndrome rather than as a human being. Thus, the psychiatric nurse must have a certain basic body of information about dealing with types of situations, but he or she must also be able to react quickly, make decisions quickly, and be able to integrate concern and creativity.

The attempt to communicate with people who are actively psychotic and are hallucinating at the time you are seeing them is very difficult. Often, in a situation like that, one's immediate belief is that the only way to become involved with the patient is to participate in the content of the hallucinations or of the delusional system. Thus, one is often tempted to speak as if one believes the patient's delusions. Almost always, this approach is anti-therapeutic in that the patient himself would be extremely suspicious of anyone else sharing his delusional system, which he covertly realizes is not based in reality.

With the actively hallucinating patient, the important approach to take is involving oneself in the patient's world without leaving reality. Thus, though the patient is having visual and/or auditory hallucinations the nurse can insert himself into the patient's world to the extent that the patient is aware of the nurse and listening to the nurse. The nurse should be reassuring, non-threatening, and non-participating in the patient's craziness.

Patients who are mute are particularly difficult to deal with. This occasionally happens in catatonic schizophrenia and in some forms of severe depression. There is often a belief on the part of the nurse or of the physician that because a patient does not communicate verbally, he or she is not really attuned to what is happening around him. In fact, many totally mute patients, particularly the schizophrenics among them, are exquisitely attuned to what is being said and done. Therefore, in spite of the fact that the patient does not indicate any wish or need for verbal communication, the nurse should continue to discuss things with the patient, to ask the patient questions, and not to talk about the patient as if he were part of the furniture.

Although mental retardation is not usually a psychiatric syndrome, it is not infrequent that mentally retarded people also have serious psychiatric problems which sometimes require intervention. The nurse's role in dealing with the retarded is to treat them as potentially responsible adults. There is often a tendency to infantilize retarded people and to treat them as little children. The nurse needs to recall that the developmental tasks of retarded people are the same as those of people with higher levels of intelligence. In fact, retarded people have very frequently managed to mature in several areas in spite of their intellectual impairment. Thus, the 30-year-old severely retarded man still has a self-concept of himself as an adult and would be offended by the suggestion that he play, that he might enjoy going for a ride on a swing, etc.

Very dependent patients with other psychiatric pathology are not uncommonly seen in psychiatric settings. Dependence is a complex phenomenon which derives from infancy in which we are totally dependent. A great potential problem for people in the mental health professions is that by virtue of their very profession they must care for and about patients or clients. This can often foster the dependence of an already pathologically dependent patient. One of the major dilemmas which psychiatric professionals face is the need sometimes to make a patient more dependent to satisfy the needs of the professional. Many professionals, acutely aware of this possibility, take an equally destructive tact, which is to refuse to ever meet the dependency needs of a patient who is indeed needy. Patients who have had inadequate parenting often have to become quite "pseudoindependent" at an early age. These people deny the fact that they have normal needs for dependence and attempt to be extremely independent. Often, later in life when some tragedy occurs, such as a work-related accident, such people revert to a hopelessly dependent stage.

Patients who have dependency conflicts generally think of dependence as a total rather than a partial phenomenon. Thus, they believe that they are either "dependent" or "independent." Frequently, professionals also tend to think in these terms. There is, however, nothing wrong with the normal, omnipresent need for partial dependence. A mature type of dependence is found in people who are able to gratify their dependency needs through work, marriage, etc., in a flexible way.

Patients with borderline personality disturbances also create many special ward problems, and these will be discussed in another section.

Burnham has described a type of patient or, more precisely, a type of patient-staff interaction which he has termed "the special problem patient" (1). Such patients are perhaps uncommon, but they certainly do exist and create more havoc on a psychiatric unit than any other type of patient. These are extremely appealing people who are often borderline or primitively narcissistic in their personaltiy structure. Often, such a patient begins to have a checkered hospital career before hospitalization even occurs. As Burnham has pointed out, frequently special requests are made for the patient by the referring agency or physician. Frequently, it is explained that the patient will need a private room or some other special sort of favor. When the patient arrives at the hospital, there is often a certain amount of confusion. Often, the patient will be unable to go through routine admissions procedures, will want to give a particularly long history and in so doing will manage to put the nurse or physician in the position of feeling responsible and guilty. This sort of patient continues to place people in the position of being responsible for the patient's self-esteem. Such patients are extremely destructive to all other staff-patient relationships on the floor they are hospitalized on, and the existence of such a patient-staff relationship should be ascertained very quickly and steps taken to make sure that the patient is not treated differently and to realize that the patient's excessive demands and the staff's unusual compliance with those demands is actually a manifestation of the patient's illness.

Another variant of the so-called special problem patient is the V.I.P. (2). The V.I.P. may or may not be intrinsically a difficult patient, but when a captain of politics, industry, etc., is admitted to a psychiatric unit there are many reverberations within and without the institution. The caregiver has to be aware of the fact that the V.I.P. deserves as good treatment as the other patients. This frequently means that the V.I.P. will not receive any special privileges or be held in great awe.

The type of patients described in this chapter are encountered very commonly. They are not the only patients who present special problems. The main points to be gleaned from this chapter are that every patient has some special problems which require ingenuity and inventiveness on the part of the health professionals caring for the patient. At the same time, such innovative approaches should not be discriminatory to other patients or imply any kind of "special" relationship which unconsciously colludes with the patient's own psychopathology.

Although all of us will like some patients more than others, we must view and analyze these likes and dislikes in the context of countertransference. If we are to act as professionals, we must view all our patients as V.I.P.'s but treat them all as human beings in need rather than as important people to be collected.

REFERENCES

1. Burnham, D.L.: The special-problem patient: victim or agent of splitting? Psychiat, *29:*105, 1966.

2. Weintrauk, W.: "The VIP Syndrome": a clinical study in hospital psychiatry. J Nerv Ment Dis, *138:*181, 1964.

PART 4

NURSING ROLES

26 The Practice of Psychiatric/ Mental Health Nursing

Marcia Justic and Pamela Peters

INTRODUCTION

Psychiatric/Mental Health Nursing is a specialized area within the nursing discipline. The sciences of human behavior serve as the basis for practice with emphasis upon developmental, psychodynamic, general systems, family, group and crisis theories. The practice focuses upon the delivery of nursing care to promote, restore, and maintain mental health of the individual, family, and community. Mental Health Nursing practice is not an independent, isolated entity; it is interdependent with the disciplines of psychiatry, social work, clinical psychology, general medicine, and community health.

The activities of the Psychiatric/Mental Health nurse may differ according to various mental health agencies and settings. In many of these agencies, the nursing process is utilized to deliver nursing care. This care can be psychotherapeutic by offering support, assistance in identifying and clarifying the client's current living problems, problem solving, teaching, and evaluation of coping strategies.

Two types of practitioners are delineated by the American Nurses Association: the Psychiatric Mental Health nurse and the Psychiatric Mental Health Nursing Specialist. The Psychiatric Mental Health nurse is a licensed professional nurse who demonstrates a level of performance in psychiatric nursing which exceeds general practice. This level of performance is developed through experience, continued education beyond basic nursing preparation and supervised clinical practice. Expertise in individual psychotherapy is essential with knowledge of family and group dynamics. Formal review and certification is available for the psychiatric nurse through the Division on Psychiatric and Mental Health Nursing Practice of the American Nurses Association. There are special requirements related to length of experience and numbers of hours of direct nursing practice. A written review is also involved in the certification process.

The Psychiatric Mental Health Clinical Specialist is a licensed professional who has had considerable experience in psychiatric nursing and has completed a graduate degree in Mental Health Nursing. Carolyn Garant identifies basic areas of a graduate curriculum which include psychopathology, psychodynamics, research and supervised clinical experience (1). These areas should build upon the baccalaureate program which should have included such topics as psychosocial aspects of patient care, growth and development, stress and communication theory as well as the effects of mental illness on the client, family and community (2). This knowledge base should enable the clinical specialist to provide patient care in a more thorough, creative and independent manner. The clinical specialist is expected to function in all modes of psychotherapy, including group and family. This specialization allows this nurse to function in some settings as an independent practitioner while in others, the specialist may work in a collaborative relationship with other disciplines. Indirect roles which are part of the clinical specialist's function may include supervision, education, consultation, clinical research, patient care coordination and management.

Certification of the clinical specialist is available through the same agency which certifies the Psychiatric Mental Health nurse. Requirements include a Master's or higher degree in Nursing with specialization in Psychiatric Mental Health Nursing. The American Nurses Association does give individual consideration to Master's and Baccalaureate degrees in related areas. In addition, post-Master's experience is required as well as current involvement in direct patient care. The nurse must have experience in more than one treatment modality and this experience should include previous and current supervision.

PSYCHIATRIC MENTAL HEALTH NURSE

Psychiatric Mental Health nurses most frequently deliver first-line care in hospital settings as staff nurses. The role of the Psychiatric Mental Health nurse has progressed dramatically since its early days. In 1882 and 1885 "training schools" were developed to prepare psychiatric nurses (3). As early as 1900, psychiatric nursing was recognized as an area of specialization. Nationally, the problem of mental illness began to attract concern and attention during and after World War II. Mental illness was seen as a nationwide security problem since many men could not be drafted due to mental instability. Following the war, Veterans Hospitals and other facilities began to develop and expand treatment centers. The treatments offered at this time were mainly somatic therapies. The nurse worked primarily with physicians and performed mainly a custodial role, offering medical nursing skills adapted to psychiatric patients (4).

Nursing education was not prepared to face the demand for psychiatric nurses in the post World War II era. In 1935, over one-half of the diploma nursing programs did not even offer psychiatric nursing in the curriculum (5). It was not until 1952 that psychiatric nursing was required for state licensure (6). Another important event occurred in 1952 when Hildegard Peplau's publication *Interpersonal Relations in Nursing* provided a framework for nursing practice. Many leaders in psychiatric nursing followed with psychiatric textbooks, articles, and research studies.

With the Community Mental Health Centers Act, the focus of mental health care shifted from an institutional to a community orientation (7). This evolution as well as the utilization of psychotropic drugs has resulted in the progression of the psychiatric nursing role. While at one time psychiatric nursing care was custodially-oriented, today nurses create a therapeutic milieu for the clients (8). In this milieu, both psychological and physiological needs are met through a variety of therapeutic modalities. There is now a focus on interpersonal functioning in relationships particularly within the family network (9). The client's involvement in group, family, recreational, and occupational therapies provides for a smoother reintegration into the community upon dismissal.

SCOPE OF PRACTICE OF THE PSYCHIATRIC/MENTAL HEALTH NURSE

Changes in the last few decades have had a great impact on the role identity of the psychiatric nurse. The role is more broadly defined and therefore not easily distinguishable at times from that of the psychologist, psychiatric social worker, or the variety of other therapists who work in mental health settings. Instead, various functions of these health team members may overlap so that the nurse performs many different types of activities.

Depending upon the setting, the nurse may accompany clients to the theater, arrange for follow-up care, or administer psychological tests. Psychiatric nurses continue to struggle with identity problems according to a research study, *Role of the Psychiatric Nurse*, conducted by Robert Plutchik *et al.* in 1976 (10). In this study, nurses did not rate individual, family, or group psychotherapy as nursing functions of prime importance. Instead, more traditional activities such as assessing the effects of somatic therapies and assessing the noise level of the ward rated higher. Discrepancies were revealed between a nursing group and psychologist/psychiatrist group in terms of nursing roles and functions. The psychologist and psychiatrist group rated "developing and implementing the nursing care plan" as more important than did the nurses (11).

Another change is the evolution of the team concept. This has expanded from primarily the doctor-nurse relationship to a multidisciplinary mental health team including psychologists, social workers, music and art therapists, recreational and occupation therapists (12). The team functions in a variety of inpatient settings including acute and long term treatment centers, day hospitals and night hospitals. It is apparent that the nursing role varies a great deal according to the types of setting and the roles of those other health team members.

The direct patient care activities of the Psychiatric Mental Health nurse differ from those of nursing in general hospital areas. Bathing, feeding, mouth and skin care, positioning, dressing changes, making beds, monitoring intravenous feedings and passing many medications are a few of the daily activities of a general staff nurse (13). In contrast, fewer medications are passed by psychiatric nurses, and the other activities mentioned either do not exist or are usually carried out by the patients themselves. What does the Psychaitric Mental Health nurse do? The activities of psychiatric nursing are perhaps best described by reviewing the nursing process.

ASSESSMENT

The nurse is responsible for the thorough ongoing assessment of the client from admission to discharge. Initially, the nurse conducts a psychiatric evaluation which consists of mental status exam and a psychosocial history. In collecting this data, the nurse may meet with the family as well as the client in order to gather pertinent family history and perhaps formulate a family genogram. Continuous data collection is essential since all of the pertinent information may not be available after one or two interviews. With each client encounter, the nurse assesses the client's mental status and overal response to therapy, i.e., behavioral changes, affectual change, development of insight, and improved thought processes. The documentation of this data is essential in order to communicate with other health team members. In many settings, each member health team charts in the same progress notes so that observations can be easily compared and shared.

PLANNING

The initial assessments of the client should lead to planning not only among the nursing staff but also with all other health team members. The nurse may often coordinate the meetings involving the entire mental health team (14). Such planning should focus upon goal setting as well as developing intervention strategies. The client should be involved at some phase of the planning so that he/she participates in setting goals. For some clients, their goals may be quite clear and concrete; however, other clients may define their goals in an abstract manner, i.e., "to stop having weird thoughts and feelings." In either case, the nurse can assist the client in developing concrete steps toward goal fulfillment. For example, with a client experiencing anxiety, the nurse and client may set the goal, "to feel less anxious." In attaining this goal, the nurse may help the client identify personal manifestations of anxiety and precipitating factors, as well as increase the client's awareness of these symptoms and new ways to cope with them.

The nurse should document this mutual goal setting and planning in the nursing care plan. The nursing care plan usually includes nursing diagnoses, client goals or expected outcomes and nursing orders which describe the approach and interventions which the nursing staff should implement when caring for a specific client. The mental health team should make initial attempts to identify outcome criteria in order to determine the client's progress. This helps the team to be consistent in their approach to the client and avoid completely subjective evaluation of the client's progress.

INTERVENTION

In discussing nursing intervention, it is important to note that leaders in psychiatric nursing often differentiate between nurses who practice in mental health settings and psychiatric nurses. Nurses who have had basic nursing education but no specialized psychiatric preparation or supervision perform essentially the same role as nurses in other health care settings with some adaptation for the psychiatric client (15). This includes assessment, planning, intervention and evaluation; however, intervention for such a nurse may be more limited than that of a psychiatric nurse who has had additional psychiatric preparation.

The nurse in the psychiatric setting will help create the therapeutic milieu, carry out medical orders, including dispensing medications and monitoring effects, and provide for physical needs. Other activities include participation in the special treatments and client activities, talking with clients and providing for coodination of services and referrals. Although the psychiatric nurse will engage in all of these activities, additionally, he/she functions as a member of the mental health team doing individual, group and family therapy and coordinating discharge planning (16). The psychiatric nurse may also have more expertise in dealing with acutely disturbed clients. All nurses working in a psychiatric setting participate in teaching at some level. Clients often require generalized health teaching relating to diet, exercise, specific conditions or illnesses. In addition, mental health teaching is continuous as the nurse informs the client about many areas of living, i.e., the importance of identifying and verbalizing feelings. Teaching is especially important if the client/family is involved in any specialized therapies such as electroconvulsive treatments or chemotherapy. The nurse must develop an understanding of adult learning principles and provide information for the client/family which is appropriate to his/her level of understanding.

EVALUATION

The process of evaluation is ongoing as the nurse assesses the client's progress. The expected outcomes may need to be modified depending on the rate of the client's progress. The team should also evaluate their approach to determine if specific interventions are effective for the client. The client should be included in the evaluation process. The nurse should assist the client to review the extent of his/her adjustment beyond symptom relief.

ADDITIONAL ROLES

The psychiatric nurse may function in a variety of roles which do not involve the provision of direct patient care but do affect the quality of this care. One such role is that of the nurse educator sometimes referred to as an inservice instructor. The educator is often responsible to orient new employees to the psychiatric area by providing classes and supervised clinical experiences which will prepare them to function independently. The educator may review such areas as psychotropic drugs, specialized therapies, treatment strategies, family and group dynamics, and emergency measures, i.e., nursing care for suicidal, aggressive, or acutely disturbed clients. The nurse educator is often the new employee's only identified mentor and source of support. The educator may also assess the learning needs of the nursing staff and provide formal and informal classes and seminars to meet these needs. This is a very important role since nursing practice is directly affected by the level of knowledge and expertise existent within the nursing staff. The nurse educator should have some preparation in adult learning strategies and program development.

Nursing research is another area of involvement for the psychiatric nurse. Although the Psychiatric Clinical Specialist usually identifies the topic of research and develops the proposal, the psychiatric nurse may serve an integral function in conducting and evaluating the study. This role may involve direct nursing care if the research concerns specific nursing activities or problems. Otherwise, the research may be related to nursing theory or the evaluation of nursing care. This type of research can be very valuable and may affect the quality of nursing care.

The area of nursing management provides indirect roles for the psychiatric nurse. Such roles may involve clinical supervision of the nursing staff as well as various administrative functions such as staffing, budgeting, evaluation of nursing care, and dealing with staff morale, conflicts, and discipline. Hospitals vary in the titles which they give to management functions. While some hospitals still refer to the Head Nurse, others have developed the titles of Unit Coordinators or Clinical Managers. Management functions may extend beyond one unit to a psychiatric area comprised of several individual units. These may include adult, adolescent, crisis intervention, chemical dependency, and intensive psychiatric care areas. The nursing manager at this level not only directs the units on a day to day basis, but is responsible for long term planning and evaluation. Such a position usually entails conducting business with other departments and units which are involved with the psychiatric area. These functions usually remove the psychiatric nurse quite completely from direct client care; however, a psychiatric background is important in managing a psychiatric area in order to confront nursing care issues and affect the quality of care.

CONCLUSIONS

Whether the psychiatric nurse functions mainly as a direct care provider or in more indirect nursing care roles, the role has evolved to a place where the nurse functions very independently. The nurse has a great deal to contribute to the mental health team by sharing information related to specific client cases as well as providing teaching for this team, based upon a broad theory base and experience (17). Nurses need to continue to develop confidence in their expertise as well as a level of assertion in order to share their ideas and make an impact on the quality of client care.

PSYCHIATRIC MENTAL HEALTH NURSING SPECIALIST

Although the term "clinical specialist" was initially conceptualized in 1900, its existence did not become a reality until the 1950's. At this time, nurses were considered non-professional, their practice needing to be supervised, and graduate education focused on administration, teaching, and supervision. But, as nursing knowledge became more specialized and nurses became viewed as professionals, graduate education added opportunities to enhance clinical knowledge and skills in medical-surgical, psychiatric, and maternal-child nursing. In recent years, the idea of clinical specialization, with the inherent understanding of excellence in practice, is very much accepted within nursing and is becoming better understood by consumers, employers, and by other professions (18).

SCOPE OF PRACTICE OF THE PSYCHIATRIC MENTAL HEALTH NURSE SPECIALIST

A major role of the psychiatric mental health nurse specialist in the inpatient setting involves the provision of direct nursing care to clients in such therapeutic modalities as individual, family, and group. It may include such activities as scheduled and nonscheduled interactions with clients or family members, and acting as cotherapist in group psychotherapy (19). It is estimated that clinical specialists spend one-fourth of their time in patient care (20). Nursing actions within this role may include listening, summarizing, clarifying, using behavioral modification, helping clients develop new coping methods, dealing in "here and now," sharing feelings, facilitating social interactions via client groups, and problem-solving as a joint endeavor between client and staff (21).

In many cases, the clinical specialist provides direct client care to clients who have not been admitted to the hospital primarily for psychiatric problems. Most nonpsychiatric patients are referred to the clinical specialist because of grief reactions, pain, terminal illness, suicide attempts, or drug and alcohol dependence (22). The nursing process is a vehicle to help clients and families through the "dehumanizing process of hospitalization" (23). Some creative uses of the clinical specialist's talents include meeting with families of dying or critically ill patients, or those with newly diagnosed chronic illnesses, and conducting crisis groups for families of cancer patients (24).

A major part of providing direct client care is crisis intervention. In many instances, intervention with general hospital clients falls within the framework of crisis intervention (25). The process of crisis intervention is described as a process of taking a thorough psychosocial history and interview to reveal the client's level of understanding about what he is experiencing, the adequacy of his support systems, and how well he can cope with his experience (26). Intervention can provide cognitive information for the patient, improve, create, or identify a support system, and begin to improve the patient's coping ability (27).

Educating clients is an essential component in providing direct nursing care to clients. The clinical specialist gives accurate, reliable information to clients regarding their illness, mode of therapy, alternatives for change, and discharge teaching, continually assessing the client's level of understanding and readiness to synthesize new information. Education can be useful in the prevention of recurrent mental illness. It serves as a mechanism for primary prevention as the clinical specialist provides information on developmental stages and predictable life crises.

Finally, the clinical specialist functions as a liaison person and patient advocate with community agencies. In this function, for example, she may serve as discharge coordinator in helping certain clients return home to their community. The clinical specialist may communicate directly with community agencies to arrange for services such as follow-up treatment, vocational counseling, or financial assistance.

The psychiatric mental health nurse specialist provides indirect nursing care to clients, consuming from one-half to three-fourths of his/her time. In most hospital settings, the clinical specialist serves as both clinical supervisor and consultant to the nursing staff. The activities in the consultant role include participating in nursing team conferences, interdisciplinary team conferences as well as conferences with individual nurses concerning client care. Solving ward personnel problems may be a function of the clinical specialist (28). There is, however, a disagreement in the literature regarding the provision of staff counseling by the clinical specialist. Several authors feel that staff should be referred to community health facilities for treatment of personal problems whereas others feel it is appropriate for the clinical specialist to provide short-term supportive counseling for staff members. All authors agree that it is appropriate for the clinical specialist to meet with groups of staff members to discuss feelings towards particular nursing issues or problems, i.e., death and dying.

Beyond the psychiatric setting, the clinical specialist has expanded her consultant functions to serve hospital staff in medical-surgical areas. Three formats for successful consultation have been suggested by Weinstein, *et al.* (29): regularly scheduled meetings, crisis intervention, and nursing rounds. All three formats were successful in teaching nurses to handle emotional problems of clients and to reduce staff anxiety under specific circumstances. The clinical specialist may become directly involved with clients when consulting, in addition to consulting directly with staff nurses.

To compliment consultative functions in medical-surgical areas, the clinical specialist serves as staff educator, teaching formally and informally through conferences with the patient care team and serving as a role model (30). Examples of teaching areas offered by the clinical specialist include crisis theory, the emotional response to illness and hospitalization, care of the dying patient, communication skills, and listening (31). The clinical specialist offers more specialized educational topics in the psychiatric area which may include chemical dependency and detoxification, family and group therapy, psychotropic drugs, psychodynamic theories, nursing intervention for specific client behaviors, and psychophysiology.

Another indirect function of the clinical specialist is that of research, which calls for investigation of clinical nursing problems, development, and testing of nursing theory and evaluation of the findings in relation to nursing practice. This role, although essential, seems to be receiving least priority in the time of the clinical specialist. In addition to clinically-oriented research, it is essential that research be carried out in relation to the psychiatric mental health nurse specialist role. Because the clinical specialist position is so new and because nurse clinical specialists have neglected to develop firm criteria to measure their impact in the health care delivery system in the past, research is warranted in this area. Research should be aimed at measuring the effect or impact of the role, both in the indirect consultative activities with the nursing staff and the direct care rendered to clients (32).

In some hospital agencies, the clinical specialist role may include serving as a clinical or unit coordinator. Because these institutions have not found it economically feasible to hire a clinical specialist for clinical skills alone, they have found it necessary to add management functions to the role. In these situations, the clinical specialist does not hold the traditional responsibilities of the Head Nurse. Main responsibilities include unit management and supervision of clinical staff while excluding staff scheduling and fiscal concerns. Several agencies utilize the clinical specialist as instructor for educational institutions together with unit manager functions.

The clinical specialist is an important member of the interdisciplinary team who may serve as an important link between medical-surgical and psychiatric areas. One such function of the clinical specialist is to maintain communication between medical-surgical and psychiatric units when clients are transferred from one area to another. The clinical specialist is frequently seen as psychiatry's representative, daily negotiating the boundaries between psychiatry and medicine as well as those between nurses and physicians (33). These liaison activities may expedite communication between the physician and the psychiatrist in urgent situations (34).

In the psychiatric setting, liaison with interdisciplinary members becomes more interdependent and collaborative in nature. Information is shared with chaplains, psychiatrists, psychologists and social workers to help them better understand nursing roles and functions. For example, a social worker may offer information about community resources, patients' eligibility for various types of assistance/facilities, and application procedures, whereas the clinical specialist will give information about the side effects of drugs, the prognosis for certain diagnoses, and explanations of surgical procedures and diagnostic tests (35).

CONCLUSIONS

In the general hospital setting, the Psychiatric Mental Health Nursing Specialist functions as practitioner, consultant, educator, and researcher in providing direct and indirect care to clients. Numerous functions and activities are available to the clinical specialist, depending on the specific institution, needs of the staff and creativity of the specialist. These responsibilities require that the clinical specialist have a strong background in psychiatric nursing theory and clinical experience in psychiatric and medical-surgical areas. It is apparent that a variety of needs can be met by the clinical specialist in the general hospital.

EPILOGUE

Although the Psychiatric Mental Health Nurse and Psychiatric Mental Health Nursing Specialist perform different functions, each is responsible and accountable for his/her own level of practice. Responsibility implies that the nurse is reliable, trustworthy and dependable (36). Accountability in psychiatric nursing practice is more comprehensive than the concept of responsibility in that it requires that the nurse be answerable to the patient, family, peers and supervisors for nursing activities and theoretical knowledge (37). This type of answerability includes written and/or verbal disclosure so that evaluation and change may occur to improve the nurse's own level of expertise and the quality of patient care. In developing accountability, the nurse must actively formulate methods for formal evaluation by self, peers and supervisors. The criteria for evaluation should be mutually established by the nurse, peers and supervisors. In addition, evaluation should be arranged at concrete, regularly scheduled times. It is suggested that informal evaluation be ongoing in addition to more formal evaluative methods.

In addition to peer evaluation, support from and collaboration with peers is essential. Nurses must recognize the need for peer input and feedback concerning patient care. Personal needs must also be acknowledged; such needs can be met through staff support groups, burnout seminars, and peer interaction which allow for the sharing of experiences and feelings.

Hospitals can also provide support to nurses by acknowledging quality nursing care and professionalism through promotion and career mobility. Many hospitals have developed several types of career ladders so that nurses in all areas can be recognized not only for their management qualities buy also their clinical expertise. This is extremely valuable in an area like psychiatry where nurses are interested in further development of individual, group, and family skills and often do not want to leave direct client care for advancement. The clinical ladder is usually developed on the basis of role performances, post basic nursing experience and education. The levels usually range from the new staff nurse to that of the Clinical Specialist who should demonstrate an exceptional level of clinical and research expertise, as well as supervising and teaching skills. Within that range, psychiatric nurses are recognized for their skill in all phases of the nursing process, multidisciplinary team functioning, staff teaching, peer feedback, supervision and professional growth and development.

REFERENCES

1. Garant, C.A.: The Psychiatric Liaison Nurse - An Interpretation of the Role. *Supervisor Nurse,* 75, April, 1977.

2. Fried, A. and Fried, F.: Hospital and community psychiatric nursing. *Journal of Psychiatric Nursing and Mental Health Services,* 31-36, December, 1976.

3. John, A., Leite-Rebeiro, M., Buckler, D.: The nurse in mental health practice: Report on a technical conference. Geneva: World Health Organization, 22, 1963.

4. Burgess, A.: *Psychiatric Nursing in the Hospital and Community.* Third Edition. Prentice Hall Co., Englewood cliffs, 39, 1981.

5. *Ibid.*: pg. 39.

6. Plutchik, R., Conte, H., Wells, W., Toksoz, K.: Role of the psychiatric nurse. *Journal of Psychiatric Nursing and Mental Health Services*, 38-43, September, 1976.

7. Davis, E. and Pattison, E.: The psychiatric nurse's role identity. *American Journal of Nursing*, 299, February, 1979.

8. Burgess, A.: *op. cit.* pg, 39.

9. *Ibid.*: pg.

10. Plutchik, R., *et al.*: *op. cit.*, pp. 38-43.

11. *Ibid.*: pg. 39.

12. Benfer, B.: Defining the role and function of the psychiatric nurse as a member of the team. *Perspectives in Psychiatric Care, 18:*4, 166-177, 1980.

13. Peplau, H.: Psychiatric nursing: role of nurses and psychiatric nurses. *International Nursing Review, 25:*41-47, March/April, 1978.

14. Benfer, B.: *op. cit.*, pg.

15. Peplau, H.: *op. cit.*, pg. 41.

16. *Ibid.*: pg. 46.

17. Benfer, B.: *op. cit.*, pg. 173.

18. Smoyak, S.: Specialization in nursing: from then to now. *Nursing Outlook*, 676-681, November, 1976.

19. Riehl, J. and McVay, J.: *The Clinical Nurse Specialist - Interpretations.* New York: Appleton-Century Crofts, 1973.

20. *Ibid.*: pg.

21. *Ibid.*: pg.

22. Schilp, J.: Are you especially interested in feelings? Be a psychiatric nurse specialist. *Nursing '76*, 101-103, November, 1976.

23. *Ibid.*: pp, 101-103.

24. *Ibid.*: pp. 101-103.

25. Goldstein, S.: The psychiatric clinical specialist in the general hospital. *Journal of Nursing Administration*, 34-37, March, 1979.

26. *Ibid.*: pp, 34-37.

27. *Ibid.*: pp. 34-37.

28. Riehl, J. and McVay, J.: *op. cit.*, pg

29. Weinstein, L., Chapman, M., Stallings, M.: Organizing approaches to psychiatric nurse consultation. *Perspectives in Psychiatric Care, 17:*2:66-71, 1979.

30. Nelson, J. and Schilke, D.: The evolution of psychiatric liaison. *Perspectives in Psychiatric Care*, 61-65, April-June, 1976.

31. Goldstein, S.: *op. cit.*, pp. 34-37.

32. Nelson, J. and Schilke, D.: *op. cit.*, pp. 61-65.

33. Goldstein, S.: *op. cit.*, pp. 34-37.

34. *Ibid.*: pp. 34-37.

35. Peplau, H.: The psychiatric nurse - accountable? To whom? For what? *Perspectives in Psychiatric Care, 18:* 3:128, 1980.
36. *Ibid.*: pg. 130.
37. *Ibid.*: pp. 130-131.

27 Relationships with Colleagues

Lloyd A. Wells

In the training of all mental health professionals, an enormous emphasis is placed on one's ability to establish, maintain and develop relationships with patients. For reasons probably having to do with security operations, defensiveness and countertransference, we devote very little time in any of the mental health professions to a consideration of relationships with colleagues. Often, there is an attempt to deny the existence of differences among colleagues; all mental health professionals are seen as equally competent, and all mental health professions are seen as offering the same services to patients. It is ironic that many of the people who seem to hold such a mental set in terms of their own working conditions are vociferous in their professional organizations, urging stronger assessment of competence within the particular mental health profession and urging a greater and more clearly defined role for that profession in the delivery of mental health services to patients.

Of course, we must realize that within any discipline some practitioners will be more competent than others. Similarly, we must realize that, though physician, nurse and social worker are all professionals and are all capable of autonomous practice, the type of practice, the methods of practice, and the approach to the patient are different — as they should be.

Most mental health practitioners, of whatever professional background, tend to be egalitarian people. This is a philosophical and sometimes even a characteriologic component of the majority of these professionals. At the same time, they are placed in a system in which both within their given profession and among the other mental health professions, they are placed in an extremely hierarchical setting. This causes a considerable amount of role stress. Many practitioners react to the stress by denying its existence. The person at the top of the hierarchical pyramid tries to act as if he or she and the janitor are really doing much the same sort of work. This is obviously deleterious and really a type of condescending *noblesse oblige* which has little place in the harsh reality of mental health practice.

A more common type of reaction to this role stress is for the person a bit lower on the pyramid to attempt to get higher. This can be a thoroughly benign and indeed rewarding quest, but all too often it is done by the use of backhanded, indirect, inappropriately critical maneuvers.

One must keep in mind, then, that whether for good or ill, all mental health professionals are involved in a hierarchical setting. The setting is also, fortunately, a dynamic one. The practitioner must be aware of relationships with equals, relationships with people lower in the heirarchy, and relationships with people higher in the hierarchy, both in his or her own profession and outside that profession among other mental health workers. In addition, he or she must keep in mind that this hierarchy is dynamic and changing. Finally, he or she should keep in mind — although this is probably most rarely done — that the function of any sort of mental health care system is indeed to provide care for the patient.

The particular role strain and role relationship which specifically occurs between nurses and physicians will be discussed in two other chapters in this book. Among nurses themselves, one must look at communication patterns for the presence of denial, which can be counter-productive to the care of the patient, and the presence of collusion, which is a type of identification between two professionals which gives them a sense of professional identity, often at the expense of the patient. The frequent use by psychiatric nurses of the term "inappropriate" as applied to a patient's behavior often represents such collusion.

One must look at the fact that in any profession in which there is a hierarchy — and there certainly is one in nursing — people who are below the top of that heirarchy will have some anti-authoritarian feelings. This does not necessarily represent immaturity — it is a ubiquitous phenomenon in any profession. The most helpful way of dealing with such anti-authoritarian strivings is first to be aware that they are and will be present, and second to examine the particular conflict with authority — its specifics — and ask whether it represents merely a neurotic type of conflict or whether, in fact, one is totally justified in one's approach. Almost always, the answer lies somewhere in the spectrum between those two extreme positions. It is then necessary to attempt to weigh the degree of neurotic conflict and the degree of realistic concern, and act accordingly.

Another very common role strain in psychiatric nursing is that the psychiatric nurse is often asked to supervise a great many other nurses. Unlike some of the other mental health professions, such as psychiatry and clinical psychology, the level of expertise and level of training of the psychiatric nurse tends to be very disparate. Thus, the psychiatric nurse in charge of a unit may very well be at a Master's or Ph.D. level while the nurses she supervises may range from Master's degree level to licensed practical nurses. In addition, the nursing department is often asked to supervise the work of various technicians with a widely differing level of training. This experience can, of course, be a frustrating one. One of the hazards of having to supervise such a broad group is that of becoming extremely authoritarian and condescending to those one is supervising. Such an attitude is rapidly detected and is certainly resented for obvious reasons. Another common attitude is to treat everyone as an equal. While this boosts morale, it does not boost patient care because, in fact, many of the workers will not be particularly competent.

Perhaps most important is the need to look for defense mechanisms that one uses in dealing with other professionals and to insist that one be direct, though not aggressive, in dealing with them.

The author is not suggesting from the content of this chapter that all mental health professionals offer the same services. Indeed, they do not and they need to be fully aware of this. There is certainly overlap in services offered among all these professionals and there will probably continue to be a considerable and even growing amount of bickering over who should be responsible for these overlapping areas. Nevertheless, each discipline has a distinct role to play.

Because of discrepancies and variations in training, the fund of knowledge imparted to some professionals is considerably less than will be found in others in their same discipline or profession and this needs to be evaluated on an individual basis. The philosophy of each discipline varies considerably and the types of approaches to psychodynamic issues also vary.

One of the great problems in dealing with other mental health professionals is the attitude on the part of several people in each discipline that any helping person of good intent can help the psychiatrically impaired patient. Good intentions do not make up for the lapses and lack of knowledge imparted by poor professional education. Tbe well intentioned person who is also well trained in any of the mental health disciplines can be a good clinician but the well intentioned person who is poorly trained will blunder repetitively.

In the struggle for autonomy and even supremacy which occurs among the mental health professions and among mental health professionals, one needs to be constantly vigilant that one's progress or the progress of one's discipline is not at the expense of the patient. Very frequently, in situations where different disciplines see a patient in different ways, observation and treatment of the patient will be designed by each discipline to prove itself right. This type of approach totally loses sight of the patient's individuality and often sacrifices what could be a good treatment opportunity for the purpose of professional one-upsmanship. This type of approach is extremely common in psychiatric settings where alas it has no place whatsoever. At the same time, many individual mental health professionals will deny or minimize their own important observations of and suggestions for the care of the patient in order to be perceived well by colleagues who may be more powerful. This has the same deleterious effect on the patient that the mistake discussed in the previous paragraph has and in addition it tends to split the professional off from his own peer group.

As the nurse also has to deal with other professionals outside of nursing, the situation is similar but perhaps a bit more complex because of different levels of training and different professional self-concepts.

Another area which sometimes is difficult includes relationships with students. When one is functioning as a student, there is an additional problem with the hierarchy in that one is often dealing with both an educational hierarchy and also a practice hierarchy. The interactions between those two hierarchies are rarely clear, and the role of the student is often as someone in the middle.

In the next chapters of this book, the specifics of role relationships among nurses and between the nursing profession and any other given profession are examined.

28 Nursing in a Therapeutic Milieu

Donnis Lassig and Karla Schroeder

INTRODUCTION

Today's trends in the practice of psychiatry allow innumerable opportunities for nursing to make a major impact on patient care. No longer are we bound to base our practice on custodial cares. One of the most exciting and now widely accepted treatment approaches is milieu therapy. Much has been written to define this therapy and results of this as an approach, but little on how to direct nurses in building and maintaining a therapeutic environment.

This chapter will address our adaptation of therapeutic milieu to a unit in a large, general hospital. We hope to outline the nurse's role and types of problems nurses encounter. A description of the program will also be provided.

Since there are multiple terms and definitions used to describe milieu therapy, we will clarify the definition we use throughout the chapter. As noted by Kraft, "Any program which uses environment or aspects of the environment may be classified as milieu therapy; whereas in the therapeutic community all social and interpersonal interactions in the hospital are therapeutic for the patient" (1).

We do not utilize the entire hospital as an environment in which to observe interactions. The unit is part of a general hospital and receives many diagnostic dilemmas for evaluation. Many patients find it difficult to transfer from a medical/surgical unit, to say nothing of engaging in the milieu. Unlike a classical therapeutic community we do not encourage active patient government. Since we are a short term treatment facility, the time is best used to focus on primary goals for treatment versus active challenging or restructuring of the organization of the unit. Further explanations of the program will define the mechanism for patients to air concerns and feelings in relation to the "governing" of the unit.

This unit has been organized to help patients recover from emotional disorders and cope more effectively with everyday life. The philosophy emphasizes promotion of an environment that encourages open expression of feelings and behaviors so that we might understand the pain and discomfort with which individuals are struggling. Through this, we can sometimes assist them in learning healthier modes of communication and coping.

Within milieu therapy, we focus on two primary goals.

The first is symptom relief. Certainly, we would like to alleviate all of the patient's pain, but, realistically, we hope for a decrease in the intensity of symptoms. The types of problems presented fall into the categories of neurotic disorders, eating disorders, psychomatic disorders, personality disorders and situational crises. These problems have taken time to develop. The process of helping patients to learn about the impact or correlation of their symptoms to behavior, emotions and interpersonal relationships takes time — more than is reasonable to expect of a three to four week average stay.

Our job, then, is to set up a foundation for that learning process. Symptom relief often occurs in some form just by immersing the patient in a supportive and nurturing environment, away from the sources of conflict outside the hospital. This is accomplished through a family setting for meals, many group social interactions, diversion and relaxation in activity therapy and individual attention from the physician and nursing staff. This enables the individual time and comfort to begin exploring to what his symptoms might be related. Through the exploring and teaching process of therapy, individuals begin to identify dynamics surrounding their difficulties or methods for dealing with problems. Long term goals involve integration of new behaviors and communication patterns tried out while hospitalized.

A second focus of the treatment approach is to provide a corrective emotional experience. This concept is used by Irvin Yalom in describing the curative process for long term group psychotherapy (2). Within the milieu, we take every opportunity to direct the patient into a trusting relationship, be it with the primary physician, primary nurse or group. Within the relationship the patient shares and directs content of a very deep and personal meaning. The corrective experience often occurs when the therapists or group are able to accept and respond to strong emotional reactions and yet help the individual to look at current distortions in reality as they examine whether these emotional responses are based within the current relationships or carrying over from past significant or painful experiences. Many patients achieve corrective experiences in dealing with old authority issues. The accepting and supportive environment not only allows expression of these conflicts but a mechanism to understand and learn about the nature of the reactions.

Lewis Wolberg (3) has written about short term psychotherapy and lists nine goals for therapy. These goals more specifically explain results we see through individual and group approaches utilized in the therapeutic milieu:

1. Work on patient's immediate need (band-aid effect).
2. Reduce neurotic symptoms and leave patient more hopeful.
3. Help combat feelings of loneliness and isolation as patient discovers shared difficulties.
4. Activate people socially so they can achieve better interpersonal relations and more socialized personalities.
5. Sublimation of antisocial trends.
6. Growth of mutual empathy and acceptance of others even though different.
7. Emotional re-education.
8. Orient patient more appropriately to reality so more realistic choices can be made to test his misperceptions against reality.
9. Improved self-image through feedback reactions from peers and authority figures.

THE UNIT

The unit is a 30-bed, open, self-care facility. Patients are referred by staff psychiatrists. They are, in most instances, adults who have been referred for complete psychiatric evaluations and/or short term treatment. At the time of discharge, most patients are referred to some type of follow-up care in their home communities. The treatment team consists of a staff psychiatrist-consultant, a group of resident physicians being supervised by the consultant, a social worker, recreational therapists and a primary (RN) and associate (RN or LPN) nurse. The consultant directs the focus for treatment after the team members have assessed the patient. Along with planning treatment strategies around milieu therapy, each consultant offers an emphasis on varying approaches.

They range from psychoanalytic approaches to family therapy. With the many specialties and expertise the consultants bring, the nursing staff are challenged to learn broad and eclectic treatment approaches.

Periodic changes in medical personnel are characteristic of teaching hospitals. We have found that nursing holds the key to maintaining consistency and continuity for the treatment approach while these changes occur.

The program itself encourages patients to assume as much responsibility and independence as possible for daily activities. Patients who have been unable to handle the responsibilities prior to admission are encouraged to do so gradually during the initial phase of their hospitalization, In most instances, patients are responsible for performing activities of daily living independently. These may include simple dressing changes, diabetic cares, ostomy cares, basic respiratory routines and self administration of some medication — all after an initial period of teaching and supervision. Patients wear street clothes and do their own laundry. They make their own beds, as well as change linens. The patients are encouraged to use the community meetings to organize and delegate responsibility for keeping patient lounges and the kitchen orderly, watering plants, planning and executing activities, and for discussion and resolution of problems affecting all patients on the unit.

There are no telephones or television in the patients rooms. This appears to promote socialization and gives the patients opportunities to learn constructive conflict resolution over use of communal property (e.g., telephones, television, laundry and kitchen facilities). Nurses inform patients of scheduled times for medications, vital signs and various treatments requiring nursing assistance. They are, in turn, expected to seek out their assigned nurses for assistance with these activities. When patients desire late passes or weekend LOA's it is expected that they will plan and arrange for this with their physician. During the week, patients are asked to be up, dressed and involved in planned activities. Difficulties in fulfilling these expectations become the focus of discussion, mutual goal setting and planning between the patients and their primary/associate nurse.

The emphasis on self-care is designed to mobilize patients who have become entrenched in the sick role. This minimizes the more obvious secondary gains associated with the patient's symptoms. It also helps to focus staff's attention on the healthier aspects of the patient's personality. We attempt to give the patient a clear message that he is capable of responsible, age-appropriate behavior. As individuals assume these responsibilities, their self-confidence and self-esteem often appear to improve. This is the first step in preparing individuals to function in the various roles that will be expected of them when returning home.

If one wanted to really capture the nurse's role in milieu therapy, it would start by following the patient into the hospital. Treatment begins during the patient's admission interview and introduction to the unit. Whenever possible, the patient's primary nurse conducts the nursing admission interview. The patient is encouraged to describe his problem in his own words and share any ideas he has about the development of the problem. With supportive questioning the patient is usually able to verbalize any feelings he has about the hospitalization. The patient is asked to describe his expectations of treatment and thoughts about follow-up care. The patient and available family members are given a tour of the unit. The primary nurse generally meets with any available family members and does an initial assessment of the family system. The admission process generally concludes with a discussion of unit policies, programs and expectations. Patients' reactions to this discussion vary — anxiety, apprehension, hostility, and increased somatization are common. The nurse supports the patient's and family's efforts to verbalize these feelings and reassures the patient that he will be given time to adjust to the new environment.

Several objectives are accomplished during the admission process. The nurse can make a comprehensive assessment of the patient's needs, coping mechanisms, support systems, physical status and personality strengths. In supporting the patient to verbalize his concerns, fears, and expectations the nurse begins to lay the groundwork for an effective therapeutic relationship; she gives the patient the message that he is accepted and that she is interested in his concerns. During the initial teaching about unit programs and expectations, the patient is given the message that others have confidence in his ability to function more autonomously. Finally, the admission process provides an opportunity to begin to develop a supportive relationship with the patient's family.

There are several principles to bear in mind about the initial phase of the patient's hospitalization. First, each patient must be allowed to adjust to the milieu and involve himself in the therapeutic process at his own pace. Some patients become involved in unit activities almost immediately, while others must be encouraged to do so gradually over a period of days. Second, "hooking" the patient into the environment is an active, planned process. The plan arises from the nurse's initial assessment of the patient's expectations, coping mechanisms and acceptance of psychiatric treatment. Some patients, for example, are initially permitted to regress somewhat and to act out their dependency needs until they begin to develop a sense of security and trust in the staff. They are then gently pushed to become more active and independent and to assume more responsibility in their own treatment. Third, initial milieu teaching should always be repeated. Patients are always anxious at the time of admission and as a result are often unable to attend to descriptions of programs and expectations, or to understand the rationale behind them. Finally, other patients often provide the most successful orientation to the milieu. They can identify with the new patient's discomfort, confusion and fears about treatment. They provide far more convincing reassurance than staff could as to whether they can get better. They can discuss the positive and negative aspects of the milieu from a patient's point of view. The patient group will generally do much to decrease the new patient's feelings of loneliness and hopelessness.

Following the initial phase of admission and assessment comes the most important phase of planning. Long term planning begins with the meeting of the treatment team. The patient's history is reviewed, the patient is interviewed and team members share observations and assessments. The team attempts to delineate the patient's individual needs, coping mechanisms, ability to benefit from the program and what aspects of the environment should be included in the treatment approach. The staff psychiatrist makes recommendations related to proper diagnosis, any needed medication, and directives for treatment strategies.

I cannot emphasize enough the importance of consistency and agreement in the approaches by both the medical and nursing staff. Unresolved conflicts in this area are almost always detrimental to the patient. Significant changes in the treatment plan should be communicated to the nursing staff by the primary nurse, after discussion with the physician.

Patients are both directly and indirectly involved in the planning stage. Medical recommendations are discussed with the patient in the presence of the patient's nurse and generally other members of the treatment team. At this point, the patient is encouraged to comment on the team's recommendations. In some instances, specific aspects of the plan may be negotiated in order to make it more workable to the patient. Negotiation of even small aspects of the treatment plan is also useful in helping the patient to experience a greater sense of control over the treatment process and the new environment. At times, the nurse attempts to involve the patient directly in establishing a nursing plan of care through a process of mutual goal setting. This is especially effective with highly manipulative patients, and with those who have a strong need to feel that they are in control. This approach has been most beneficial for patients who have difficulty assuming responsibility for any aspect of their treatment or those who cannot seem to focus their efforts on any specific concerns or goals. Planning and replanning for treatment approaches are ongoing processes that always follow continuous reassessment of the patient's progress.

Following the planning stages, one would find the nurse very busy with patient teaching. This is an important aspect of every nursing care plan. Areas and methods of teaching are individualized and based on the nurse's ongoing assessment of patient's learning needs. In the course of their hospitalization, most patients are exposed to learning experiences in the areas discussed below. It is important to remember that our patient teaching is not confined to solely one-to-one interactions or didactic presentations. Much teaching is done in group settings and in many instances is done by other patients. Informal teaching takes place on an ongoing basis in any therapeutic milieu and there are "teaching" aspects to most therapeutic interventions made in individual therapy.

COMMUNICATION

Teaching about communication skills focuses on both the development of basic social skills and upon increasing the patient's awareness of communication patterns. The feelings and needs behind the patterns and the way in which they affect relationships and one's self-esteem are equally important. Many patients have never developed the basic social skills one needs to function adequately within the family and community or to establish reasonably satisfying interpersonal relationships. Other patients have forgotten how to use these skills as they have withdrawn from interpersonal contacts and become increasingly preoccupied with their symptoms. The therapeutic milieu provides the patient with the security and support he needs to gradually assume the risks associated with interacting. The type of support needed varies with the patient and may require gentle pushing and insistence that minimal expectations be met related to the amount of time he must spend out of his room in a social setting. As interpersonal activities increase, the nurse teaches communication skills through role modeling, role playing, and helping the patient verbalize feelings and concerns about talking with others. The nurse provides objective feedback about the patient's social skills and discusses nonverbal behavior. It is very important to support the patient's efforts to improve social skills. The nurse uses her relationship with the patient to encourage him to practice these skills in relationships with other members of the milieu and eventually in activities outside of the hospital. Development of social skills is an important aspect of many of the group programs to be described later. Because all of the patients have an increased interest in communication processes and skills, considerable teaching and experimentation takes place within the patient group. Patients can be very constructively supportive of one another's efforts to develop social skills.

For patients with adequately developed social skills, teaching is focused on helping them learn more about how they communicate with people in the environment and how these communications are involved in the problems that led to hospitalization. In the process of discussing this, the nursing staff would help the patient to focus on specific difficulties in communicating. For example, there may be new awareness of problems with authority figures or with persons who appear helpless or dependent. Focusing on the feelings he has in these situations helps to increase his understanding of the needs or conflicts that support the patterns. Patients are encouraged to look at how these patterns emerge in significant relationships outside the hospital. The nurse uses her relationship with the patient to increase his awareness of the impact of these communication patterns on her and others by providing direct feedback. This is on the basis of her own reactions and by supporting patient efforts to seek out similar feedback from group members, other patients and staff. Gradually, patients become aware that the messages, feelings and needs they intend to communicate are not necessarily those perceived by others. As they become more aware of others' reactions to their communication patterns and the internal factors that perpetuate the patterns, they can frequently be encouraged and supported to experiment with new ways of relating. The ultimate goals of teaching and nursing interventions at this level is to enable the patient to change the way he relates to other patients in group, the milieu, at home and in the community. As he experiments with these changes, he is generally able to gain an understanding of the interpersonal meaning of his presenting symptoms.

All teaching about communication involves teaching about basic mental health principles. Many patients have never been told that it is normal to experience "negative" feelings such as anger, envy, hatred, disappointment, etc. Others have never learned that there are acceptable ways of expressing feelings directly. Nursing staff discuss the consequences of attempting to hide feelings and the indirect ways in which "hidden" feelings are expressed. Other teaching is direct toward increasing awareness of basic human needs and the importance of verbalizing these directly and appropriately.

RELATIONSHIPS

A great deal of time is spent focusing on the patients' relationships. They learn a lot about interpersonal relationships in the process of initiating, developing and terminating friendships with other patients and working therapeutic relationships with nursing and medical staff.

Most specifically, patients are encouraged to define the expectations they have of themselves and others in the relationships they establish in the milieu, with co-workers, in the family and their community. Nursing staff assists the patient to explore relationships they develop on the unit and in group, in an effort to learn more about the needs they try to fulfill. The feedback of group members, primary nurses and physicians helps to increase patient awareness of these needs and the ways the patient attempts to influence others to fulfill them. The nurse works to help the patient identify basic assumptions about how emotional needs are met. The common sources of the assumptions (e.g., family, society, mores of various ethnic groups) are identified and patients are helped to see how these affect their behavior in group and other important relationships. The goals of these efforts are to make the patient more aware of how the assumptions and expectations interfere with his ability to recognize and fulfill needs in appropriate ways, to increase awareness of the ways symptomatic behavior enabled him to fulfill emotional needs, to help the patient identify more effective and satisfying ways to meet needs. The patient is supported and praised for experimentation with new interpersonal behaviors that can aid him in achieving relationships with greater meaning and satisfaction.

Learning about interpersonal relationships involves learning how to handle conflicts. Nursing attempts to teach patients that conflicts are part of life and that numerous problems may arise when conflicts are denied, avoided or smoothed over. As conflicts occur between patients, or patients and family, the nurse avoids becoming directly involved in the conflict. Rather, she intervenes to help the patient explore his feelings and thoughts about the conflict, to plan strategies for resolving the conflict, and she supports the patient's efforts to assume responsibility for handling the conflict. When patients have some success with conflict resolution, they often experience an increase in self-confidence and self-esteem. A similar approach is taken with conflicts arising among members of therapy groups. When conflicts involve several members of the community, patients are encouraged to voice their concerns during the bi-weekly community meeting. If patients have an opportunity to experience conflict resolution in a group setting, they frequently are more willing to acknowledge and address family conflicts, as well as those between co-workers and friends.

TEACHING AND EXPLORING ROLES

Many patients are experiencing considerable difficulty fulfilling the expectations of various social roles. In some instances, patients find themselves in roles for which they have little preparation from society or their family of origin. An example would be the young woman reared in a seriously dysfunctional family system who is now having difficulty fulfilling expectations associated with the roles of wife and mother. Some patients experience difficulty adjusting to significant changes in their social roles (e.g., recent divorce, retired corporate executive, middle aged woman with "empty nest" syndrome). Others have abandoned social roles as their presenting symptoms became more severe and disabling. Certain patients react to feeling "trapped" in roles they find intensely dissatisfying. The primary nurse must assess the nature of new patients' role-related difficulties and address these in the care plan.

Nursing staff may intervene with some basic instruction in parenting skills or typical developmental problems in family or marriage. While this is currently done on an individual basis, providing this teaching in a systematic group setting is sometimes a good alternative. The nurse may request the assistance of various community resources which focus on role-related problems. Frequently, the patient's discharge plans include on-going contact with appropriate community agencies.

Patients are also encouraged to explore their feelings, needs and expectations associated with their social roles or changes in those roles. Much of this discussion is initiated in one-to-one sessions between the patient and nurse. However, the concern is carried over to group sessions and other informal discussions with patients and staff.

The group discussions offer a good arena for working out these concerns. Patients are able to identify with the feelings expressed by others struggling with similar conflicts. The groups also increase patient awareness of the emotional needs that arise in an effort to fulfill role expectations. The group works to help individuals identify ways of meeting the needs identified.

The therapeutic milieu's emphasis on independent functioning and personal responsibility is helpful in motivating patients who have abandoned all role responsibilities. Patient peer pressure is an important factor here, as is support from staff for any efforts to assume more responsibility. Successful role assumption on the unit prepares the patient to assume appropriate role responsibilities at home and in the community.

IDENTIFICATION OF STRENGTHS

Nurses can be very helpful in assisting patients to focus attention on their strengths and abilities. By the time the patient's symptoms have become so severe and disabling that hospitalization is suggested, he has typically experienced a significant loss of self-esteem. He feels powerless and lacks a sense of self-worth. He frequently speaks of having no purpose or meaning in his life. Ironically, the feelings of worthlessness, poor self-esteem, etc. often involve the patient's denial of actual weaknesses. Thus, many nursing interventions are directed toward using the milieu to help the patient recapture a sense of self-esteem.

The therapeutic milieu, itself, promotes the development of self-esteem. Patients are encouraged to assume responsibilities in which they will achieve some success. As they become involved in unit activities, they receive feedback which assures them that their presence and contributions are important to the functioning of the whole group. In both individual and group meetings the patient learns that he is not alone with his feelings and concerns. All of these factors decrease feelings of isolation and increase feelings of effectiveness and self-worth.

Through individual and group work, the patients are helped to acknowledge and accept human and personal weaknesses and to make realistic assessments of their strengths. Sometimes, just discovering that they can complete a ceramic project in activity therapy or organize a weekend social activity offers a great source of reward. Moreover, discovering that they are valued by persons with whom they have shared their imperfections offers a healing and strengthening effect.

Effort is made to help patients identify relationships that perpetuate feelings of worthlessness and helplessness and self-defeating behaviors or communication patterns. The milieu is a valuable arena in which all of these difficulties can be played out. Role-playing alternatives can teach patients healthier methods of dealing with these difficulties and can sometimes leave them with a greater sense of strength and self-respect.

It is important to offer the patient positive reinforcement for efforts to change self-defeating behaviors. Typically, this support comes from other patients, as well.

As the patient becomes more aware of his strengths and weaknesses, self-esteem improves. He is better able to make realistic plans for handling the stresses he will encounter upon leaving the hospital.

REALITY TESTING

We think it is important to make note of the nurse's role in assisting the patient with reality testing. In a general sense, all of the nursing interventions previously described promote reality testing. We tend to think of reality testing as helping psychotic patients to see and hear reality more clearly. However, the whole teaching approach of nursing to expand the patient's perception of appropriate or normal feelings and reactions helps to broaden the rigid definitions of "normal" behaviors and feelings that the patients perceive. The nurse provides direct and ongoing feedback and models less rigid interpretations of "healthy" communication. Behaviors can be modified, and expectations of self and others can become more realistic when the milieu invites more creative and flexible expression. Patients discover that all human beings have feelings and needs and that there are acceptable and satisfying ways of expressing them.

LIMIT SETTING

A final area in which nursing is quite involved is limit setting. This is crucial in helping to keep the milieu a therapeutic one. That is not to say it is a mechanism for staff to practice rigid control, but rather that it can be a mechanism to let patients know that we won't let the environment or themselves get out of control.

Generally, limit setting is necessary when: (1) the patient's behavior is dangerous to himself or others; (2) the patient's behavior seriously disrupts the milieu, and (3) the patient's behavior reflects a temporary need for more structure than is typically available. *Dangerous* is rather loosely defined in this instance and refers to compulsive, ritualistic behavior that threatens the health of the patient, as well as physically aggressive and self-destructive behaviors. If ignored, impulsive or severely anxious and agitated behavior can seriously disrupt the milieu and can lead to the development of more severe symptoms in the patient. The same is true in regard to severe somatic and pain behaviors. At times, reasoning, teaching, peer pressure or support of staff and patients is not sufficient to help the patient control these behaviors. It is in these situations that the nursing staff must find ways of providing external controls until the patient develops the internal resources to apply internal controls. (The interventions discussed do not exclude the possible need for medication to assist the patient in controlling his behavior.)

Limit setting occurs in a variety of forms. One currently popular form involves the use of a contract in which both patient and staff agree that specific behaviors will result in specific consequences. To be most effective, the contract is made only after there is significant trust between the patient and those he is contracting with. The contract may be for short intervals at a time or extended periods. While this form can be effective, it is not without problems. For example, patients may be asked to contract with staff to report any self-destructive impulses or acting out. In many instances, the consequences of approaching a nurse with this information are not specified. Even if they are specified, they may be frightening to the patient (e.g., greater controls, such as seclusion) that he is reluctant to follow the contract. The patient is placed in a double-bind situation in which he fears unacceptable consequences whether he abides by the contract or not. This type of contracting does not promote the development of open and trusting therapeutic relationships. If the patient cannot follow through with the contract, he suffers the guilt and shame of letting down the staff. It can also curtail meaningful discussion of issues if the patient fears consequences for talking about poor control of impulses. Contracting can be useful in the more compulsively manipulative behaviors, such as one sees in patients with certain eating disorders.

Structuring a patient's time and activity can be a very effective means of limit setting. Severely anxious patients often need assistance in organizing their time and planning activity for a purposeful outcome. They may also require some persuasive and supportive external controls to insure that basic needs for nutrition and rest are not ignored. Significantly regressed patients and those who have become withdrawn and immobilized by somatic concerns or chronic pain may require assistance in structuring time and activities. With these patients, it is helpful to place limits on the amount of time they can spend in bed and in talking about their pain with staff. The nurse should anticipate angry responses as limits are placed on these patients.

An effective means of limit setting for self-defeating behaviors can be accomplished by limiting the amount of time and attention given in response to these behaviors. This is frequently the approach taken with patients who exhibit a variety of somatic and dramatic pain behaviors, or chronically manipulative patients threatening self-destruction. There are three important points to make about this method of limit setting. First, the overall physical and emotional condition of the patient should be carefully assessed on an on-going basis. While we want to avoid reinforcing self-defeating behaviors, we must also avoid failing to respond to legitimate physical symptoms or serious suicidal ideation. Secondly, these patients must be receiving attention and time in response to their efforts to engage in more appropriate behaviors. It is easy to become so involved in the ways that we should or should not respond to the symptomatic behavior, that we forget about supporting and nurturing healthier aspects of their personalities and behavior. Thirdly, when we limit the interest we show in something as subjectively important as patient's symptoms, we must look for ways in which we can convey our interest and concern for the patient as a person. This can be done by spending time with the patient and supporting him as he pursues a new activity or demonstrates efforts to modify unhealthy behaviors.

When a patient's behavior is chronically irresponsible, limit setting may take the form of restricting privileges within the environment. For example, patients who chronically abuse open ward or pass privileges, may have passes retricted until they can demonstrate the ability to act responsibly. It is important to specify the reasons for restricting the patient's privileges. If his behavior is having a detrimental impact on others or preventing him from engaging in his own therapy, this should be carefully explained to him. The limit setting is therapeutic only if the patient is helped to understand that it will promote his efforts to feel better or to establish more satisfying relationships. It should never by a punishment or means for staff to "vent" their own anger at the patient.

Limit setting is difficult for many nurses and it is therefore important to remember that in addition to being necessary for the unit, it can be therapeutic for the patient. Some patients need concrete assurance that we will protect them (and others) from loss of control before they can begin taking the risks that are part of therapy. In helping the patient to set limits on agitated, compulsive and manipulative behaviors we help him preserve some of the energy he needs to engage in therapy. The process of limit setting can increase the patient's awareness of the impact of his behavior on others. Similarly, the patient learns that all behaviors have consequences and that, ultimately, he must assume responsibility for both the behavior and its consequences.

Equally important are teaching and modeling for patients. Within the milieu, the patients watch staff to see how they deal with annoying behaviors of various patients. They will use nurses as examples, good and bad, and they will often begin experimenting with new approaches themselves. Many areas of conflict in therapy often center on individuals' inability to say *no* or to set limits on others' requests and demands. This may be centered on past significant authority figures and, in turn, carries over to many other conflicts in current reality. As the patient learns that it is normal and acceptable to limit unreasonable authority, he begins to practice this in the milieu with the nursing and medical staff. Though difficult to deal with at times, it can be the beginning of new autonomy and self-esteem as the patient learns to limit or reject unreasonable expectations, demands, and authority. This is a healthy step towards greater independence for the patient.

Many of the previous nursing interventions are related to individual work with patients and alluded to therapeutic groups in which similar interventions occur. Group programs are an integral part of our milieu. The following is a brief description of the groups we currently use as part of the milieu approach. They were developed to provide a well-rounded experience for the patient's hospitalization. While social workers, activity therapists, and physicians are active in several of these groups, our description focuses on the nurse's role in group programs.

COMMUNITY MEETING

These are held at least twice weekly and include all patients, nursing staff and activity therapists. Each week a chairman, secretary, and exercise leader are elected by the patient group. A staff nurse is appointed to work directly with the group. The chairman delegates responsibility for other tasks (e.g., watering plants, arranging transportation for patient activities, organizing a cooking activity, distributing mail) to members of the "community." The meetings provide a forum for the discussion of any problems or concerns that are occurring on the unit, and provide an opportunity to practice working cooperatively with peers and "authority figures" in decision making and problem solving. The meetings are also used to plan patient activities. The activity promotes the idea that each individual plays an important part in the functioning of the whole community. It promotes development of various social and communication skills. The chairman is given a notebook outlining details of running the meeting. This leadership position has helped many patients to recapture a sense of worth and esteem through successful organization and leadership skills.

This activity requires active, positive nursing involvement to be successful. Patient interest and attendance dwindle when nursing enthusiasm and attendance taper. This is an opportunity for nurses to reinforce their support of the milieu approach. The staff in the meetings must be able to model effective communication and problem solving skills. They must be sensitive to the needs of the particular patient group as well as individual needs. They need to feel secure enough within themselves and their role to handle patient criticism constructively, and to promote active problem solving and decision making by the group. To accomplish these goals, the nursing staff must show that it can give up enough control and promote healthy strengths within the group to suggest changes and independent projects and activities.

Nursing staff have frequently held extra community meetings when some type of crisis (acting out, vandalism, suicidal gestures) has occurred. The purpose of such a special meeting is to provide an open supportive atmosphere in which the group can discuss their reactions to the crisis and the way it was handled, and can hopefully gain a sense of confidence from staff that the environment is secure and under control.

ASSERTIVENESS GROUP

This group meets weekly in a two-session group in which patients learn to be more assertive in their interactions with others. During the first session, a member of the nursing staff presents a didactic lecture defining and describing the differences among passive, aggressive, and assertive behavior. Patients are encouraged to consider and share examples of their own passive, aggressive, or assertive behavior. Much emphasis is placed on the types of responses these various behaviors tend to elicit from others and in the various feelings that tend to accompany each type of behavior. Patients are encouraged to become more aware of the needs and feelings they are trying to communicate to others. They are taught to consider both the verbal and nonverbal aspects of their communication. The second session involves role playing by the patients and the nursing staff. Patients are encouraged to describe actual situations in which they have behaved passively or aggressively. They are then helped to role-play the situation in a more assertive manner. The role playing allows the patient to experience some success with a new type of behavior. It also provides an opportunity for patients to discuss their reactions to their partners' passive or aggressive behavior. This often stimulates thoughts about others' reactions to their own behavior.

Nursing staff must be sensitive to the needs and resistances of each particular group and must often creatively approach these needs and resistances to get the role-playing started. If they are successful in this attempt, patients generally consider this group beneficial. They frequently return each week to the role-playing session for further practice, or will ask their individual nurse to role-play difficult situations with them.

DISCHARGE GROUP

This group is facilitated by two nurses and includes patients who will be dismissed in the coming week. The purpose of the group is, first, to answer any specific questions regarding dismissal and, second, to give patients an opportunity to discuss concerns they have about their pending discharge. Common areas of discussion include: feelings about going home, concerns about what significant others will expect of them and what they can expect from important family members, changes that they have made in the hospital and what it will be like to incorporate changes outside of the hospital, concerns over what to tell family and friends about the hospitalization and plans for follow-up care. Nursing staff attempt to give each patient support for and specific feedback about risks taken and changes made during his hospitalization. Patients are also given the message that ambivalent feelings about discharge are common and apprehension is to be expected. The possibility that the patient might experience a mild recurrence of symptoms initially, is discussed openly. Patients are encouraged to share their ideas for coping during this period of adjustment. Nurses discuss and model the importance of terminating important relationships that have been established on the unit.

INTERPERSONAL SHARING GROUPS

This refers to a variety of structured group activities led by nursing staff two to three evenings a week. The specific goals of each activity vary, but all are designed to promote socialization and interpersonal learning. All patients and interested family members are invited to attend. The groups are most beneficial when nursing staff carefully assess the needs and characteristics of the particular patient group, and selects an activity to meet those. The facilitators attempt to create an accepting and supportive atmosphere which promotes sharing of feelings and ideas. The activity allows the staff to establish closer relationships with all patients. It gives staff the opportunity to assess the varying social skills of each patient.

These groups allow for creativity and multiple types of media to base the activity on. Examples of the groups might be dividing the large group into groups of 3 and 4 and providing them with magazines, scissors and glue to build collages representing their major goals or feelings at this time. Another group could be an activity geared towards "ice breaking" when there is a large group of newly admitted patients. We have utilized music, clay, exercise and other such vehicles on which to base the activity. All of these allow a different focus for attention, while helping the group to relax and begin to share.

LEISURE EDUCATION

This is a four session group conducted by the activity therapy staff. The patient's attention is focused on his use of leisure time and how he can plan leisure activities to more effectively meet his needs. Nursing staff attend the group as participants, as well as observers. During these sessions, patients often become aware of needs, work habits that they perceived as leisure and the scarcity of time spent relaxing and enjoying leisure time. Issues identified in this group are then taken back to individual sessions with the doctor and nurse. Nurses can be instrumental in providing the encouragement patients need to follow through with some of the plans established in leisure education.

DAILY THERAPY GROUPS

For a thirty-bed unit, we have two insight oriented groups and one support group, each of which meets for one hour each day, Monday through Friday. Registered nurses with additional training in group dynamics, resident physicians, social workers and activity therapists act as co-therapists for the groups. Groups are observable through a one way mirror. This facilitates on-going supervision for the therapists and gives physicians and staff an opportunity to observe and assess their patients' interpersonal functioning. Insight oriented groups are designed to help patients become more aware of the way in which they interact with others, the impact of their behavior on others and the ways in which others' reactions to their behavior influences their self-esteem. The group helps the patient to become aware of the interpersonal meaning of his symptoms and offers the patient alternative methods of handling basic needs. Patients are encouraged to examine and modify their expectations of themselves and others. Honesty, direct communication of feelings and opinions, empathy, non-judgmentalism, active listening and mutual respect and support are modeled and reinforced by co-therapists and more experienced group members. The group is directed to focus on here and now issues; members are then helped to explore the ways in which they handle similar conflicts and situations outside of the hospital, with family, friends and employers.

The support group is a more structured group designed for patients who need special assistance in social integration, reality testing and supportive encouragement to share feelings and discuss problems.

All groups are heterogeneous in terms of both areas of conflict and the personality traits of the members. The groups are open ended and members are, therefore, expected to make ongoing adjustments to changes in the composition of the group. While both factors can hinder the development of group cohesiveness, they also recreate situations which the group members will be expected to handle outside the hospital. Emphasis is placed on helping group members explore their responses to change, individual differences, and experiences of loss — all of which characterize open-ended heterogeneous groups. If they are to be helpful, therapists must develop the ability to accurately assess the needs and capabilities of each patient group, as well as the flexibility to adjust expectations and interventions accordingly. The input of nursing staff who work individually with group members and the feedback received from staff observing group facilitate this process.

FACILITATED REPLAY

Ideally, each therapy group participates in one replay each week. Group members are always informed that the group is being videotaped and are encouraged to verbalize any discomfort they feel about the process. The replay is held the same day that the group is taped. The session is conducted by a nurse, activity therapist, or physician, all with group training. The replay therapist is always separate from the group co-therapists. The therapist attemtpts to focus the group's attention on group process, while the members view the tape. The replay therapist must be sensitive to the discomfort patients can feel when observing themselves at the same time he is confronting the individual behaviors and group patterns visible on the videotape.

Patients are often quite apprehensive about video replays, and nursing staff play an important role in helping the patient work through his fears, while enabling him to learn from the experience. Individualized teaching prior to the replay can address particular concerns and make the experience less threatening. This experience may be the most directly confrontive of all therapies, though frequently noted by patients to be very helpful.

MODIFIED PSYCHODRAMA

This is a weekly, one and one-half hour group for all patients who are members of a therapy group. It is considered a part of the group experience, and expectations for attendance are the same as daily group. Group co-therapists plan and conduct the sessions according to individual and group needs. Staff nurses and activity therapists attend as participants to promote enthusiasm and to act as participant observers. The purpose of the group is to help patients become more aware of their feelings and the manner in which they are expressed. This is accomplished through the use of theatrical exercises, role playing, improvisations and by acting out short scenes from a variety of plays. The scenes focus on affects and conflicts frequently occurring in relationships with family members and friends. Patients often experience an initial fear related to "inability to act." It is essential that adequate teaching prefaces each session to help the group relax and understand that no one is assessing acting abilities. The important point is to create a light and active atmosphere that will promote risk taking. Patients have frequently practiced expressing anger more directly and meaningfully, through playing the part of an angry individual. They are encouraged to play opposite parts from a character they may sympathize with, so as to feel what the other person is experiencing. This group requires strong leadership and energetic facilitators for reasonable success.

PSYCHOTHERAPY ORIENTATION

This group meets periodically when the need is identified in several patients. Facilitated by a nurse, it is started with a relaxed, real life videotape of a patient entering her first visit with a psychiatrist. The tape captures the typical confusion and fear that patients experience about what to say to a psychiatrist. It demonstrates what psychotherapy is all about and gives concrete examples to guide patients into therapy. Following the 15 minute tape, the nurse encourages expression of fears and questions among the group members. Further explanation and direction are offered by the nurse to help the patient get the most out of his psychotherapy. A key point is that the nurse conveys an understanding that this is a difficult and often new experience for the patients, but offers hope and encouragement for them to actively engage in the therapy process.

MARITAL CONJOINT THERAPY AND FAMILY MEETINGS

Nursing staff frequently function as co-therapists with resident physicians and social workers in marital conjoint sessions and family meetings. The meetings are arranged for the following purposes:

1. Assessment and history gathering, with special attention to learning how the identified patient's symptoms affect the marriage/family.
2. To prepare the couple or family for the patient's discharge and return home.
3. Teaching about basic mental health concepts, the patient's illness, communication skills, parenting skills, family relationships, medications, follow-up care.
4. Promote effective communication in the family and offer support to family members.
5. Conduct short term marital/family therapy.
6. Introduce the couple or family to therapy sessions to prepare them for long term care in a home community.

It is important to note that this represents only the formal involvement for the nursing staff. Ongoing support and assessment of the family is part of the day to day approach. It is important to watch the identified patient as he interacts within the family system and to incorporate the observations into assessment and revised approaches. Since many of our patients are from out of state, we do not have the opportunity to work consistently with their families. Whenever possible, the family is included in evening activities and encouraged to offer input and observations. Nursing must be familiar with family dynamics to understand the reactions family members have. Efforts are made to meet with various family members at their request as they struggle to understand the conflicts.

Milieu therapy offers an exciting and creative role for nursing. Along with it, however, come some problems. We have identified several areas of potential difficulty for staff. Our best results have been achieved by anticipating and planning for these problems with the staff, through educational programs and care conferences.

THE NEED TO BE LIKED

The profession of nursing, historically, has promoted the image of an all-giving and self-sacrificing woman in white. With due respect for Florence Nightingale, times have changed a bit with males joining the ranks, and current expectations of nurses are more realistic. Nevertheless, we seem to retain the image of a very giving profession. Many of us entered nursing because of the reward and gratification from helping others, and look for positive reinforcement and satisfaction as a result of it.

In a psychiatric setting, the nurse has been responsible for maintaining safety, administering medications and providing physical comfort. With the acceptance of milieu therapy, we are called upon to turn our skills to building an environment in which people feel free to express their pain from emotional discomfort, and yet learn more satisfying ways of behaving and communicating. With that comes a requirement to establish therapeutic relationships, set limits, confront unacceptable behaviors and be understanding of feelings directed at the nurse, though not necessarily based on the reality of the relationship.

This is a definite change in types of expectations for the psychiatric nurse. The nurse's need to be liked must be assessed by her individually to determine how strong that need is. Certainly, we all have it to a certain extent, if we have entered a helping profession. Working in the milieu means delaying one's gratification as we wait to see if our teaching and listening will help the patient. This delay is quite different from the sense of well being and appreciation a nurse feels after administering treatments or direct care that could immediately ease discomfort.

In supervising psychiatric nurses, we believe we need to guide and direct nurses in assessing their own needs to feel liked by the patient. Working as a psychiatric nurse often means waiting to see results, and perhaps even then only the most minor behavioral changes. We need to counsel nurses in an honest way to seek other areas of practice if they experience chronic frustration or are unable to set their own needs aside in order to work with patients.

When the nurse's need to be liked and accepted takes precedence over the patients' needs we see some of the following problems:

1. Inability of the nurse to set limits.
2. Interference with the ability to give constructive feedback.
3. Interference with the ability to be a healthy role model.

These problems tend to overlap. When a nurse is required to set limits, she also must give meaningful feedback about the unacceptable behavior. The limits set may be unclear or inconsistently carried out. The problems may surface as affection or sympathy for some patients. I recall an incident in which a middle-aged woman was admitted with a conversion reaction. Her time out of bed was spent in a wheel chair. She was quite challenging and hostile in her communication with staff, ordering us about and demanding that we care for her. As plans to move her from the wheelchair to a walker progressed, she became more hostile and refused to work with the staff, except for two nurses. These were "the only nurses who really understood" her. The apparent needs of these nurses to feel special and needed seemed stronger than the need to move the patient's treatment plan along. The two nurses became engaged in requests to delay the goals for the walker and often stated the staff and physicians were being harsh and rigid. This problem surfaced very quickly as the staff split and began bickering about expectations for the patient. Through several care conferences, we addressed the difficulty nurses had in setting reasonable time limits with the patient, as well as how uncomfortable they felt in confronting her demanding behavior. When the staff agreed upon target goals and utilized consistency in both limits for time and attention, and direct feedback for unacceptable behaviors the patient again began to progress. Certainly, there was discomfort in withstanding her angry outbursts related to limit setting, but this was a necessary phase in her progress toward greater autonomy.

In both individual and group interactions, nurses need to provide constructive and direct feedback. It may be even more uncomfortable with groups, in which the nurse runs the risk of upsetting many patients. One of the most difficult criticisms that patients give a nurse is the statement, "You don't understand." This statement is an easy defense which can prevent the nurse from offering the feedback which needs to be given. This too, will prevent the patient from learning about the impact of his behavior on the nurse, as well as other patients and family members. If the patient is to engage in more meaningful behavior for improved interpersonal relationships, we must help them to see what is getting in the way of that engagement, putting our own needs aside.

Patients need to be able to depend on the nursing staff to model healthy expression of positive feelings, anger, conflict resolution, and acceptable social behaviors. All of these require a level of self-confidence within the nurse, as well as insight into her own needs and methods of communicating. The need to be in favor with the patient will always create a barrier to meaningful functioning of the nurse. We find that addressing this potential problem with each new nurse early in her employment helps to keep her aware of this hazard.

RECONCILING PERSONAL NEEDS vs. PATIENT NEEDS vs. NEEDS OF THE PATIENT GROUP

So that she can maintain a therapeutic relationship with patients, the nurse needs to be taught to question and reflect on the scope of feelings she encounters through all stages of the nurse-patient relationship. As she works to establish therapeutic boundaries in the relationship, it is helpful to teach her to ask, "Will this intervention satisfy my needs or the patient's?" The recognition of particularly intense feelings, whether positive or negative, is usually an indication that the nurse should review the relationship with a peer in formal supervision and get objective feedback on the appropriateness of the interventions.

A new nurse's struggle to find appropriate boundaries in the relationship will often lead her to share bits of personal information or do special favors for the patient in an attempt to ease initial anxiety and find acceptance with him. This is more typical of a social, friendly relationship than a therapeutic nurse–patient relationship. The supervisor can help the nurse by assuring her that it is normal to feel anxious in the initial stages of getting to know the patient. Teaching nurses the stages of a relationship and various phenomena that occur in each will help them to anticipate patient reactions and plan for more appropriate interventions. We have often watched nurses struggle in both the working and termination phases of the relationship. The nurse may want to help the patient so much that she forgets to plan goals according to what the patient verbalizes as needs, instead of what she would like him to achieve. One particular situation comes to mind in which a nurse was working with a forty-year-old man admitted with headaches. Behaviorally, he demonstrated passivity in situations with other patients as well as his wife. Consequently, his marital discord had reached major proportions, and his ward relationships were characterized by others exploiting him. He complained of loss of control frequently and that no one paid attention to what he said. The nurse set a goal for him to confront the other patients and his wife about the exploitation and domination. In her enthusiasm for him to gain greater control over his life through more assertive behaviors, she failed to see all of the sympathy and secondary gains he achieved through his passivity. He safely avoided greater responsibility both at home and on the unit. The nurse's need to have him change was far greater than his and she suffered chronic frustration and eventual anger at him. These types of difficulties for nurses are decreased through their constant evaluation of whose needs are really met by the care approaches. This can be accomplished through discussions with peers, as well as care conferences to review approaches.

One particular area to watch is the staff's need for control. Giving up control is sometimes very difficult for the staff. Because patients usually come to us in a helpless and dependent state, it is easy to assume that the nurse should make decisions for them and direct them. This undermines one of the most important treatment goals, and that is to help the patient reach as high a level of autonomy as he is capable of. The nurse must learn to constantly reevaluate each patient's need for direction and assistance and learn to step back and let the patient problem-solve on his own. The timing of this becomes an important skill for the nurse to learn in milieu therapy.

Personal needs of the nurse can overshadow less clearly defined patient needs in the process of terminating the relationship. This seems to be an area that causes more difficulty for the psychiatric nurse. Perhaps the fact that there are not cures, but rather some relief of symptoms or behavior changes in psychiatric patients creates more struggle for the nurse to let go of a relationship. The nurse works very hard and often waits to receive gratification from moderate results. For whatever reason, the nurse may be blind to difficulty in terminating. This may be evidenced by ongoing phone calls or personal visits following the patient's discharge, steady mail correspondence or even relinquishing of the therapeutic role to a social friend-type relationship while the patient is still hospitalized. If the nurse is blind to her own ambivalence about termination of either a very positive or negative relationship, she may leave for a vacation or days off without saying goodbye, totally avoid the issue in the individual sessions, or find a less significant reason to be angry with the patient. I have supportively teased many nurses who "by accident," left goals for the discharge and termination process off the care plan. Again, letting nurses know through educational approaches that it is natural to feel both ambivalent and angry about a termination can be helpful. Some patients have a way of making the nurse feel very valued because of her nurturing responses and patient responses to them. That can be hard to give up. And, realistically, the nurse may have done outstanding work and feel great satisfaction from the relationship. The key is to teach her to share her satisfaction and ambivalence in a constructive way with the patient in order to model effective termination. The patient learns from hearing direct positive feelings expressed, as well as sincere sadness over the ending of a meaningful relationship. This is an experience that he will face many times over in his life.

Along the line of assessing and reconciling needs are the problems that occur when nursing has to intervene with a patient or group of patients after determining that behavior of one is destructive for the other. An example of this occurred as a 21-year-old female continuously disrupted interpersonal sharing groups and informal social groups on the unit. She continuously challenged and argued with patients' responses in the group or jeered at the interpersonal content they shared. In the patient lounge, she often changed the television channel from one currently being watched and mumbled sarcastic remarks in low tones. This created a great disruption in the milieu while fulfilling the chief complaint of the young patient that no one liked her and that she could not express her ideas and feelings directly without negative results. On the one hand, the nurses wanted her to learn more socially acceptable skills in communicating which necessitated social interaction within the milieu. On the other hand, the needs of the larger patient group were consistently interfered with because of her hostile and disruptive behavior.

This example points out the need for nurses to be constantly aware of both needs of individual patients and the larger group.

There are two general characteristics of milieu therapy that guide the types and timing of interventions by the nursing staff:

1. Concern for and interest in what happens to individual patients and to a group of patients over a 24 hour period.
2. Takes into account the individual patient's needs in relation to the needs of the group of patients with whom he will be interacting throughout the day (4).

Problems occur in the milieu when nursing staff does not maintain the milieu with sensitivity to needs of both. Most often, the use of limit setting is the most effective intervention to manage these problems.

DEPENDENCE / INDEPENDENCE

If there is one thing that is certain about the role of the psychiatric nurse, it is that it requires the ability to allow patients to transfer intense dependence needs to the nurse. Whenever we hear a nurse complaining of fatigue at the end of a day, it usually proves to be a sign that she is struggling with the demands and needs of some very dependent patients. Nurses can be best prepared for this with a frank discussion about expecting patients to be very dependent on the nurse. Patients generally come to the hospital unable to carry out their roles in jobs and families, along with a suffering self-esteem. They need to sense that it is acceptable to let down and lean on someone else who is not afraid of their needs. The patients need to know we will help them to regain a sense of independence and self-confidence.

Some common requests and signs of dependency needs are demonstrated to the nurse through excessive demands of time and attention, difficulty terminating a session and getting out of the room, requests to see the nurse for one more thing, special assistance with activities of daily living not warranted by physical limitations, requests for frequent advice and direction, and asking permission for many activities.

Helping nurses to cope with intense dependency needs is crucial to insuring the patient's independence. Problems arise when nurses do not recognize the demands as dependency needs or when they have difficulty accepting them. The acceptance is eased by being prepared to anticipate the experience as well as by the individual nurse's level of maturity. The nurse who can put aside her own needs to be liked by the patient and tolerate reactions without personalizing them handles the experience with greater ease.

We can recollect a situation in which a nurse was angrily telling us she did not know why a specified patient was allowed to continue his hospitalization since he was not even trying. In discussing the situation with her, we discovered that she was angry at the patient for continuously asking her to bring his medication to his room and trying to get her to plan and structure his day for him. What, in reality, was happening was that the nurse had demanded that he function more independently. His repeated efforts to gain assistance from her was a message that he was not feeling capable of functioning at the level of independence asked by the nurse. His repeated dependency needs made the nurse angry with him. We frequently lingered about the conference room to listen to nurses discuss their planning and interventions. We noticed many indications of anger at dependency needs of patients and tried to promote discussion and further understanding of the patients' psychodynamics.

Another area for potential conflict centers around fostering of unhealthy dependence of patients on the nurse. If the nurse lacks the faith that these patients can achieve more autonomous functioning, he is apt to keep expectations too low and take over excessive direction and decision making for the patient. When this occurs, the nurse may be blind to the actual gratification she is experiencing from the patient needing her so much. This situation is usually revealed when another nurse works with the patient and he can function with less direction. The nurse's peers and supervisor are the best answer to point out the situation and help the nurse examine her own needs and motives in the relationship.

There is no ideal recipe or approach that ensures a well balanced relationship of dependence and independence for the patient and nurse. In the course of the relationship, the patient is apt to experience many periods of ambivalence. One day he needs the nurse's assistance with multiple activities and the next day he does not want to talk to her. An understanding that this is normal as the patient struggles to identify a level of autonomy he is comfortable with should be taught. The nurse needs to plan goals with the patient, starting at the level of dependence he is currently functioning at and gradually moving up. This can mean that the nurse may need to utilize limit setting interventions on his demands for time. Occasionally, a patient needs to learn that his needs may be unrealistic for any one person to meet. He then needs support and exploration to understand that and a realistic approach for planning more gratifying need satisfaction. The reality of this occurring in a relationship with the nurse can be a valuable tool to draw correlations to current conflict within his own family system.

Successful transition of a very dependent patient to a more confident and independent one should become a source of reward and satisfaction for the nurse. Allowing a patient the freedom to need the nurse less and yet to praise and enjoy this autonomy is a sign of a therapeutic relationship.

ANGER WITH PATIENTS

Probably the most important lesson we ever learned about being a psychiatric nurse is that we are human beings and have feelings, too. That means we should expect to feel angry at times because we will be dealing with some very difficult situations.

Our experience with psychiatric nurses is that they often feel that they should not get angry with their patients because they are sick and cannot effectively manage their emotions . . . and anyone knows that the nurse can always keep her feelings under control! Nevertheless, nurses do get angry, and the anger is manifested in many ways. The subtle signs most frequently observed are being late for meetings with the patient, making them wait for medications, delaying answering their call light, forgetting to give the doctor their message, refusing to care for the patient, goals and expectations set too high for the patient to meet, and short visits or dozing off during the session. These expressions of anger represent a sign that nurses seem to have some difficulty accepting that anger and directing it in a more straightforward manner.

Since we know that situations will always exist in which nurses feel angry with patients, it is essential to teach them to handle their anger in a more constructive manner.

There are many reasons why nurses get angry with patients. In our experience they have fallen into the following areas:

1. *The patient is not controlling his symptoms.*

It is easy to understand why a nurse might feel annoyed at listening to a patient ruminate about his back pain day after day. However, the patient came for help with the symptom. Often, limiting the time he is allowed to discuss pain and then redirecting the conversation to other issues will help this. Along with that, the nurse needs to be tactfully direct to let the patient know she is frustrated by the fact that the only thing she knows about him is his pain. This allows the nurse to handle her frustration in a direct way, as well as teaching the patient about the impact of his behavior on their relationship. It demonstrates the nurse's interest to get to know the patient better.

2. *The patient is not willing to explore at the depth of introspection the nurse expects.*

This type of problem generally means the nurse's expectations have been set too high for the patient. She will no doubt need to reassess his condition and determine whether she set goals too high or whether the patient is not motivated to work at this time. Patients' resistance may be pain avoidance or a sign that adequate trust has not been established to allow sharing at a deeper level.

3. *The patient is too dependent or independent.*

This problem was previously addressed. I include it in the list because it surfaces as a common area in which nurses get covertly angry with patients.

4. *The patient makes the nurse feel helpless.*

A nurse feels useful and important when she can provide some source of comfort, ease pain or teach a new skill. Although the nurse may work very hard to explore conflicts, offer support and provide feedback, the patient may repeatedly say that nothing is helping. This type of patient often has a lifelong pattern of rejecting help to fulfill his own fears that no one truly understands him or can help him.

Nurses give many reasons for feeling angry with patients. This is best handled by the nurse acknowledging the anger to herself and a peer or supervisor. The nurse's peers may be the ones to alert the nurse to the subtle signs they may be observing. A discussion to understand the anger can be very beneficial. In the case of unreasonable and difficult patients it is wise to build in acceptance of a support group or care conferences in which a nurse can feel free to vent and receive support. Another consideration is to rotate the assignment of the patient to 2 or 3 nurses, rather than just one. This can decrease the intensity and help to make the care of that patient more tolerable. A third option is to plan interventions to direct reasonable expression of anger to the patient if it serves an objective to help him in his struggle to understand difficulties in his interpersonal relationships. This should never be used solely for the nurse to relieve her own anger. The nurse should have a clearly defined objective for directing her anger and enough understanding and control of her own emotional reaction to avoid an explosive outburst.

ACCEPTANCE OF LIMITED GOALS

In our setting, we have experienced problems with setting our expectations too high, at times. It is easy to forget that a short-term treatment center does not allow pursuit of all needs identified and assessed by the initial history. Occasionally, it is helpful to remember that we do not provide cures. By providing limits for goals that may be achieved in three to four weeks we can avoid feeling overwhelmed by many goals and frustrated by setting ourselves up to accomplish too much with the individual.

We have found that nurses generally blamed themselves and felt disappointed for not reaching all goals and expectations set. We must realistically address other factors, however. The patient may not be motivated to change. For whatever reason, one needs to look at possible secondary gains involved which make behavioral changes less attractive for the patient. If a patient is not uncomfortable enough with the symptoms to work with the milieu for changes, nursing needs to be ready to accept that without personalizing it as failure.

As previously mentioned, if all nursing approaches are meeting with resistance, that is a good cue to reassess and lower expectations so that the patient can achieve success from the approaches for treatment. This has frequently occurred with very regressed patients who could not utilize the milieu in its entirety, but after lowering our expectations, to perhaps just participating in activity therapy and sitting in the group lounges the patient achieved satisfaction and improved self-worth from limited goals.

Finally, the nurse can avoid some problems by listening carefully to what the patient presents as his problem and what he hopes to accomplish through hospitalization. Each patient brings a different perception of what his health and "feeling normal" means. Family members can offer invaluable information to help clarify what is normal for the identified patient. if we plan our approaches and goals around what the patient presents as a problem the success of the nursing interventions will be greater.

In summary, we have reviewed one way of structuring programs and activities to provide a successful therapeutic milieu. The nursing role provides many opportunities for creativity and an exciting practice for the nurse who is mature and responsive to individuals suffering from emotional pain. In planning a program to utilize milieu therapy it should meet the needs of the patient population utilizing your hospital. For us, this means that the environment should be flexible enough to accommodate a wide range of patients with varying capabilities. The nursing staff should be aware that each group of patients is different and those differences offer new and exciting challenges.

The problems encountered in milieu therapy are diminished by teaching staff to be honest and direct in expressing their feelings and concerns about their patient-nurse relationships. The staff should be taught to rely on one another for support and direction in planning meaningful interventions and maintaining therapeutic relationships.

The success of milieu therapy can be largely determined by the competent and well prepared nursing staff supporting it.

REFERENCES

1. Kraft, A.M.: The Therapeutic Community: In Arieti, S. (ed.) *American Handbook of Psychiatry* (Vol. 3), New York: Basic Books, Inc., 542-551, 1966.

2. Yalom, I.D.: *The Theory and Practice of Group Psychotherapy,* Second Edition. New York: Basic Books, Inc., p. 25, 1975.

3. Lewis, R., Wolberg, L.: *Short Term Psychotherapy,* New York: Grune and Stratton, 1965.

4. Holfing, C.K., Leininger, M.M., Bregg, E.: *Basic Psychiatric Concepts in Nursing,* Second Edition. Philadelphia: Lippincott, p. 87, 1967.

29 The Role of the Nurse on a Consultation-Liaison Team*

Sondra K. Stickney and Richard C.W. Hall

Abstract: The authors report on the role and functions of a nurse-consultant on an expanding psychiatric consultation–liaison service. One hundred consecutive requests for intervention by a nurse were compared with 100 consecutive requests for psychiatric intervention. Psychiatrists saw 3½ times as many patients on critical care units as did the nurse-consultant. Patient withdrawal and depression were the prime reasons stated for requesting consultation with the nurse, but 24% of the cases seen by the nurse focused on issues of death and dying or on the need for staff or family support, areas in which formal psychiatric intervention was not routinely requested.

While psychiatric consultation–liaison services date back to the early 1930's, when they were instituted in five university hospitals with the aid of funds from the Rockefeller Foundation (1), it is less than 20 years since references to the psychiatric nurse-consultant began to appear in the literature (2). Therefore, it is not surprising that "growing pains" and role conflicts still abound for the nurse involved in consultation–liaison programs.

The role of the nurse-consultant evolved in response to requests from nursing staff members for assistance in defining and planning care for "difficult" patients (3). Previously, psychiatric consultation had been confined to the evaluation of psychotic behavior.

Even though the health care system has attempted to de-emphasize the "sick role," in actual practice patients are often expected to be dependent, allowing the hospital to assume responsibility for them. In view of these divergent expectations, it is not surprising that the behavior of patients has caused management problems. The resulting requests for consultation often have

*Reprinted with permission from *Psychosomatics, 22:*224-235, 1981.

reflected complex issues involving not only the patient but also his family, his physicians, nurses, other caretakers, and the hospital system (4). Such staff and system concerns highlight the need for the consultation team and the liaison nurse to function in concert, rather than working separately or competitively.

The ideas presented here are based on a two-year cooperative effort between the psychiatric consultation–liaison service of a university medical school department of psychiatry and the consultation–liaison nurse in the department of nursing at the university's teaching facility, Hermann Hospital. The psychiatric consultation department expanded from one part-time physician to a team of three full-time physicians, a resident, and a full-time research specialist at the same time that the hospital instituted the position of nurse-consultant. Therefore, the development of a comprehensive consultation service was the mutual goal of all concerned. All members of this team had worked together previously, and their relationships were trusting and friendly.

DEVELOPING THE NURSE'S ROLE

In the past, nurse-consultants have, in general, functioned in one of four basic ways: 1) as a part-time consultant with full-time responsibility on a psychiatric unit and availability for other hospital services if necessary (4); 2) as a member of a specialty team geared to manage patients with specific problems, such as rape or hemophilia; 3) as a full-time member of an interdisciplinary consultation–liaison team representing a department of psychiatry or an outside agency; or 4) as an independent hospital practitioner supervised and backed up by psychiatrists and peers as needed (5).

In developing the role of the liaison nurse for our purposes, we combined the best elements from each of these modes of practice. Although the nurse-consultant reported to the director of psychiatric nursing, her job description provided both autonomy and flexibility. She served as consultant to the various psychiatric units and to any other unit in the hospital when necessary. Also, she attended weekly head-nurse meetings in psychiatry to keep abreast of departmental policy changes and to serve as a resource for procedural issues. The nurse-consultant's relationship to the psychiatric liaison team was flexible and based on mutual need. She attended administrative meetings regarding the functioning and development of the service. Team members were available to supervise or help her.

Because the nurse-consultant had worked with several members of the consultation team in the past, good working relationships had been developed prior to the institution of her new role. These relationships were considered of paramount importance in the development of a comprehensive consultation–liaison service.

Each day, the liaison nurse attended the consultation-team rounds, at which time patients in common, as well as those treated separately, were discussed. Over time, this give-and-take of information was found invaluable in providing a comprehensive approach to patient care. When the psychiatrist felt specific staff intervention was needed or staff-patient relationship problems existed, the liaison nurse was able to use this information as a basis for assisting the nursing staff with the planning and implementation of appropriate care. Conversely, the nurse was often able to provide the consultation team with information regarding their patients that was lacking in the formal consultation request. In addition, she frequently generated her own requests for psychiatric consultation.

The nurse's presence at rounds was considered educationally beneficial for medical students rotating on the serivce. As has been previously noted (6, 7), such involvement assists students in gaining an understanding of ward management problems from the nurse's point of view and helps them to appreciate the staff's expectations of the nurse. They learn to view the nurse as a worthy collaborator rather than as a separate or competitive entity.

TEAM EFFECTIVENESS

The overall success of a psychiatric liaison team relies heavily on two factors — its availability and visibility. The nurse's association with our consultation team enhanced both of these. By virtue of her hospital employment, she had accessibility to members of the nursing staff not routinely available to other members of the consultation–liaison team. In this way, she was able to expand the referral base for the psychiatric service to include all members of the nursing staff. Also, her daily ward rounds and high visibility on the various hospital units contributed not only to an increased number of referrals, but also to an increased number of requests by the staff for information on liaison services. The ability of the liaison nurse to provide direct liaison service often saved the consulting physician time and allowed him to see newly referred patients. The institution of "Kardex rounds" (i.e., a review of the nursing care plans developed for each individual patient) on various units helped to uncover problems and promote early intervention by the consultation-liaison team.

Intervention by the nurse-consultant was requested almost exclusively by staff nurses and focused predominantly on managing psychological problems (such as withdrawal, manipulation, aggression, hostility), the need for family support, and issues surrounding death and dying. In some cases, the nurse-consultant was asked to ascertain the extent of the problem and to suggest appropriate nursing care. If her evaluation revealed a need for further psychiatric intervention, the nursing staff would ask the attending physician to request formal psychiatric consultation. When the needs of a patient were unclear or the patient refused psychiatric consultation, the director of the liaison team was available to the nurse-consultant for guidance as to how she should intervene.

STUDY OF REFERRALS

In an effort to differentiate the types of problems resulting in requests for intervention by the nurse rather than by the psychiatrist, 100 consecutive referrals for nursing consultation were compared with 100 consecutive referrals to the consultation-liaison team over a 16-month period. One difference became apparent immediately, and that was who was seen. While the physician saw every patient referred, the nurse saw only 58% of patients referred and/or their families. This finding stems from several factors, the prime one being the nurse-consultant's responsibilities as an educator as well as a caretaker. As a result, she delegated the task or intervention to the nursing staff in some cases. In other cases, her intervention was provided as support to staff members experiencing frustration or loss or as mediation when they were in conflict regarding a patient's care.

Tables 1, 2 and 3 compare psychiatric and nursing consultations according to the hospital area in which the request originated, the reason for the consultation requests, and medical problems. Several findings shown by these tables warrant comment, even though they are abased on a relatively small sample.

TABLE 1
CONSULTATION REQUESTS BY HOSPITAL AREA

	Nursing Consultations (N = 100)		*Psychiatric Consultations (N = 100)*
	With Staff Nurses Only	*With Staff & Patient*	*Total Requests*
General medical/surgical units	25	42	39
Critical care units	1	6	22
Specialty units			
Oncology	3	14	5
Orthopedics	7	8	4
Burns	1	13	8
Neurology	3	10	8
Nephrology	–	–	6
Postpartum	1	1	3
Alcoholism	1	1	–
Outpatient clinics	–	5	5
	42	100	100

TABLE 2
STATED REASON FOR CONSULTATION REQUESTS

	Nursing Consultations (N = 100)		*Psychiatric Consultations (N = 100)*
	With Staff Nurses Only	*With Staff & Patient*	*Total Requests*
Withdrawal, depression	8	22	17
Confusion	2	4	17
Agitation	–	–	6
Anxiety	–	4	13
Hallucinations	1	1	9
Aggression, hostility	4	7	1
Manipulative behavior	12	15	6
Regression	1	3	5
Demanding behavior	5	6	5
Death and dying concerns	4	17	–
Family/staff support	3	7	–
Suicidal assessment	1	1	12
Evaluation	–	11	1
Other	1	2	8
	42	100	100

TABLE 3
CONSULTATIONS CATEGORIZED BY BODY SYSTEM AFFECTED OR CONDITION

	Nursing Consultations (N = 100)		*Psychiatric Consultations (N = 100)*
	With Staff Nurses Only	*With Staff & Patient*	*Total Requests*
Gastrointestinal	12	24	17
Neurologic	5	15	17
Musculoskeletal	9	11	13
Renal	2	3	7
Cardiovascular	2	3	7
Endocrine	1	1	5
Respiratory	2	3	9
Reproductive	4	5	2
Dermatologic (including burns)	2	15	11
Cancer (multiple metastases)	3	20	5
Overdose	–	–	7
	42	100	100

Members of the consultation-liaison service saw almost 3½ times as many patients in critical care units as did the nurse-consultant. This finding was explained in two ways 1) the patients in these areas suffered predominantly from organic brain syndromes and required evaluation for the need for psychotropic medication, and 2) the nurse-consultant regularly conducted support groups for staff members in some of the critical care areas and was, therefore, viewed as a resource for staff, rather than for their patients.

While withdrawal and depression were the prime reasons given for requesting nursing consultations, 24% of the cases referred for such consultation involved concerns about death and dying or the need for staff or family support. This finding alone points out an area of patients' needs for which formal psychiatric intervention is not routinely requested, as does the fact that the nurse was sought for consultation for cancer patients four times as often as was the psychiatrist. Manipulative behavior, predominantly a ward-management issue, was another reason for consultation with the nurse, which was requested 2½ times more often than was psychiatric consultation for this problem.

The nurse-consultant, by virtue of her nonthreatening title and role, was in a unique position to pave the way for both staff and patient acceptance of psychiatric consultation. Also, the nurse's affiliation with the nursing staff and her close alignment with the liaison team allowed her to cross staff and disciplinary boundaries. This ability facilitated a coordinated approach to patient care that had not previously been in operation. The following case study exemplifies this unified approach.

CASE REPORT

A 24-year-old man was hospitalized after being struck by an automobile while he was bicycling. He was transferred to the orthopedic service following a six-day stay in the intensive care unit. Both tibiae were fractured, and a spinal-cord injury resulted in paraplegia. Ten days after his admission to the orthopedic service, the nursing staff contacted the nurse-consultant because of the patient's alternating withdrawn and abusive behavior.

His initial contact with the nursing staff revealed two major problems: 1) Many of his nurses, close to his age, felt it was "unfair" that he had lost the use of his legs. Therefore, feeling that in some ways his behavior was justified, they did not confront him about it. 2) The staff was angry with the patient's mother, who was present 24 hours a day and would not allow her son to do even the simplest tasks for himself. She refused to accept the extent of his injuries and directed her anger toward the staff, accusing them of being cold and uncaring.

Following discussions with the unit's head nurse, the patient's primary nurse, and his mother, the psychiatric nurse-consultant scheduled a conference to discuss his care with the nursing staff and the social worker assigned to the unit. The staff members ventilated their frustration and then considered a unified plan of care. They decided that the social worker would provide support for the mother and schedule appointments with her during the patient's lunch period. This would encourage him to assume some responsibility for his own care, since he would have to feed himself. It was also decided to ask the attending physician to request a psychiatric consultation to assess the patient's depression and to comment on the possible need for medication and psychotherapy. A follow-up conference was scheduled to take place the following week.

The second conference was attended by the patient's primary physician, his occupational therapist, and a member of the consultation-liaison team, in addition to the nursing staff and social worker. Since the previous conference, the patient's sleep pattern had improved with doxepin hydrochloride and, when his mother was not present, he was more cooperative and willing to initiate some self-care. The major staff complaint was now the omnipresence of his mother. He was moved to a semi-private room, which would limit the times his mother could visit. At the family's request, the nurse-consultant arranged a meeting with the psychiatrist. The nursing staff was then able to develop a nursing-care plan giving the patient more control and more active involvement in his own care.

During the course of his hospitalization, his case was discussed during liaison rounds, when the nurse-consultant reported on the patient's progress from the nursing staff's point of view. She met frequently with the primary nurse, providing support and making management suggestions. The psychiatric nurse-consultant coordinated the social worker's interactions with the patient's mother with those of the nursing staff, and she met with the patient's girlfriend, who was in the position of competing with the patient's mother for his attention. Throughout the patient's hospitalization, the nurse-consultant remained the pivot for the give-and-take of information regarding his care. This coordinated approach had not been previously available.

CONCLUSION

Over time the role of the liaison nurse has evolved in response to increased hospital awareness of the emotional impact of illness not only on the patient, but also on his family and caretakers (8). In an effort to meet these needs at Hermann Hospital, the nurse-consultant instituted staff support groups in several critical care units. A family group was established on the oncology unit, and plans are in process for establishing a similar group for the families of patients with neurologic disorders.

Because of the nurse's assessment skills, the liaison team was better equipped for preventive intervention; and patients at high risk, such as those receiving long-term intravenous hyperalimentation therapy, were more likely to be thoroughly evaluated.

Based on our experience, we feel the nurse-consultant can be a useful and valued member of the consultation liaison team. Her attachment to the nursing service of the hospital can give her the support of and access to the nursing staff not available to other members of the team. Her familiarity with hospital policies and procedures facilitates all aspects of the consultation process. In our experience, the visibility and availability of the nurse-consultant greatly increased the referral base for the team as a whole.

Finally, and perhaps most important, we feel that the collaborative program we developed was a success because good working relationships had been established between various members of the team prior to the expansion of the service. Therefore, all participants were comfortable with the interdisciplinary approach to care and were not driven by interests in power or control toward mutually exclusive goals.

REFERENCES

1. Nelson, J., Schilke, D.: The evolution of psychiatric liaison. *Perspect Psychiatr Care, 14:*61-65, 1976.

2. Johnson, B.S.: Psychiatric nurse consultant in a general hospital. *Nursing Outlook, 11:*728-729, 1963.

3. Jackson, H.A.: The psychiatric nurse as a mental health consultant in a general hospital. *Nurs Clin North Am, 4:*527-540, 1969.

4. Garant, C.A.: The psychiatric liaison nurse — An interpretation of the role. *Supervisor Nurs, 8:*75-78, 1977.

5. Goldstein, S.: The psychiatric clinical specialist in the general hospital. *J Nurs Admin, 9:*34-37, 1979.

6. Wise, T.M.: Utilization of a nurse consultant in teaching liaison psychiatry. *J Med Educ, 49:*1067-1068, 1974.

7. Barton, D., Kelso, M.: The nurse as a psychiatric consultation team member. *Psychiatr Med, 2:*108-115, 1971.

8. Bilodeau, C.B., O'Connor, S.O.: Role of nurse clinicians in liaison psychiatry in Hacket T.P., Cassem, N.H. (eds.): *Handbook of General Hospital Psychiatry.* St. Louis, C.V. Mosby, 508-523, 1978.

30 Community Mental Health Nursing

Judy Kycek-Nishimura

INTRODUCTION

After one has spent six years as a psychiatric nurse on a psychiatric unit in a private general hospital, it is assumed that much knowledge about mental health has already been acquired and assimilated. Nevertheless, the transition from hospital based nursing to my practice at a community mental health center led to an awareness of many differences and pinpointed a great many variations in nursing roles and practice. The purpose of this chapter is to look at the community mental health nurse and his or her relationship with the community as a whole.

When one starts to work in a community mental health setting, one immediately becomes involved with numerous other professions. Such centers cannot function without a multidisciplinary team. The nurse finds that these other co-workers and their sense of cohesiveness are the keys to the quality of care provided to the patient. As one looks at this team and the specific nursing role, he or she can gain a broader perspective of the patient, his problems and how they are handled.

In this chapter, I shall address some of the positive and negative aspects of a career in community mental health nursing, some of the qualifications for this type of work and an attempt at a broad overview of the field.

COMMUNITY MENTAL HEALTH NURSING

Although it seems topical to interchange the terms "community mental health" and "psychiatric," there are major differences and in this chapter the title "community mental health nurse" will be used to stress the fact that these differences exist and to stress the community oriented aspects of this type of nursing practice.

The setting of a psychiatric hospital provides the security and comfort needed by a great many patients. The psychiatric nurse in such a hospital setting has the advantage of the safety and protection which are needed to provide adequate care to the patient. When in this type of system, the nurse can feel free to use a variety of psychiatric approaches, collaborate with the physician regarding medication and other therapeutic approaches and allow the patient to feel as ill as he needs. It gives the psychiatric nurse a chance to assess the patient's interpersonal relationships because he is on a unit with peers. Therapy is ongoing and intense in that it begins in the morning and continues through the evening. If there are problems and the patient becomes actively suicidal, for example, there are other workers as well as the medical facilities to handle such an emergency. The patient may become quite dependent in such a situation and let himself regress for some time. While such a setting can be highly therapeutic to patients, it cannot be used in a community center because of the lack of structure and ambulatory nature of the practice. Thus, the community mental health nurse must change his entire approach to the patient.

There are evident similarities between a community mental health nurse and a public health nurse. Frequently, both public health nurses and community mental health nurses are involved with emotional problems and mental illnesses that occur in the community. The interaction between community mental health nurses and public health nurses remains to be studied, and liaison between these two professions will probably be an area of active interest in the future.

Nursing is becoming holistic in that it looks at the individual as a whole and is not compartmentalized. Rather than defining an individual as having schizophrenia, for example, one looks at that person from a social, psychological and physical standpoint. If that schizophrenic patient is withdrawing into his home and not eating or sleeping, there is physical danger also. Thus, while one can specialize in mental health nursing, it is always necessary to be cognizant of physical and social factors impinging on each patient. Community mental health nurses who divorce themselves from social and physical factors may well cheat themselves and their patients of quality care.

The community mental health movement has been called the third mental health revolution. It initially represented discontent with antiquated ideas of separating chronically mentally ill patients from the community. Such old ideas are rapidly fading and the community now has a new frame of reference which includes such modalities as crisis intervention, walk-in treatment and a multitude of outreach programs (1). With the advent of many new programs came the necessity of a community mental health nurse.

THE NURSE'S UTILITY IN THE COMMUNITY MENTAL HEALTH SETTING

Community mental health nurses have been found to be positive additions to community mental health facilities. While many of the other professionals employed in a community mental health center have highly specialized training, the nurse often has the advantage of a highly eclectic education (2). This education is quite specialized in some areas and yet rather general. Such a nurse has been exposed to psychiatric knowledge but also has received a considerable contribution to her education from medical, scientific, social and spiritual disciplines. The nurse may frequently need consultative assistance from other members of the team, but he has received a solid foundation to get a general impression of the patient. The medical or technical segments of the nurse's knowledge can be utilized in administration of drugs, evaluation of pharmacologic side-effects and assessment of physical illness. The nurse's social training can help to elucidate the patient's financial problems, relationships and support systems.

Nurses, too, are frequently more able than some other members of the team to deal with individuals on a realistic and practical level. Rather than deal with profound insights or in-depth tasks, the nurse is able to look at some practical ways of changing situations. When there is discomfort and pain, there should be an attempt to decrease these affects and to promote comfort and happiness. Certainly, there is a major place for profound insights and in-depth tasks in treatment of many patients, but the nurse should not be defensive about his attempt to promote comfort and happiness being referred to as a "bandaid effect" as it often is. This approach can be immediate and pain reducing.

The nurse through past training in hospital settings is often more willing than other professionals to work with less tangible results. He has on many occasions seen people get well who might have died. He knows that it is frequently impossible to determine what medication, what medical know-how, what other interventions may have been the key to improvement: the nurse has seen patients get well. The nurse continues to have hope without needing the constant reinforcement of relentlessly positive results. Therefore, the nurse can symbolize stability in a community mental health setting and also show a high frustration tolerance and an extremely pragmatic approach. The hospital experience also brings the nurse an ability to work with a variety of professions, and this ability is educational and rewarding. The "medical model," "case oriented" training and experience in management of other professionals are also a part of the nurse's background.

Schools of nursing now have a public health nurse training program which can be very helpful also to the community mental health nurse. This background can lead to some degree of comfort in public health knowledge and is extremely valuable when community consultations are required of the community mental health nurse.

Perhaps the most positive aspect of the nurse's role in a community mental health center is that he or she can provide "educated caring" (3). From the nurse's training and experiential background, he can provide care which is of such a quality that it can encourage new behaviors and controls in the patient. Caring can be a primary curative factor. If one has the ability to show this caring it is extremely therapeutic.

CHANGING ROLES OF THE PSYCHIATRIC NURSE

Community mental health nursing is a relatively new profession. Psychiatric nursing has roots in the 19th century. There have been many changes in psychiatric nursing during the past decade. Traditionally, the role of the psychiatric nurse was that of a very secondary supportive provider of care (4). Frequently, such a nurse was found in a state hospital or, more recently, in inpatient psychiatric systems. In many community mental health programs, however, the psychiatric nurse has been required to assume many of the functions of a primary provider. The tasks and functions of the psychiatric nurse in a mental health center are often indistinguishable from those performed by other workers there. This role variety is quite outstanding in the case of a psychiatric nurse.

The high degree of independence and role diffusion can make it difficult to specify the activities such a nurse will be involved in. Each mental health center may have different goals and objectives for the mental health nurse according to the needs of the community. The nurse, too, has an individual conceptual framework which may indicate the role she will be fulfilling.

THE ROLE OF COMMUNITY MENTAL HEALTH

A frequent and difficult problem is the determination of whether the community or the hospital is the more appropriate place for the treatment of the patient. Many patients with chronic mental illness and frequent hospitalizations are able to adapt well in the hospital environment with some resolution of the symptoms of the illness. Making the transition to the community leaves the patient faced with important decisions and many stresses and it is frequently the role of the community mental health center to help that patient adapt or arrange for rehospitalization.

Although the majority of situations faced by patients can be handled at the outpatient level, the following problems require rapid assessment and hospitalization:

1. Serious suicidal or homicidal tendencies. The community mental health worker frequently needs to rely on his "Gestalt" reaction and to the subjective and objective data received from the patient. A suicidal plan, apparent inability to control behavior, and the explicit and implicit request for a certain amount of structure and restraint are all clues to serious suicidal potential.

2. Active psychosis with paranoid and/or persecutory delusions. If the patient is hallucinating it is helpful to get an idea of the content of the hallucinations. It is helpful to see how the patient is handling himself when divorced from reality and important to keep the patient and the nurse safe and protected.

3. Extreme forms of psychophysiologic, psychosomatic and neurotic illnesses. Hospitalization may quickly need to be the plan of action when physical illness which may be stress induced accompanies the emotional problems. Some psychosomatic illnesses such as anorexia nervosa are potentially life threatening and in this situation hospitalization will frequently be required. Serious obsessive compulsive illness with ritualistic behavior is extremely difficult to treat in a community setting as are extreme forms of phobic anxiety syndromes and agoraphobia.

4. Family crisis: The hospital may serve as a temporary shelter for a family member who may be physically or sexually abused or extremely anxious in relation to some family difficulty.

Hospitalization may be an excellent intervention in the psychiatric illnesses of many people. The community mental health nurse needs to evaluate and assess whether his or her patients will need this type of care. One of the goals with many patients, however, is that they might be kept out of this setting and encouraged to be functioning at a relatively more independent level in the community. The nurse, therefore, provides a great deal of supportive encouragement to such patients. The nurse needs to structure settings to prevent patients from becoming increasingly fragile or disjointed and the realization that after the session the patient will again be out in the community. The nurse has no control over what happens outside the office when the patient is gone. To give such a patient as much support as possible, the community mental health nurse becomes a contact person with many other community resources. He or she consults these agencies and refers the patient to them. Such referrals are not an effort to rid oneself of the patient but rather to get the patient involved in more than one support system. It is important to realize that many chronically mentally ill patients who come to community mental health centers have no other support systems in their lives: the community organizations and agencies become their sole source of support. The community mental health nurse then may have a very important supportive role in caring for the patient but it is clear that that responsibility is two-fold. It involves not only the strong supportive measure but also the development of a program which can address and hopefully satisfy the needs of the patient.

SPECIFIC ROLES OF THE COMMUNITY MENTAL HEALTH NURSE

Specific roles for the nurse vary from community mental health center to community mental health center. At one such center the nurse is involved in the following:

1. **Assessment.** It is important for the nurse to assess the pathology, intervene in crisis and arrange hospitalization. Many hospitals request that patients be seen at a mental health center prior to hospitalization. Part of the role of such assessment can be to reduce some of the patient's anxiety through the knowledge

that an assessment is being done and an intervention will be arranged.

2. **Therapy.** The nurse frequently assumes the role of therapist. In addition to assessment, the role of therapist takes priority at this mental health center. Therapy might be individual, group, marital or family. Fragile patients as mentioned above need supportive therapy. Patients who can benefit from more firm constructive feedback are often candidates for insight oriented psychotherapy.

Supportive therapy may take the shape of encouraging a highly inconsistent and unreliable patient to appear at the sessions on a weekly basis. Specific goals in a situation like this may not be accomplished but the patient is showing some capacity to respond to firmness, structure and continuity.

Some helpful forms of therapy can occur in specialized groups. For example, at this center, a women's support group has been extremely helpful. In this group, 6 to 7 women meet on a weekly basis to discuss problems and learn more about interpersonal relationships through their interactions in the group. The community mental health nurse and the cotherapist, a psychologist, facilitate the women's dealing with these troubling issues more directly.

3. **Community Education.** Educational programs in the community provide many opportunities for prevention of serious psychosocial problems. Opportunities for community education include giving workshops and lectures at schools, churches, community organizations such as Senior Citizen's and Red Cross. The media can also be an effective method of communication. For example, a 20 minute talk show on the radio can provide important information on emotional problems of everyday life. This service has been particularly appreciated by many elderly people.

4. **Consultation.** As mentioned, it is not uncommon to have patients who need involvement with more than one human service agency. The goal of such agencies is to work as a team to meet the needs of the patient. The community mental health nurse may develop a course of action in which each agency has individual goals. Without continuity each agency might go in opposite directions leaving patients confused and poorly served. Facility with the resources and personnel of other agencies can also be extremely helpful in arranging rapid hospitalization and other emergency interventions.

5. **General Medical Nursing.** Perhaps surprisingly, the nurse's basic knowledge of medical nursing proves useful in the context of a community mental health center. Many patients who come to such centers have not been seen for physical examinations for many years and the nurse can frequently recognize the need for medical evaluation and intervention. One cannot begin to look at emotional aspects of illness until physical factors have also been addressed.

From his or her training, the nurse is able to gather medical data such as skin color, weight, nail bed color, respirations, etc. The nurse can get a thorough drug history. Proper referral to a medical center for suspected medical illness can prevent weeks of improper diagnosis and treatment.

6. **Pharmaceutical Knowledge.** Frequently, the nurse will handle questions and calls regarding medications. He or she should be knowledgeable about psychotropic drugs, their dosage, administration and side-effects. Consultation with a psychiatrist regarding drugs is a frequent responsibility. Dispensing medications per physicians' orders is also a part of one's medical training which is important in the community mental health setting. One becomes adept at giving injectable Prolixin to many long-term schizophrenic patients.

7. **Resource.** Information providing referral and awareness of available resources is a major function of the community mental health nurse. Again, one agency may not be sufficient to handle all the needs a given patient presents. The mental health nurse is, therefore, responsible to help the individual find appropriate facilities. He or she needs to be well informed of what the community has to offer. It is essential for the nurse to constantly revise files and resource manuals to have current information. It is not uncommon for a nurse at such a center to get calls asking for information such as whether the community has a cancer support group or whether there is a workshop on stress being held in the city. While one cannot be aware of all such activities, knowledge of as many of them as possible is very helpful.

8. **Program Planning.** Whether or not the community mental health nurse has a particular interest in administrative planning, some time will almost certainly be devoted to plans and policies of the center. The nurse must constantly be aware of his or her role on the multidisciplinary team and its constant state of flux with revision of old programs, and expansion in new directions.

Peer review committees, personnel committees and community board meetings are all important administrative duties with which the nurse may well be involved. The community mental health nurse is also involved in a great deal of role transfer. There is a frequent shift from one clearly defined role to another without changing disciplinary identification. While stressful, the need for this flexibility and the ability to shift roles seems a unique aspect of this type of work.

MULTIDISCIPLINARY TEAM

The team approach to patients can be a great asset when working at a mental health center. One gets a variety of ideas from many disciplines regarding approaches to specific patients and problems.

The old adage that two heads are better than one is not always true, but it frequently has some validity, particularly when dealing with difficult and time consuming problems. There is a great variability among the people staffing a mental health center. Personnel usually include psychiatrists, psychologists, social workers, child and family therapists, chemical dependency counselors, and other mental health nurses.

Much contact is made with the psychiatrist, for this professional assumes primary responsibility for the patient. Consultation with the psychiatrist may involve treatment plans, referral possibilities, and medication programs.

The psychologist may take the role of the co-therapist in groups that will be responsible for testing and may be an active member of the team offering many skills and techniques to the treatment setting.

Social workers are extremely helpful in assessing social situations and planning social intervention. They frequently function as group co-therapists.

Frequently, in a family therapy situation, a nurse and a family therapist will co-facilitate. Each professional again brings inherent skills and individual knowledge.

The chemical dependency counselor and the nurse see patients and their families together. The counselor is frequently able to assess the nature of the chemical dependency problem more accurately while the nurse is more able to intervene helpfully in the family situation.

It is sometimes a relief to know that there is a chance to get immediate consultation with colleagues from different disciplines. Immediate or crisis problems are frequent in the setting of the community mental health center and need rapid assessment and sound judgment. A good treatment team is invaluable in providing these necessities.

THE PATIENT

The care of the patient is the reason for being of a mental health center. Attention is focused on him, his family and the immediate social sphere. Too often, however, professionals have focused on the identified patient alone without any consideration of his environment. Since the review of the nation's mental health needs undertaken by the Joint Commission on Mental Illness and Health in the 1950's, many changes have occurred with development of new programs to assure quality patient care.

Often times, the mental health center is able to serve rural populations because of accessible satellite clinics in small towns. It is easier for rural patients to get to a nearby facility than one in a distant city. It is also easier for many rural people to receive psychiatric treatment in a setting which is familiar and comfortable. To many people, psychiatry is still somehow taboo and connotes either a severe mental illness or weakness. Frequently, in a satellite mental health clinic, therapists are housed in a church, physician's office, or social service building. These locations are far less threatening than a large mental health center or psychiatric hospital and hopefully they decrease the stigma which is attached to seeking psychaitric help.

Community mental health centers tend to get more low income, young and chronically ill people than private centers.

Many people without insurance who cannot pay large fees, are able to attend a mental health center where they are billed on a sliding fee scale taking into account their gross income, the number of people in their family, their insurance coverage, Social Security benefits, Medicare or Medicaid, whether the individuals are in school and their general ability to pay. The majority of patients are able to meet the standards of payment.

Payment is difficult for young families in particularly. The adjustable fee scale almost seems to be a necessity. There is the added convenience of outpatient treatment for young family members. They are normally quite involved with work, families and their home life and they prefer treatment which will not disrupt these other goals and demands. Of course, the severity of the problem has to be the final decision maker and not the flexibility of the program.

The chronically mentally ill patient often sees the community mental health center as a focal point in his life's journey. There are several reasons for this. First, it is common procedure for mental health centers to work closely with state hospitals. Referrals and authorized patient information usually flow freely within the two systems. Once the patient is able to function outside the hospital, the state hospital will send recommendations about care and medication. The mental health center follows this plan, making any necessary adjustments. Secondly, the mental health center is familiar ground since usually the chronically mentally ill patient has been referred there previously. The patient has certain ties with this system and sees old friends. Thirdly, the patient is aware that the mental health center will work closely with other agencies such as social services, public health nursing, sheltered workshops, vocational rehabilitation and halfway houses to provide continuity in care and effective management. There is thus a sense of security. Finally, the mental health center is affordable for such patients.

One should not be misled, however, by the stereotype of patients at mental health centers being chronically ill or very impoverished. The average caseload includes many middle class people with adequate salaries and stable jobs who feel that their needs can best be met by a community facility. Each carries a different set of problems.

DISORDERS OF THE PATIENTS

There are many types of disorders seen in community mental health nursing.

Personality disorders are very common and perhaps most commonly seen are personality disorders in the passive dependent/passive aggressive category. Hysterical and sociopathic personality disorders are also seen commonly and borderline personality disorder is increasingly seen.

Affective disorders are also seen frequently. Major depressions are common. Situational depressions are also very frequent and well suited to treatment in the community mental health center.

Many of our long-term chronically ill patients are coping with schizophrenia in its chronic forms.

Anxiety disorders including phobic reactions and somatizing disorders are seen frequently at the community mental health center.

Adjustment disorders such as reactions to divorce, occupational changes and marital difficulties are problems seen in abundance.

Chemical and drug dependence are very common in this society, and it is sometimes difficult to assess them. The multidisciplinary team can be very helpful in assessing and treating this condition.

Child and adolescent issues are also addressed at most community mental health centers. Here, are seen school problems, child abuse, parenting difficulties and family discord. The nurse may be involved frequently as a co-therapist in such a case.

NURSE-PATIENT RELATIONSHIP

The nurse-patient relationship is a bond between two people, and both of them bring something to that relationship and acquire something from it. The patient brings problems and needs for caring; the nurse brings professional skills and the need for a measure of success and satisfaction in her role (6).

At times, the psychiatric nurse may question and doubt the above statement. He or she may feel empty and "always in doubt." To listen, assess, comment and question can be a very draining and demanding experience. People who are troubled and lonely have no reserve supply of love or attention and sometimes make a final and massive attempt to fill that need in the nurse's office. It can be overwhelming to deal with such a patient — imagine a very angry, extremely paranoid, yet very dependent person and the conflicting responses the mental health professional will have in attempting to deal with this person.

To meet that need, even temporarily, can be rewarding and satisfying. Using one's knowledge and experience to help the patient rebuild his life to a more functional level, has long range satisfaction for many professionals.

To work with any of these areas and see change and growth the psychiatric nurse can find it helpful to set the following criteria for treatment:

1. The patient wants to change. He is uncomfortable and in pain.
2. The patient is motivated to change.
3. The patient has some support systems.
4. The patient has some record of positive steps and relationships.
5. The patient has some life goals.

CASE STUDIES

Some idea of the scope of community mental health nursing is illustrated in the following case examples.

Case 1

Presenting data: Jane and Bill are a couple in their early 30's who came to the mental health center requesting help with their stormy relationship. Jane is divorced and has a daughter, Sherri, age 3. Bill, also divorced, has described himself as a loner. All three people live together in a small rented house outside the city. Bill stays at home with the little girl while Jane, a secretary, commutes to a nearby job. Jane and Bill began to live together three weeks after they met. Both expressed feelings of loneliness and the need for companionship. Initially the living arrangement seemed to meet everyone's needs. As the three became aware of each other's vulnerable points, however, turmoil grew. Violent arguments between the couple resulted in verbal and physical abuse of each other, and the daughter would become frightened, anxious and rejecting of Bill while clinging and dependent on Jane. In the months to come, Sherri would become irritable, sarcastic, and difficult to control. The family system was no longer functioning. Jane and Bill were asking for some type of intervention. Both were feeling as if they needed to make a decision to end the relationship or begin to work on mutual goals.

Treatment plan: The key issues needing immediate attention were:

1. The physical abuse occurring between Jane and Bill. There was the strong possibility that if the arguments continued someone would be in physical danger.

2. The emotional confusion in the family and the indirect messages perceived by Sherri.

Plan:

1. Encourage Jane to move out of the house with her daughter. She would be given the option to move temporarily to a local women's shelter.

2. Encourage Jane and Bill to continue counseling.

3. Have Sherri evaluated by the center's child psychiatrist to assess the emotional impact of the family situation on her.

4. Encourage Bill and Jane to become involved in their own individual hobbies and interests.

5. Encourage each to make a list of positive and negative aspects of the relationship.

Outcome: Jane and Bill came to four sessions at the mental health center. The primary goal was that of deciding regarding continuation of the relationship. After the first session, the assumption was that they enjoyed the companionship and feared losing the security which had developed. This did not outweigh the feelings of stress, anxiety, and fear. More open communication would be a key to improvement.

Sessions 2 and 3 continued to focus on communication of uncomfortable and unhappy feelings. The couple was optimistic about the progress they had made. They were no longer having boxing matches in the living room. Sherri still felt distant from Bill but there appeared to be a steady decline in her sarcasm and demanding behavior. Bill resumes thinking about marraige which had been put on hold by Jane several times. For the first time, Jane was admitting that marriage might be a good alternative.

A therapist can feel quite powerful and omniscient after several productive sessions, but a word of caution is in order. One should proceed slowly and carefully, for the bubble may soon burst. It was probable that this couple had taken an "excursion" into health. Such a defense would prevent change.

Prior to the fourth session, Jane called to say that she had had to contact the police because of a resumption of physical abuse in the home. She stated that she would come to the session alone, for she was separating from Bill.

Jane stated that the last abusive episode had closed to her mind any possibility of reconciliation. Bill was moving to a city several hundred miles away. Jane with Sherri would continue functioning as before. Support was offered to strengthen Jane's self-esteem and prevent further involvements such as this in the future. The case was then closed with no further contact.

Case 2

Presenting data: Tom is a 26-year-old unmarried man with a diagnosis of chronic paranoid schizophrenia. He has been hospitalized at several state hospitals, usually having at least one admission per year. On discharge from the hospital, he is referred to the mental health center for continued monitoring of his medication regime.

Tom's past treatments have included electroconvulsive therapy, chemotherapy, individual and group therapy and industrial-vocational therapy. While hospitalized, Tom habitually improves. He becomes active and involved with a job at the local sheltered workshop. The persecutory hallucinations and delusions diminish. He feels less depressed about his situation and becomes more accepting of his disability.

Usually, however, after about a month out of the hospital Tom's life again takes a drastic switch. He comes into the office hallucinating, suspicious and remarking on the loss of his most recent job. He has usually stopped taking his medication. His day is now spent in total withdrawal and isolation. He admits feeling confused and scattered yet sees no need for intervention because "things will only be the same." He is unable to see that his appearance voluntarily at the mental health center demonstrates some ambivalence about the need for intervention.

Treatment plan: How does one handle such a chronic problem? It is obvious that Tom is indirectly asking for some more permanent type of inpatient setting. His dependence is great and the reasons for it obvious. Thus far, the hospital setting has been the only hope for some improved level of functioning.

Immediate goals:

1. Encourage Tom to return to the hospital voluntarily. At this time he is potentially harmful to himself and others. Keep the intervention firm but nonthreatening. Let Tom know that commitment is one alternative that could be used.

2. Call the social services agency to send a case worker to accompany Tom into the hospital.

3. Call the hospital and the admitting psychiatrist and inform him of the situation and its urgency.

4. Document Tom's visit in detail.

Intermediate goals:

1. Plan consultation with the sheltered workshop. Attempt to find a job that might be more challenging and worthwhile for Tom. Include Tom in the session.

2. Encourage Tom to come to the mental health center once a week for a half-hour. This structure might develop consistency and stability in his erratic life style. It may keep him more regular in his use of medication also.

3. Encourage Tom to attend a local support group for people with emotional problems.

4. Help Tom set specific goals for himself. Keep them basic and attainable. For example, he might go shopping at the grocery store for himself once a week.

5. Encourage Tom to seek out someone when he feels as if he wishes to quit his job.

Outcome: Difficulties with Tom continue. One can only offer alternatives with the hope that eventually Tom may be motivated to make some healthy changes. Tom is currently working at his job but has intervals when he would like to terminate it. As long as he can acknowledge these feelings and share them with someone, he is still one step ahead. He is active with his small support group — this somewhat makes the long evenings shorter and less lonely to him. Medication is always a problem because Tom feels he should handle his life stresses without the help of drugs.

POSITIVE ASPECTS OF COMMUNITY MENTAL HEALTH NURSING

As with all occupations, community mental health nursing has both positive and negative features.

Community mental health nursing has much to offer the nurse and some of these benefits and satisfactions are listed below.

First, this type of nursing allows one to have a high degree of independence, responsibility and autonomy. The environment of the mental health center allows freedom to practice various approaches. One assumes more responsibility for the patient since the mental health center provides little structure and few controls. In fact, the nurse should be quite insistent about not taking full responsibility for the patient although this can be very difficult to maintain in a crisis sort of situation.

As mentioned above, one works as part of a multidisciplinary team. It is always helpful to know that one has access to trained professionals who can be consulted at any time. Additionally, these people carry theory and knowledge form a variety of schools. The combination of ideas should add to the optimal care of the patient.

A third satisfaction is the wide range of patients and problems. The diversity of pathology seen in the community is stimulating and challenging for the therapist. This exposure to such a wide range of patients encourages further study and research in unfamiliar areas and prevents the boredom which can accompany repetitious tasks.

There is usually an opportunity to expand one's work in areas of particular interest such as writing, communicating via the media and teaching. With an increased desire to improve the mental health of the community and practice primary prevention the mental health nurse can teach skills which will help the community to deal with stress and everyday problems. If one has an interest in geriatric psychiatry, he or she can work as a consultant to nursing homes and special focus can be placed on lectures and workshops involving geriatrics.

The nurse will acquire a good understanding of resources in the community and how agencies work cooperatively together.

There is excellent opportunity to enhance one's professional growth. Continuing education including attending workshops, lectures and seminars are a major part of the job. This educational effort helps to prevent stagnation and professional burnout. It can also help the nurse constantly reassess the efficacy of the program at his or her mental health center.

Another major benefit is that hours can be flexible. There is definitely a 9 to 5 working schedule but this can be changed to some degree. Some mental health centers have specific programs in the evenings. Patients find it easier to meet after regular working hours. The therapist may run some of these programs and may enjoy such a schedule, welcoming some free time during the day.

Usually, too, there is a chance for professional advancement. This must be a personal decision. One can stay completely on a clinical level or become involved in administrative responsibilities. Working at a mental health center offers experience, knowledge and background which will be deemed valuable at any job change.

Finally, there is an excellent opportunity to follow patients long-term. In a hospital setting one may see the patient for several days to several months but after that other agencies take responsibility for the patients or the patients are sent out on their own. The health care invested by the nurse in the hospital situation is difficult to evaluate and the patient relationship is evanescent. On the outpatient basis, the nurse can keep the trust growing as the relationship develops. The nurse can then monitor how the patient progresses socially, vocationally and emotionally.

DIFFICULTIES OF COMMUNITY MENTAL HEALTH NURSING

Undoubtedly, after reading about the many positive, exciting and encouraging aspects of community mental health nursing, many readers are about to make a career change. One needs to be realistic, however. No job is perfect and there are certain problems that are inevitable in community mental health nursing. Indeed, in every professional position there are aspects which can be major hindrances.

In community mental health nursing, there is a definite increase in responsibility, decision making and autonomy. The individual must enjoy working on problems independently and have the ability to make rapid decisions about high risk problems. While there is a team approach, it is not uncommon to find oneself needing to make an immediate and important decision. Often, other staff members are at community consultations or satellite clinics which leaves fewer people from whom to acquire help or information.

There is also an increased need to handle crisis intervention. Patients attempt to handle crises by themselves. Rather than hospitalize the patient, an initial attempt is usually made on an outpatient basis. The nurse may be involved in many emergency visits which will require assessment, information giving and rapid referral. Such cases require the nurse to constantly update her resource information, knowledge about referral, and abilities to make concise and realistic judgments.

Thirdly, there is frequently minimal control or structure for the patient. The community mental health center setting allows much freedom and flexibility. The nurse works around the patient's social, vocational and family schedule. For instance, it may be difficult to involve a patient in a structured weekly support group when the employer allows only bimonthly visits.

Similarly, it is difficult to monitor a patient's schedule once he leaves the office. If he has suicidal feelings, there is always the possibility he will act on them whether or not he has made a verbal contract with the therapist. Indeed, such verbal contracts may be reassuring to the therapist, but they are inadequate means of preventing suicide. The nurse has no control over anyone's actions. He or she can involve other support systems and other community agencies but often such involvement has little impact. Thus, the risks are high, with much of the responsibility falling on the therapist.

Another potential problem is the multidisciplinary team. The benefits of such a team have been previously outlined. When various personalities meet in an intense environment, however, interpersonal problems almost inevitably occur. There are different schools of thought in any mental health center, all of whose professionals have specialized ways of handling problems; these approaches may not be in agreement. Another problem often encountered is irritability and frustration with co-workers. Frequently, this is a projective defense related to difficulties with patients, work load or personal problems. The co-worker becomes the scapegoat and needs to deal honestly and directly with his feelings about that role.

A fifth hazard of this particular professional role is the need to relate to a variety of patients within a short time. This shifting of gears can be confusing and tension producing. An hour is spent with a patient who is very paranoid and psychotic, and one devises a plan which is non-threatening, supportive and low key. The next hour is spent in a women's support group consisting of six bright, insightful and talkative women. One needs to rapidly reframe one's perspective with these rapid shifts in patient types.

A sixth problem is the large case load. As a therapist one must limit oneself to a specific number of patients or one can quickly become overloaded, and indeed the probability of over-extending oneself is very high. The therapist must settle within himself the priorities he has chosen which hopefully will include family, hobbies, friends and health. The need for mental health services is so great the nurse must set specific limits on the case load; otherwise, the list would be endless and highly stressful. Even with such limitations, hours may be long and late. This can be an individual type of decision depending on programs and areas of interest. Participation in a three hour evening workshop may cut into personal and family responsibilities but if appropriate arrangements are made and this type of schedule is desired, it can be fulfilling.

Frequently, mental health centers have satellite clinics for which the therapist travels to area communities. This time spent traveling can also cause problems when there are other priorities.

QUALIFICATIONS

Obviously, adequate preparation is necessary to fulfill the role of a community mental health nurse. Three specific categories which need to be assessed prior to entering this field include personality traits, past experience and academic background.

The nurse's character is an important factor when determining qualifications. The role of the nurse demands a capacity for relationship. The nurse should possess many of the following traits: authenticity, honesty, candor and directness, care, support and sensitivity, a good sense of reality, self-awareness, self-discipline, flexibility with stability, personal life, principal of unconditional caring (which does not mean condoning antisocial actions), confidence in her own ability to produce health, confidence in her own judgment, the ability to cope with stress or find new ways of coping, good insight and a sense of humor (7). Not all nurses can display these character traits all the time; this would make us perfect, and, in fact, all we can do is strive to be good enough. Reviewing character traits and capacities, however, can be a method of self-assessment at certain points in one's career. It also gives some idea of how we relate to our patients.

Life experience can be a major positive aspect in chosing one's career. The relationships one has had with people, the way one has handled responsibility and the coping mechanisms one has for stress are important in letting us assess our abilities. Having encountered many personal problems can be a positive aspect in helping others but self-disclosure can be hazardous for the nurse-patient relationship as can attempting to overcome one's personal problems by going into this kind of work.

Past employment in psychiatric nursing can be an excellent benefit when finding a job in a mental health center. Specialty areas such as geriatrics, work with the retarded and child care will be helpful additions.

The theoretical framework one develops sets the basic groundwork for one's job; from there the clinical practice becomes increasingly important. Each and every case carries with it a uniqueness which cannot be found in a textbook. The nurse must develop a style which works to meet the needs of each patient. To consistently use a stereotyped framework will prove disastrous to the nurse relationship. The nurse's style grows with increased experience. The combination of this developing style and increasing knowledge helps from a competent mental health nurse.

Education is important when chosing this particular field. The requirements are constantly changing but the profession is slowly becoming a specialty area. Most mental health centers require a Bachelor of Science degree in nursing with at least 2 to 3 years experience in the mental health field. These are minimal standards which change frequently due to constant revision of state laws, policies and funding. In many centers, the mental health nurse will need a Master's degree in nursing with at least 2 years clinical experience. Obviously, the nurse also needs licensure by the state (8).

SUMMARY

The role of the community mental health nurse has hopefully been brought into focus in the preceeding pages. This role is unique in that it differs from the public health nurse or hospital psychiatric nurse. This new and expanding role carries with it much independence and responsibility. Along with the added autonomy, there is access to a multidisciplinary team which adds enrichment educationally and emotionally.

Each mental health center has different concepts of what the nurse's role should be. Much depends on the needs of the community. On the whole, the nurse will be involved in individual, group and family counseling. Assessment and crisis intervention will also be major priorities.

There are positive and negative aspects in taking on such a position. The freedom to practice one's own therapy style comfortably and to see a wide variety of problems can be highly rewarding. Drawbacks center on the intensity of the work and its high level of responsibility. The variety of patients and problems has been noted as has the minimal control over the patients, which can be very anxiety provoking for the nurse.

The qualifications necessary for this job vary in each center but usually include a generous amount of clinical experience and a minimum background as a Bachelor of Science in nursing.

The community mental health nurse has become an important part of the multidisciplinary team. By adding the nurse's ideas, goals and concepts, the mental health center will continue to change, develop and provide improved mental health care to patients.

REFERENCES

1. DeYoung, C.: *The Nurse's Role in Community Mental Health Centers: Out of Uniform and Into Trouble.* St. Louis: C.V. Mosby, p. 10, 1971.

2. *Ibid.*, p. 75.

3. *Ibid.*, p. 75.

4. Davis, E.: The Psychiatric Nurse's Role Identity. *American Journal of Nursing.* February 1979, Vol. 79, 298-299.

5. *Ibid.*, p. 298.

6. Mereness, D.: *Psychiatric Nursing — Developing Psychiatric Nursing Skills.* Dubuque, Iowa: William Brown, 192-199, 1971.

7. Rowan, F.: *The Chronically Distressed Client — A Model for Intervention in the Community.* St. Louis: C.V. Mosby, 198-205, 1980.

8. Gardner, K.: Levels of Psychiatric Nursing in an Ambulatory Setting. *JPN and Mental Health Services,* Vol. 15, 28-29, 1977.

31 The Doctor-Nurse Game*

Leonard I. Stein

The relationship between the doctor and the nurse is a very special one. There are few professions where the degree of mutual respect and cooperation between co-workers is as intense as that between the doctor and nurse. Superficially, the stereotype of this relationship has been dramatized in many novels and television serials. When, however, it is observed carefully in an interactional framework, the relationship takes on a new dimension and has a special quality which fits a game model. The underlying attitudes which demand that this game be played are unfortunate. These attitudes create serious obstacles in the path of meaningful communications between physicians and nonmedical professional groups.

The physician traditionally and appropriately has total responsibility for making the decisions regarding the management of his patients' treatment. To guide his decisions he considers data gleaned from several sources. He acquires a complete medical history, performs a thorough physical examination, interprets laboratory findings, and at times, obtains recommendations from physician-consultants. Another important factor in his decision-making are the recommendations he receives from the nurse. The interaction between doctor and nurse through which these recommendations are communicated and received is unique and interesting.

THE GAME

One rarely hears a nurse say, "Doctor I would recommend that you order a retention enema for Mrs. Brown." A physician, upon hearing a recommendation of that nature, would gape in

*Reprinted with permission from *Arch. Gen. Psychiat., 16:*699, 1967.

amazement at the effrontery of the nurse. The nurse, upon hearing the statement, would look over her shoulder to see who said it, hardly believing the words actually came from her own mouth. Nevertheless, if one observes closely, nurses make recommendations of more import every hour and physicians willingly and respectfully consider them. If the nurse is to make a suggestion without appearing insolent, and the doctor is to seriously consider that suggestion, their interaction must not violate the rules of the game.

Object of the Game

The object of the game is as follows: the nurse is to be bold, have initiative, and be responsible for making significant recommendations, while at the same time she must appear passive. This must be done in such a manner so as to make her recommendations appear to be initiated by the physician.

Both participants must be acutely sensitive to each other's nonverbal and cryptic verbal communications. A slight lowering of the head, a minor shifting of position in the chair, or a seemingly nonrelevant comment concerning an event which occurred eight months ago must be interpreted as a powerful message. The game requires the nimbleness of a high wire acrobat, and if either participant slips, the game can be shattered; the penalties for frequent failure are apt to be severe.

Rules of the Game

The cardinal rule of the game is that open disagreement between the players must be avoided at all costs. Thus, the nurse must communicate her recommendations without appearing to be making a recommendation statement. The physician, in requesting a recommendation from a nurse, must do so without appearing to be asking for it. Utilization of this technique keeps anyone from committing themselves to a position before a sub rosa agreement on that position has already been established. In that way open disagreement is avoided. The greater the significance of the recommendation, the more subtly the game must be played.

To convey a subtle example of the game with all its nuances would require the talents of a literary artist. Lacking these talents, let me give you the following example which is unsubtle, but happens frequently. The medical resident on hospital call is awakened by telephone at 1 a.m. because a patient on a ward, not his own, has not been able to fall asleep. Dr. Jones answers the telephone and the dialogue goes like this:

This is Dr. Jones

(An open and direct communication)

Dr. Jones, this is Miss Smith on 2W — Mrs. Brown, who learned today of her father's death, is unable to fall asleep.

(This message has two levels. Openly, it describes a set of circumstances, a woman who is unable to sleep and who that morning received word of her father's death. Less openly, but just as directly, it is a diagnostic and recommendation statement; i.e., Mrs. Brown is unable to sleep because of her grief, and she should be given a sedative. Dr. Jones, accepting the diagnostic statement and replying to the recommendation statement, answers.)

What sleeping medication has been helpful to Mrs. Brown in the past?

(Dr. Jones, not knowing the patient, is asking for a recommendation from the nurse, who does know the patient, about what sleeping medication should be prescribed. Note, however, his question does not appear to be asking her for a recommendation. Miss Smith replies.)

Pentobarbital mg 100 was quite effective night before last.

(A disguised recommendation statement. Dr. Jones replies with a note of authority in his voice.)

Pentobarbital mg 100 before bedtime as needed for sleep, got it?

(Miss Smith ends the conversation with the tone of a grateful supplicant.)

Yes I have, and thank you very much doctor.

The above is an example of a successfully played doctor-nurse game. The nurse made appropriate recommendations which were accepted by the physician and were helpful to the patient. The game was successful because the cardinal rule was not violated. The nurse was able to make her recommendation without appearing to, and the physician was able to ask for recommendations without conspicuously asking for them.

The Scoring System

Inherent in any game are penalties and rewards for the players. In game theory, the doctor-nurse game fits the nonzero sum game model. It is not like chess, where the players compete with each other and whatever one player loses the other wins. Rather, it is the kind of game in which the rewards and punishments are shared by both players. If they play the game successfully they both win rewards, and if they are unskilled and the game is played badly, they both suffer the penalty.

The most obvious reward from the well-played game is a doctor-nurse team that operates efficiently. The physician is able to utilize the nurse as a valuable consultant, and the nurse gains self-esteem and professional satisfaction from her job. The less obvious rewards are no less important. A successful game creates a doctor-nurse alliance; through this alliance the physician gains the respect and admiration of the nursing service. He can be confident that his nursing staff will smooth the path for getting his work done. His charts will be organized and waiting for him when he arrives, the ruffled feathers of patients and relatives will have been smoothed down, his pet routines will be happily followed, and he will be helped in a thousand and one other ways.

The doctor-nurse alliance sheds its light on the nurse as well. She gains a reputation for being a "damn good nurse." She is respected by everyone and appropriately enjoys her position. When physicians discuss the nursing staff it would not be unusual for her name to be mentioned with respect and admiration. Their esteem for a good nurse is no less than their esteem for a good doctor.

The penalties for a game failure, on the other hand, can be severe. The physician who is an unskilled gamesman and fails to recognize the nurses' subtle recommendation messages is tolerated as a "clod." If, however, he interprets these messages as insolence and strongly indicates he does not wish to tolerate suggestions from nurses, he creates a rocky path for his travels. The old truism "If the nurse is your ally you've got it made, and if she has it in for you, be prepared for misery," takes on life-sized proportions. He receives three times as many phone calls after midnight than his colleagues. Nurses will not accept his telephone orders because "telephone orders are against the rules." Somehow, this rule gets suspended for the skilled players. Soon he becomes like Joe Bfstplk in the "Li'l Abner" comic strip. No matter where he goes, a black cloud constantly hovers over his head.

The unskilled gamesman nurse also pays heavily. The nurse who does not view her role as that of a consultant, and therefore does not attempt to communicate recommendations, is perceived as a dullard and is mercifully allowed to fade into the woodwork.

The nurse who does see herself as a consultant but refuses to follow the rules of the game in making her recommendations, has hell to pay. The outspoken nurse is labeled "bitch" by the surgeon. The psychiatrist describes her as unconsciously suffering from penis envy and her behavior is the acting out of her hostility towards men. Loosly translated, the psychiatrist is saying she is a bitch. The employment of the unbright outspoken nurse is soon terminated. The outspoken bright nurse whose recommendations are worthwhile remains employed. She is, however, constantly reminded in a hundred ways that she is not loved.

GENESIS OF THE GAME

To understand how the game evolved, we must comprehend the nature of the doctors' and nurses' training which shaped the attitudes necessary for the game.

Medical Student Training

The medical student in his freshman year studies as if possessed. In the anatomy class he learns every groove and prominence on the bones of the skeleton as if life depended on it. As a matter of fact, he literally believes just that. He not infrequently says, "I've got to learn it exactly, a life may depend on me knowing that." A consequence of this attitude, which is carefully nurtured throughout medical school, is the development of a phobia: the overdetermined fear of making a mistake. The development of this fear is quite understandable. The burden the physician must carry is at times almost unbearable. He feels responsible in a very personal way for the lives of his patients. When a man dies leaving young children and a widow, the doctor carries some of her grief and despair inside himself; and when a child dies, some of him dies, too. He sees himself as a warrior against death and disease. When he loses a battle, through no fault of his own, he nevertheless feels pangs of guilt, and he relentlessly searches himself to see if there might have been a way to alter the outcome. For the physician a mistake leading to a serious consequence is intolerable, and any mistake reminds him of his vulnerability. There is little wonder that he becomes phobic. The classical way in which phobias are managed is to avoid the source of the fear. Since it is impossible to avoid making some mistakes in an active practice of medicine, a substitute defensive maneuver is employed. The physician develops the belief that he is omnipotent and omniscient, and therefore incapable of making mistakes. This belief allows the phobic physician to actively engage in his practice rather than avoid it. The fear of committing an error in a critical field like medicine is unavoidable and appropriately realistic. The physician, however, must learn to live with the fear rather than handle it defensively through a posture of omnipotence. This defense markedly interferes with his interpersonal professional relationships.

Physicians, of course, deny feelings of omnipotence. The evidence, however, renders their denials to whispers in the wind. The slightest mistake inflicts a large narcissistic wound. Depending on his underlying personality structure the physician may obsess for days about it, quickly rationalize it away, or deny it. The guilt produced is usually exaggerated and the incident is handled defensively. The ways in which physicians enhance and support each other's defenses when an error is made could be the topic of another paper. The feelings of omnipotence become generalized to other areas of his life. A report of the Federal Aviation Agency (FAA), as quoted in *Time Magazine* (Aug. 5, 1966), states that in 1964 and 1965 physicians had a fatal-accident rate four times as high as the average for all other private pilots. Major causes of the high death rate were risk-taking attitudes and judgments. Almost all of the accidents occurred on pleasure trips, and were therefore not necessary risks to get to a patient needing emergency care. The trouble, suggested an FAA official, is that too many doctors fly with "the feeling that they are omnipotent." Thus, the extremes to which the physician may go in preserving his self-concept of omnipotence may threaten his own life. This overdetermined preservation of omnipotence is indicative of its brittleness and its underlying foundation of fear of failure.

The physician finds himself trapped in a paradox. He fervently wants to give his patient the best possible medical care, and being open to the nurses' recommendations helps him accomplish this. On the other hand, accepting advice from nonphysicians is highly threatening to his omnipotence. The solution for the paradox is to receive sub rosa recommendations and make them appear to be initiated by himself. In short, he must learn to play the doctor–nurse game.

Some physicians never learn to play the game. Most learn in their internship, and a perceptive few learn during their clerkships in medical school. Medical students frequently complain that the nursing staff treats them as if they had just completed a junior Red Cross first-aid class instead of two years of intensive medical training. Interviewing nurses in a training hospital sheds considerable light on this phenomenon. In their words they said,

> "A few students just seem to be with it, they are able to understand what you are trying to tell them, and they are a pleasure to work with; most, however, pretend to know everything and refuse to listen to anything we have to say and I guess we do give them a rough time."

In essence, they are saying that those students who quickly learn the game are rewarded, and those that do not are punished.

Most physicians learn to play the game after they have weathered a few experiences like the one described below. On the first day of his internship, the physician and nurse were making rounds. They stopped at the bed of a 52-year-old woman who, after complimenting the young doctor on his appearance, complained to him of her problem with constipation. After several minutes of listening to her detailed description of peculiar diets, family home remedies, and special exercises that have helped her constipation in the past, the nurse politely interrupted the patient. She told her the doctor would take care of the problem and that he had to move on because there were other patients waiting to see him. The young doctor gave the nurse a stern look, turned toward the patient, and kindly told her he would order an enema for her that very afternoon. As they left the bedside, the nurse told him the patient has had a normal bowel movement every day for the past week and that in the 23 days the patient has been in the hospital she had never once passed up an opportunity to complain of her constipation. She quickly added that if the doctor wanted to order an enema, the patient would certainly receive one. After hearing this report, the intern's mouth fell open and the wheels began turning in his head. He remembered the nurse's comment to the patient that, "the doctor had to move on," and it occurred to him that perhaps she was really giving him a message. This experience and a few more like it, and the young doctor learns to listen for the subtle recommendations the nurses make.

Nursing Student Training

Unlike the medical student, who usually learns to play the game after he finishes medical school, the nursing student begins to learn it early in her training. Throughout her education she is trained to play the doctor-nurse game.

Student nurses are taught how to relate to physicians. They are told he has infinitely more knowledge than they, and thus he should be shown the utmost respect. In addition, it was not many years ago when nurses were instructed to stand whenever a physician entered a room. When he would come in for a conference the nurse was expected to offer him her chair, and when both entered a room the nurse would open the door for him and allow him to enter first. Although these practices are no longer rigidly adhered to, the premise upon which they were based is still promulgated. One nurse described that premise as, "He's God almighty and your job is to wait on him."

To inculcate subservience and inhibit deviancy, nursing schools, for the most part, are tightly run, disciplined institutions. Certainly there is great variation among nursing schools, and there is little question that the trend is toward giving students more autonomy. However, in too many schools this trend has not gone far enough, and the climate remains restrictive. The student's schedule is firmly controlled and there is very little free time. Classroom hours, study hours, meal time, and bed time with lights out are rigidly enforced. In some schools meaningless chores are assigned, such as cleaning bed springs with cotton applicators. The relationship between student and instructor continues this military flavor. Often their relationship is more like that between recruit and drill sergeant than between student and teacher. Open dialogue is inhibited by attitudes of strict black and white, with few, if any, shades of grey. Straying from the rigidly outlined path is sure to result in disciplinary action.

The inevitable result of these practices is to instill in the student nurse a fear of independent action. This inhibition of independent action is most marked when relating to physicians. One of the students' greatest fears is making a blunder while assisting a physician and being publicly ridiculed by him. This is really more a reflection of the nature of their training than the prevalence of abusive physicians. The fear of being humiliated for a blunder while assisting in a procedure is generalized to the fear of humiliation for making any independent act in relating to a physician, especially the act of making a direct recommendation. Every nurse interviewed felt that making a suggestion to a physician was equivalent to insulting and belittling him. It was tantamount to questioning his medical knowledge and insinuating he did not know his business. In light of her image of the physician as an omniscient and punitive figure, the questioning of his knowledge would be unthinkable.

The student, however, is also given messages quite contrary to the ones described above. She is continually told that she is an invaluable aid to the physician in the treatment of the patient. She is told that she must help him in every way possible, and she is imbued with a strong sense of responsibility for the care of her patient. Thus she, like the physician, is caught in a paradox. The first set of messages implies that the physician is omniscient and that any recommendation she might make would be insulting to him and leave her open to ridicule. The second set of messages implies that she is an important asset to him, has much to contribute, and is duty-bound to make those contributions. Thus, when her good sense tells her a recommendation would be helpful to him she is not allowed to communicate it directly, nor is she allowed not to communicate it. The way out of the bind is to use the doctor-nurse game and communicate the recommendation without appearing to do so.

FORCES PRESERVING THE GAME

Upon observing the indirect interactional system which is the heart of the doctor-nurse game, one must ask the question, "Why does this inefficient mode of communication continue to exist?" The forces mitigating against change are powerful.

Rewards and Punishments

The doctor-nurse game has a powerful, innate self-perpetuating force — its system of rewards and punishments. One potent method of shaping behavior is to reward one set of behavioral patterns and to punish patterns which deviate from it. As described earlier, the rewards given for a well-played game and the punishments meted out to unskilled players are impressive. This system alone would be sufficient to keep the game flourishing. The game, however, has additional forces.

The Strength of the Set

It is well recognized that sets are hard to break. A powerful attitudinal set is the nurse's perception that making a suggestion to a physician is equivalent to insulting and belittling him. An example of where attempts are regularly made to break this set is seen on psychiatric treatment wards operating on a therapeutic community model. This model requires open and direct communication between members of the team. Psychiatrists working in these settings expend a great deal of energy in urging for and rewarding openness before direct patterns of communication become established. The rigidity of the resistance to break this set is impressive. If the physician himself is a prisoner of the set and therefore does not actively try to destroy it, change is near impossible.

The Need for Leadership

Lack of leadership and structure in any organization produces anxiety in its members. As the importance of the organization's mission increases, the demand by its members for leadership commensurately increases. In our culture human life is near the top of our hierarchy of values, and organizations which deal with human lives, such as law and medicine, are very rigidly structured. Certainly some of this is necessary for the systematic management of the task. The excessive degree of rigidity, however, is demanded by its members for their own psychic comfort rather than for its utility in efficiently carrying out its mission. The game lends support to this thesis. Indirect communication is an inefficient mode of transmitting information. However, it effectively supports and protects a rigid organizational structure with the physician in clear authority. Maintaining an omnipotent leader provides the other members with a great sense of security.

Sexual Roles

Another influence perpetuating the doctor-nurse game is the sexual identity of the players. Doctors are predominantly men and nurses are almost exclusively women. There are elements of the game which reinforce the stereotyped roles of male dominance and female passivity. Some nursing instructors explicitly tell their students that their femininity is an important asset to be used when relating to physicians.

COMMENT

The doctor and nurse have a shared history and thus have been able to work out their game so that it operates more efficiently than one would expect in an indirect system. Major difficulty arises, however, when the physician works closely with other disciplines which are not normally considered part of the medical sphere. With expanding medical horizons encompassing cooperation with sociologists, engineers, anthropologists, computer analysts, etc., continued expectation of a doctor–nurselike interaction by the physician is disastrous. The sociologist, for example, is not willing to play that kind of game. When his direct communications are rebuffed the relationship breaks down.

The major disadvantage of a doctor–nurselike game is its inhibitory effect on open dialogue which is stifling and anti-intellectual. The game is basically a transactional neurosis, and both professions would enhance themselves by taking steps to change the attitudes which breed the game.

Mrs. Gertrude Hermsmeier, RN, Mrs. Joyce McCollum, RN, Arnold M. Ludwig, MD, and Arnold J. Marx, MD, of Mendota State Hospital, aided in this report.

32 The Psychodynamics of the Nurse-Psychiatrist Relationship

Barbara Chamberlin

The professional relationship between nurses and psychiatrists is a complex interplay of tangible and intangible factors in countless permutations and combinations that reflect individual traits and idiosyncrasies. It is somewhat of a miracle that, through it all, most professionals do succeed with the ultimate goal of quality patient care.

Psychiatric patients present some unique and challenging care problems. The defensive or paranoid patient needs special understanding and frankness. The dependent patient often demands extra personnel time and support. Overtly psychotic patients need repeated interpretations of reality and of circumstances in their environment. Suicidal patients may need to be physically restrained to prevent them from harming themselves. All of these needs are superimposed on the requirements of routine medical care. Meeting the challenges posed by patients' concurrent medical and psychiatric care needs requires substantial creativity and flexibility as indicated in the following vignette.

> **Example:** A 55-year-old recently widowed woman experienced repeated anxiety-panic attacks requiring both medication and extensive attention and reassurance from the nursing staff. Her exaggerated helplessness and dependency evoked rescuing actions from staff. She admitted that she felt unable to control her actions or take responsibility for the consequences.
>
> The nursing staff mobilized to offer the patient support, but on a limited basis and in combination with interactions designed to encourage her to take more responsibility.
>
> In the midst of her hospitalization, with her psychiatric nursing care plan well underway, the patient developed an acute psychotic reaction, apparently secondary to isoniazid administered for recently diagnosed pulmonary tuberculosis. The psychiatrist-

nurse team shifted their approach immediately to include antipsychotic medications, increased environmental structure, and closer nursing supervision, while temporarily de-emphasizing the therapeutic goals related to increased dependence.

A second shift toward a more "medical" approach was later necessitated when the patient developed nausea and vomiting with elevated liver enzymes, also secondary to isoniazid.

Both nurses and physicians are expected to continuously monitor and understand their own psychological reactions to patients and patient care situations. Exposure to the psychiatric patient's tenuous ego integration, with its fine border between psychotic and nonspychotic thought processes, is often personally threatening for physician and nurse alike. Experiences with psychotic patients can reawaken basic dependency and security needs; raise or revive issues of authority, power, and control; stir repressed aggressive and sexual drives; and arouse primitive fears and feelings of vulnerability, loneliness, and abandonment.

Example: A 35-year-old businessman was hospitalized with a two year history of depression and agitation following financial losses. His mood fluctuated markedly and he demanded much one-to-one attention. He manipulated and controlled therapy group time, refused to take prescribed psychotropic medications, and rejected all therapeutic suggestions from nurses and psychiatrists, while at the same time complaining that no one was helping him.

In a staff discussion, the psychiatrist and nurses on the unit shared their increasing feelings of frustration and hostility toward this patient, and many of the staff admitted that they hoped he would elect to leave the hospital. On this same morning, the patient attempted suicide by hanging in his hospital room. Lengthy resuscitation efforts were finally successful. The intense grief, guilt, and anger mobilized in the work team by this episode were never fully resolved, although the patient eventually responded to antidepressant medication and returned home.

Racial, sexual, and religious stereotypes can be causal or contributory factors in some cases of emotional illness. Many argue that societal and interpersonal oppression are important sources of depression and problems related to low self-esteem among women and minorities. Thus, a goal of psychiatric care is to help patients explore the fallacies of prejudice and validate reality. This goal, however, is predicated on the assumption that the psychiatric professionals have a foundation of insight into their own biases and presupposes that they have acted to alter their own stereotypical behavior. An indicator that this is not always the case is provided by the male physician and female nurse who evolve and accept roles based on unconscious expectations of traditional sex role stereotyeps that lead to a clear splitting of power, authority, and dependency.

Miller has written eloquently of the dangers of dominant-subordinant role division (1). The dominant group defines acceptable behavior for the subordinants, and in time both groups accept their "job descriptions" as "normal," performing the required tasks with the required attitudes. To accept these role descriptions complacently is to be "well-adjusted," and any alternative to the domination-subordination process may be viewed as illness. The mirroring of dominant-subordinant roles by psychiatrists and nurses implies that this behavior is healthy and desirable. In essence, such behavior on the part of mental health care providers suggests that societal oppression is not real and the patient's problems stem entirely from intrapsychic conflicts. Such attitudes and role modeling can obviously be destructive to the patient's emotional health.

> **Example:** A male psychiatrist, accompanied by his entourage of residents and nurses, entered a woman patient's room on morning rounds. He began conversation with the patient by complimenting her on her shade of lipstick and her hairstyle and then, in an attempt at humor, suggested that she might have some advice to share in these areas with the female nursing staff.
>
> Both the patient and the female nurse were puzzled by their angry reactions to this apparently harmless social chat. Neither they nor the psychiatrist consciously recognized the demeaning implications of his focus on appearance and the hostile, competitive nature of his comparison of the patient and the nursing staff.

Job and social status are also powerful dictators of interactions. Nurses continue to struggle to redefine their professional image, which is associated with less prestige and power than that of the physician. The presence on psychiatric units of medical students and residents in training further obscures the hierarchy of status and power, and there are often many mixed messages about division of responsibility. Is the nurse mentor to the resident, or vice versa?

Certain expectations seem more common between psychiatric physicians and nurses than among nonpsychiatric work teams. Because the daily emphasis is on receiving and responding to emotional needs, psychiatric professionals often expect similar understanding and sensitivity from each other. Each may be angered and offended when the other fails to perceive and satisfy dependency and nurturance needs, and the work team can become disabled by preoccupation with the perceived insensitivity of a team member.

> **Example:** The psychiatric work team had functioned well until a pleasant but psychologically unsophisticated medical resident joined them for a six-week rotation. He was irritatingly oversolicitous, appeared insincere, and had some difficulty observing and appropriately interpreting psychopathology in patients. Other team members labeled him as superficial and became preoccupied with his mistakes. If he arrived five minutes late or did not know some minor detail about his patients, he was confronted in front of the entire team. The attending psychiatrist began to review the resident's charts, looking for errors. On rounds, the team scrutinized the resident's patients, often leaving no time to spend with patients cared for by the other residents and the medical students on the team.
>
> The ultimate irony was the realization at the end of the resident's rotation that his patients had progressed reasonably and as rapidly as those cared for by other team members.

The tangible issues that affect the interactions of the psychiatrist–nurse team may be equally complex. An example is the question of malpractice liability, which represents a special preoccupation for both groups of professionals. Most physicians and nurses are confused about the boundaries of their own respective liability. Some physicians are unaware that nurses have their own legal liability and often carry malpractice insurance. In general, the physician may be liable in cases that conform to the Respondent Superior Principle of Law. That is, the physician who has the power, supervision, and control over the nurse during the period of the nurse's services may be liable for any nursing errors (2). Because the nurse may simultaneously serve more than one employer (hospital and physician), the physician may be liable even though the nurse is a hospital employee (borrowed servant doctrine). (2).

Regardless of the physician's power of supervision, the nurse is considered liable when performing nursing tasks that do not require medical skills (sponge counts, enemas, etc.) (2). The law also requires that nurses make independent judgments about the validity of medical orders and exercise reasonable care to safeguard patients from danger. A nurse may be liable if she does not thoroughly understand medical orders before administering them (3). Thus, there are few situations in which physician and nurse do not *both* have significant liability. This shared liability adds pressure to the decisions about division of responsibility in the work team.

Sherard has described differences in work concepts and structure that can lead to misunderstandings in nurse-physician relations (4). Physicians are viewed as having a "holistic" global approach to care and an enduring sense of time, resources, and responsibility. They are not paid by the hour or scheduled on eight-hour shifts, and they do not need to consider supply availability in making treatment decisions. Nurses must budget their time, and they may prefer regimens that fit in eight-hour schedule blocks (e.g., routine vitals versus q3h vitals). Because nurses organize their work by tasks (blood pressure, daily weights, etc.) rather than by patient, they may appear to lack an integrated sense of the relationship between task and patient. Physicians also are often unaware of the many nonmedical tasks that take up nurses' time.

> **Example:** The psychiatrist member of a work team fumed angrily as he waited for the nursing team members to join him for rounds. They were several minutes late and were in an intense discussion with other nurses in an adjacent room. As the team members finally left their discussion and joined the psychiatrist, he mentally prepared a mild reprimand. However, before he could deliver the criticism, a nurse apologized, explaining that the unit was short staffed, that a patient needed to be taken across town for testing in another hospital, the morning ECT on the ward was about to begin, a transfer patient from another ward was expected imminently, and a patient-family conference with nurse participants was about to begin. The psychiatrist admitted that he had not been aware that the nurses had such varied responsibilities, including time-consuming non-nursing tasks like escorting patients for testing.

The nurse's task-oriented division of labor, hourly wage, and eight-hour shift can also contribute to a limited sense of mastery (4). This is in direct opposition to the physician's holistic approach, which provides a strong sense of mastery and control. Perhaps as nursing administrators increasingly turn to flexible schedules (e.g., seven days on followed by seven days off; four ten-hour days per week), nursing concepts may be able to shift to a more flexible and holistic approach.

Physicians and nurses often lack a shared understanding of the details of one another's educational backgrounds. Few physicians are aware of the specifics of nursing education, the courses and types of degrees available, and the level of skill such degrees imply. As a consequence, the physician may use the "least common denominator" approach in assessing the competence of an individual nurse. Conversely, nurses often equate the medical degree with omniscient knowledge in all areas of medicine. Such attitudes demean the nurse and burden the physician with unrealistic expectations.

> **Example:** A nurse's aide entered a patient's room to remove a bedpan. Although this woman was clearly dressed in an aide's uniform, an unobservant physician who was perusing a chart asked her to assist him in a lumbar puncture he was about to perform. The aide became nervous and left the room saying, "Just a minute." Minutes later an RN arrived and provided competent assistance. Yet the physician, still uninformed, assumed that he had been abandoned by an incompetent nurse rather than an appropriately trained aide.
>
> The same physician later encountered similar difficulties when he asked an LPN to start an IV. Fortunately, this time the nurse educated him by explaining the limitations of her skills and called an RN.

In recent years, nursing concepts have changed to include the patient as a consumer of services with the nurse as a patient advocate. Organized medicine in general has not adopted this consumer orientation, and the role change in nursing has puzzled many physicians. Some have felt that the nurse has "changed sides" and is now working against the physician. Some nurses may have contributed to this misunderstanding by appearing to use the advocacy role in an adversarial manner to challenge the doctor and to gain power.

Example: The 55-year-old woman described in the first example was known to have pulmonary TB on admission to the psychiatric ward. The admitting nurse, acting as advocate for the other patients, immediately notified the nurse epidemiologist without first contacting the admitting physician. The nurse epidemiologist instructed her to place the patient in strict isolation. The psychiatrist felt undermined and embarrased when he arrived minutes later to do the initial work-up and found isolation precautions. Although he did not argue the necessity of special measures, he felt displaced from his role as decision maker. He was puzzled by the nurses' unilateral action, which he viewed as implying that she did not consider him a patient advocate.

The patient advocacy role on the surface appears to challenge the traditional privileged doctor-patient relationship. While confidentiality of doctor-patient communication protects the patient's privacy, it also contributes to nurse-physician-patient misunderstanding. The nurse who must care for psychiatric patients without the knowledge of important facts related to their illness is at a disadvantage and may receive the message that his or her nursing skills are superfluous. The patient who is unaware of the confidentiality rule may draw the same conclusions about the nursing staff, further undermining their efforts to care for the patient. Further, the physician who tends to forget that the nurse is operating without certain information may make inaccurate assumptions about the nurse's competence.

Example: A 17-year-old female patient had been admitted to an open psychiatric ward for long-term psychotherapy, with a chief complaint of depression and a history of multiple past suicide attempts. Concealed razor blades were found in her room during a routine nursing search. As the intensity of her therapy increased, she became more dependent on her psychiatrist and spoke less with the primary nurse. She began again to express suicidal ideation on the ward and broke a window in her room immediately after a therapy hour. The nursing staff, who were uninformed about the details of therapy because of confidentiality rules, had little information with which to evaluate the seriousness of the patient's aggressive behavior or her suicidal potential. They felt their only recourse was to transfer her to a closed ward. The psychiatrist resisted this recommendation because she felt comfortable with the patient's progress and felt such a move would interrupt therapy goals. She tried to reassure the staff while protecting the patient's privacy. Yet without details that would allow them to make a competent nursing assessment, the nurses remained understandably anxious and concerned about the patient. The situation remained uncomfortable for all involved until the patient's suicidal ideation ceased.

The behavioral expectations between hospital nursing and administrative personnel may also have an intense effect on the physician-nurse relationship. Spencer (5) has written an angry, challenging comment on the divided loyalties and goals of nursing directors. Perhaps because they occupy that tenuous middle ground between hospital administration and nursing staff, nursing supervisors often seem rigidly conscious of the hierarchy of job descriptions and concomitant powers. They may appear to adhere inflexibly to prescribed roles and may seem to resist any fluidity and sharing of responsibility. They may be scapegoated by nurses, administrators, and physician staff as the source of obstruction to team work (5).

Example: The nursing supervisor was privy to hospital financial information and was aware of the economic importance of maintaining full-bed capacity. She was also aware that the psychiatric ward always had a lengthy waiting list. This was in part due to chronic staff shortages which made it difficult to deliver quality patient care at full-bed capacity. Should she support more admissions with the possibility of reduced care quality and the risk of malpractice? Or should she risk the economic problems of a less than full ward which might lead to a cost-cutting decrease in the number of beds and thus to an even longer waiting list?

Farther up the ladder of power and control is the hospital administration with its preoccupation with efficiency and financial solvency. As illustrated in the vignette above, these concerns often contrast markedly with "front line" concerns about patient care (5).

CONCLUSIONS

From this discussion, it should be clear that there are no simple solutions to the difficulties that can arise in psychiatric work teams. The risks inherent in a simplistic approach to the complicated psychodynamics of nurse-psychiatrist interaction are multiple. Primary among these is the temptation to "scapegoat," i.e., to blame one or the other profession for difficulties that exist in their interactions. Such obviously counterproductive attitudes can adversely affect both staff morale and the quality of patient care. Strict adherence to predefined "job descriptions" and hierarchichal role behavior with the hope of eliminating stress by increasing predictability is another danger. The flexibility that is so important to the care of psychiatric patients obviously cannot develop in such an environment. Further, this desire for stability and predictability, while understandable, can also lead to the preservation of traditional role stereotypes and the continuation of the consequences associated with them.

What, then, can be done to facilitate productive and mutually satisfying professional relationships in the psychiatric work team? Such popular trends as flexible scheduling, communication skill classes, committee shared assignments, and restructuring of formal job descriptions are helpful but they are unlikely to be totally successful in achieving this goal. What is more essential is the development and reinforcement of flexibility, sensitivity, patience, insight, and understanding at the many interpersonal levels that are involved in the delivery of quality patient care.

Development of such skills must begin with awareness of the antithetical traits of insensitivity, impatience, rigidity, and rudeness. For example, it would be appropriate for the male psychiatrist described earlier, who compared his patient's and nurse's grooming habits, to be privately reminded of the insensitivity implicit in such a comparison and tactfully educated about his responsibility for the consequences of such comments. It is also the responsibility of the nurses and physicians alike to educate one another about not only their special skills and abilities but the limitations of their training. An obvious prerequisite here is demonstrating the ability to rise above the personal power-control struggles inherent in any open discussion of abilities, responsibilities, and limitations.

Perhaps most important in the development and reinforcement of flexibility, sensitivity, insight, and understanding is the modeling of these traits. Psychiatrists and nurses have a responsibility to their students, patients, and co-workers to act as mentors, tutors or guides, through the maze of interpersonal relationships that both foster and impede quality patient care. In daily rounds, patient care assignment meetings and case conferences, the psychiatrist-nurse team must routinely address interpersonal aspects of patient care. This role modeling of concern and acceptance of the psychodynamics of the psychiatrist-nurse team is the best hope for survival of the team concept and quality patient care.

REFERENCES

1. Miller, J.B.: The Effects of Inequality on Psychology. *Psych Opinion*, 29-32, August, 1978.
2. Veazey, M.F.: Physician Versus Nurse Liability. *Med Legal Bulletin*, 1-7, Richmond, Virginia, August, 1976.
3. How to Avoid Liability in Administering Drugs. *California Nurse*, December 8, 1978. Reprinted from *Malpractice Digest*, July-August, 1978.
4. Sherard, T.: The Structure of Conflict in Nurse-Physician Relations. *Supervisor Nurse*, 14-18, August, 1980.
5. Spencer, C.E.: Nurses Need Liberation - But From Whom? *RN*, 63-69, July, 1979.

PART 5

THE FUTURE

33 Major Trends in Psychiatric Nursing

Lloyd A. Wells

Because of its rapidly changing nature, psychiatric nursing cannot be considered as a static entity. An appreciation of its past helps us understand its current position, but that position will be changed even while this book is going to press. A consideration of the future of psychiatric nursing should be a major consideration for every psychiatric nurse.

It goes without saying that most of our current predictions will be seriously in error with the hindsight provided by 20 years or so. Nevertheless, only by thinking about these predictions and making one's own can one hope to actually shape the future of psychiatric nursing.

I see eight major trends in psychiatric nursing. The first of these is a continuation in the trend toward diversity. The profession will become even more stratified, with many different roles for the psychiatric nurse. A major role, however, will continue to be the provision of bedside nursing to hospitalized psychiatric patients. No one is qualified to do this better than a nurse, and it would be regrettable if this task were eventually left to technicians or aides.

A second trend will be the further integration of psychiatric nursing with other mental health professions, including psychiatry and psychiatric social work as well as clinical psychology. There are areas of overlap in all these disciplines. These areas need to be identified so that what is unique to each discipline can be preserved for it and what is common to all the disciplines can be improved by healthy interaction.

Independent practice of psychiatric nursing will become increasingly commonplace. At the same time, the techniques, goals and appropriate areas for such practice will be much more completely defined than they are at present. The practitioner will offer that which is common to all the mental health professions as well as what is specific to psychiatric nursing. Obviously, such a practitioner will have a great deal more training than many other psychiatric nurses.

Another major trend in psychiatric nursing of the future will be more research by psychiatric nurses. Again, the research will be partially in areas common to all the mental health professions but will be more specific to areas unique to nursing. What those areas are will remain somewhat controversial, however. One major aspect of the research will focus on relationships, both among patients and nurses and between nurse and nurse, and nurse and other professionals.

The education of psychiatric nurses will continue to be multi-tiered. In general, most nurses will enter the profession with a baccalaureate degree. Nurses will function with Bachelor's degrees, Master's degrees and Ph.D.s in nursing, and it is possible that Master's and doctoral level programs in a more broad-based mental health science will also be developed. The level of education will be roughly equated to the level of practice, but it will be possible to practice at a higher level than one is technically educationally qualified for.

In general, inpatient psychiatric units will continue to be the psychiatrists' domain, but the nurse will have a greatly expanded role here, too. The nurse will often have independent responsibility in individual psychotherapy, group psychotherapy, family and conjoint therapies, and will be accepted much more as a professional, co-equal to the physician.

Along with all these improvements in the status of the nurse will come a great many regulations from government, insurance companies and the nurses' own professional organizations. These regulations will be greatly lamented by many nurses but will probably be welcomed by somewhat jealous, over-regulated colleagues.

Finally, the already admirable credentials and certification process initiated by the American Nurses Association will continue to be reviewed and revised.

In sum, the future of psychiatric nursing will be exciting, and the years ahead should generate controversy and much thought.

34 Current and Future Professional Realities

Denise M. Wells

As is stated or implied elsewhere in this volume, any predictions about the future of the profession of psychiatric nursing will be risible to any reader who happens to glance at this book 20 years from now. Nevertheless, it is useful for any profession to attempt to predict the future because such a prediction underlines some of the happier as well as less fortunate trends in the profession at present. To discuss the future of psychiatric nursing seriously, we must examine the overt and subtle realities which affect the profession today and which will very possibly have impact on it in the future.

One not so subtle reality is the fact of a major nursing shortage throughout the United States. It has been argued that there is not really a nursing shortage but that there is an enormous decline in quality of current nursing students, considerable disaffection with nursing as a career, and an enormous dropout rate. Data indicate, however, that there is a very real shortage and that fewer competent and intelligent people are entering the ranks of nurses than was the case during the preceding two decades. Nursing historically has been a career which provides upward mobility for bright women of middle class origin. Opportunities in other fields have mushroomed for such women in recent years. The deficit in bright, competent people entering training for nursing is compounded by the gross inconsistencies in training programs. Training programs for nurses all teach some psychaitric nursing but their psychiatric programs range from those which offer a comprehensive introduction to psychodynamics and psychopathology to far less defined programs which foster superficial knowledge, a false sense of security, frequent misinformation and inaccurate facts. The premise of such programs often seems to be that anyone who is well intended does some good.

There is little governmental involvement in monitoring the quality of academic programs in nursing, and formal accreditation does not guarantee a solid program. Indeed, many shaky programs gear all their effort toward insuring accreditation and technically meet the requirements while providing students with a very poor educational experience. Without governmental assessment and with technical assessment only by nursing accreditation organizations the faculty and clinicians in psychiatry in such programs need to evaluate one another's work. Such a process can become a vicious cycle of positive feedback in which each peer keeps a focus on the *patient's* unwillingness to work or lack of motivation rather than the incompetence of the helping person. There continue to be many programs in this country which employ clinical instructors with minimal — sometimes no — actual experience in caring for hospitalized psychiatric patients. Recent legal decisions have also undermined the candor of clinical assessment of student expertise in some institutions. The ever present threat of suit and liability have made it extremely difficult to delete nursing incompetents. Indeed, some formal evaluations of nursing students are incredibly bland in order to prevent instructor liability. Clearly, no well motivated nursing training program wishes its instructors to react in this manner, but instructors are human, and many of them do. Thus, we see poor nursing role models prevalent both in the educational and clinical areas.

The second reality which will impact on the future of psychiatric nursing is its current state of flux. With all the rapid changes in this profession over the past decade and a half, it is understandable that its identity is diffuse and many of its most able practitioners are insecure about its identity — and theirs. The wide range of competencies among psychiatric nurses perhaps encourages many of them to project their own professional difficulties and the difficulties of psychiatric nursing to external sources: paraprofessionals or the medical profession itself.

Although it seems sexist to dwell on it, it nevertheless remains a fact that most psychiatric nurses are women, and the dramatic impact of the feminist movement has certainly been reflected in the identity issues which are found in psychiatric nursing. There has been very often a move away from the very important maternal, nurturing role of the psychiatric nurse to competition for medical treatment with the physician. Nurses are uncomfortable with this move but many of them certainly participate in it because of peer pressure. In attempting to define a more "masculine" role and in keeping with the competitive issues, the profession has begun to implement its own jargon by redefining psychiatric terms. In fact, we now term the patient, the *consumer* or *client*. We need only reflect briefly to feel the impact of that change.

Confusion, disorganization and identity diffusion of psychiatric nurses and psychiatric nursing are necessary concomitants to the growth of the profession. They offer the profession and its members an opportunity to turn inward and gain insight to better develop expertise, but often instead of this inward turning we find psychiatric nurses wrestling with the medical profession to take over part of its job description to better demonstrate the role of psychiatric nursing as an effective one. The question should be, effective for whom? There is a need for psychiatric nurses to continue to provide a nurturing environment. There is no need to be defensive about caring and structuring an empathic milieu. It is tragic to relinquish that role to less qualified individuals.

The third reality is more subtle. As we review the history and social perspectives of psychiatric nursing, we begin to question how the role of the professional psychiatric nurse has evolved. In the past, nurses were educated in programs specifically designed and taught by physicians. The actual content which was taught was limited, but a caring attitude was mandated (see chapter 3). This attitude was sincere and nonjudgmental. Its essence emphasized each individual's personal dignity. There was far less likelihood than exists today for the nurse to initiate change directly, but, rather, the necessity of a safe, trusting atmosphere and identification and implementation of the patient's needs were emphasized. These attempts were often superficial, and certainly the same unconscious agendas that undermine many interventions today probably were in effect back then, but, overall, the complexities of each individual were acknowledged more than is the case today. Furthermore, in the 1800's nursing students could be and frequently were deleted if their attitude was inappropriate or if the academic content seemed too difficult for them. Today, there is far less quality control. Aggressive individuals may use the profession of psychiatric nursing to meet their needs. The growing emphasis on assertiveness in psychiatric nursing and the lessening emphasis on a caring attitude can lead an aggressive individual with much repressed hostility to provide patient care which is actively harmful to the patient.

One role of the psychiatric nurse is to act as a facilitator of "corrective emotional experiences" (see chapter 26). In the nurse-patient relationship, the nurse attempts to develop trust and honesty which encourage self-esteem and self-acceptance. We gauge our responses to each individual within a basic framework of psychiatric knowledge, hoping to encourage the growth of healthy interpersonal responses in the patient. The nurse's perspective is drawn from his or her knowledge of normal growth and development, frequently emphasizing various highly theoretical developmental models. Accordingly, the nurse's knowledge of psychopathology is broken down into syndromes and disease entities with specific and often oversimplified proposed treatment regimens. Within this perspective the nurse can begin to lose sight of the totality of each individual being more than the mere sum of his parts.

In some situations, too, nurses encourage patients to deal with feelings — but not with the nurse! We insist that a patient has the right to be angry, and we encourage the patient to express angry feelings toward other patients, his family and his physician. Frequently, however, nurses reject anger which deals directly with them. As with children, the goal for patients still seems to be the well-behaved, appropriately controlled individual. Separation, which must include a break with the psychotherapeutic team, is sometimes difficult for the staff to endure. While we should be encouraging separation and individuation, we sometimes unconsciously encourage pseudomutuality. Thus, the future of psychiatric nursing should address itself to a growing sophistication in dealing with individual patients without applying a cook book kind of care plan and remediation based on syndrome, and it must also address itself to understanding and further defining the conscious and unconscious attributes and weak areas of the individual nurse. Should the profession be successful in these areas of necessary growth, its practitioners will indeed become more sensitive and will provide great service to individual patients. Should the profession be unsuccessful in these two areas of needed growth, it seems to me that the nurse will become more and more an administrator or a technician.

When any patient is admitted to a ward, professionals working on that ward, including the nurses, have a natural tendency to view the patient as representative of an illness: this makes the patient seem more comprehensible and less threatening to us and is to be expected. We end up visualizing the patient *as* an illness in terms of our theoretical expectations, and we sometimes fail to realize that we are using a model for dealing with the patient. We sometimes fail to listen to the experiences, feelings and reality of the patient. Our treatment care plans then take on the rigidity of entrenched steps through which the patient must work to insure getting better. Approaches may vary from dealing with the "here and now" to encouraging the patient to verbalize affects, particularly anger. None of these approaches *per se* is wrong, but if they are all we provide we are doing nothing more than performing within the textbook description of treatment of specific psychiatric syndromes; we have taken a complex human being's life and simplified his totality into the mere confines of an illness.

In discussing the more abstract and far less tangible reality, we must now begin to focus on the verbal and non-verbal messages that nurses can communicate to patients. Frequently, the professional's scope becomes so narrow that he or she denies the existence of universal human attributes, particularly dependency and narcissistic needs. Frequently, nurses view the emergency of dependence or narcissism in a patient as inappropriate because the nurses — and all other human beings — have difficulties with their own needs in these areas. We fail to comprehend that every human being is dependent to some degree or the very reality of any relationship would be nonexistent. Yet, I have frequently seen nurses and other professionals communicate hostile messages to patients and their families whose dependencies seem temporarily overwhelming. This is not to say that dependence should be fostered as a virtue, but rather that a degree of dependence is a basic need for us all. Indeed, the vicissitudes of dependence, particularly in their pseudoindependent form, are particularly common in nurses and other medical professionals.

Likewise, many professional nurses have areas of conflict in working with some adolescents and young adults. It is very difficult to retain one's perspective or even one's self-esteem in a situation where one's control is constantly being tested. This is particularly difficult when the nurse is himself of herself not too far removed from adolescence. For the nurse to use the authoritarian role to emphasize who is adult and who is child, however, is little more than role reversal.

One of the principle thrusts of psychiatric nursing in the future should be ascertainment of the type of milieu nurses should provide for the patients they try to help. Identification of individual and group defenses which militate against patient recovery should be systematically pursued, written about and communicated to nurses and supervisors.

Another principle thrust in the future of psychiatric nursing should be a systematic, unemotional study and delineation of relationships between nursing and other mental health professions and an attempt to identify methods of providing a healthy environment in a collaborative team setting which lacks the current covert agendas played out by professionals who unwittingly use patients as their pawns.

Some predictions and trends in the field of psychiatric nursing include a proliferation of open ended programs — the chance to move from the one year LPN to the two year associate degree RN to the tacking on of a couple of extra years for a later baccalaureate. While such programs will allow some career enhancement, many of them will also yield a simplicity to theoretical tenets and constructs which is not valid. The student leaves a program at whatever level feeling that he or she has something to offer, but really knows far less than he thinks.

In many educational programs, there will be a decrease in the amount of clinical exposure of students to psychiatric patients. It has become difficult in many settings to provide good clinical experiences appropriate to the students' needs.

Third, the deletion of incompetent nurses by their peers is a necessary part of the professional growth of the field. This is particularly so of incompetents in teaching ranks. The current certification process is an excellent step in the right direction, but perhaps there should be more checks and balances in the lower ranks of the system as well. Similarly, the uneven quality of various nursing programs throughout the country needs at some point to be addressed, and many more quality control efforts will need to be made.

The profession will need to develop an enhancement of nursing continuing education and graduate programs. Many highly educated and intelligent nurses actually switch fields because of the lack of intellectual stimulation provided by academic nursing. This may not be true in some centers, but it is certainly true in a great many.

Institutional credentialing of psychiatric nurses for specific talents and areas of expertise should grow, and perhaps some kind of interinstitutional credentialing could also be an outgrowth of this process. It is tragic for a psychiatric nurse with 20 years experience as a group therapist to move to a different hospital or geographic area only to find that she is no longer "qualified" to do group therapy.

A *caveat* about credentialing is in order, however: as nursing — or any other profession — initially establishes credentialing and self-policing activities there is a tendency to legislate too much. It would be wonderful if, as we develop such techniques in psychiatric nursing, we can continue to prefer ability to formal credentials!

* * * * *

Decisions will have to be made in the near future about whether psychiatric nursing is to be a profession or a trade, if collective bargaining with hospitals *versus* individual contracts with them will be preferred.

More men will need to be involved in nursing and as more men become involved with nursing there will be less of a strident need to prove that psychiatric nursing is not merely a feminine profession. Paradoxically, a growing number of men in the ranks will allow psychiatric nurses to be more "feminine."

Many of the trends listed in this chapter are alarming. Clearly, they represent the view of one individual and are not shared by everyone, or even very many. I shall suggest two further trends which seem to be unfortunate. One is the increasing use of gimmicks in psychiatric nursing. There are an increasing number of "programs" which attempt to plug an individual into a given set of psychodynamics and psychotherapeutic efforts, many of which are trendy and some of which may actually help some patients. Nevertheless, there is a movement away from addressing the specific and unique needs of the individual patient to finding "programs" to meet the needs of a particular type of patient. Gimmicks and machines can sometimes be helpful but they can also lead to an enormous distancing of the nurse from the patient.

A second major unfortunate trend, and one that will never be bucked, is that everyone wants to be a practitioner and no one wants to be a care-giver.

* * * * *

In spite of the generally cynical tone of this chapter, I should like to emphasize the continued need for an expanded cohort of psychiatric nurses — expanded both in quantity and very much in quality. The last two decades of this century will show an increasing amount of narcissistic psychopathology in Western society.

Psychopathology will become even more complicated by the seeming withdrawal of family involvement from the children of that family. There is a growing tendency for both parents to work and a growing tendency to find alternative child caretakers to take the place of parents. The process of separation and individuation *is* difficult, and usually more difficult when the mother is not the primary caretaker. Regardless of a patient's station in life or stage of life, his introjects and familial constellation continue to be of paramount importance. No amount of self-esteem or security will be generated when early childhood needs failed to be met. The lack of familial closeness will not allow patients to develop the kinds of interpersonal skills to reach emotional maturity. Thus, the future will pose a far greater challenge than has ever been posed before to the specific role of psychiatric nurses in providing caring and nurturing. A proliferation of stress workshops, communication workshops, hypnosis, biofeedback, support groups, and psychic soothsayers is with us. While some of these approaches may meet some patients' needs, it is frustrating to sit by and view an individual as he progresses through each such therapy with little long-term relief. The profession of psychiatric nursing continues to be necessary. Grappling with and coping with the long-term challenge of the next two decades in a creative *versus* a mechanistic way could lead psychiatric nursing to major professional status.

Index

C

D

R

S

T